Dentofacial Anomalies

Abdul-Latif Hamdan
Robert Thayer Sataloff
Valerie Trollinger • Mary J. Hawkshaw

Dentofacial Anomalies

Implications for Voice and Wind Instrument Performance

Springer

Abdul-Latif Hamdan
Otolaryngology, Head and Neck Surgery
American University of Beirut
Medical Centre
Beirut
Lebanon

Robert Thayer Sataloff
Otolaryngology – Head and Neck Surgery
Drexel University College of Medicine
Philadelphia, PA
USA

Valerie Trollinger
College of Visual and Performing Arts
Kutztown University of Pennsylvania
Kutztown, PA
USA

Mary J. Hawkshaw
Otolaryngology – Head and Neck Surgery
Drexel University College of Medicine
Philadelphia, PA
USA

ISBN 978-3-030-69108-0 ISBN 978-3-030-69109-7 (eBook)
https://doi.org/10.1007/978-3-030-69109-7

This Springer imprint is published by the registered company Springer Nature Switzerland AG
The registered company address is: Gewerbestrasse 11, 6330 Cham, Switzerland

To our families.

Preface

This book is intended for otolaryngologists, laryngologists, speech-language pathologists, voice teachers, professional voice users, wind instrumentalists, instrument teachers, arts medicine physicians, physical therapists, orthodontists, and other dentists as well as members of the general public who are concerned about their voices and/or wind instrument playing.

The prevalence of dentofacial anomalies is very high worldwide, involving 39–98% of the population. Despite this high prevalence and the known vocal tract anatomic variations associated with these anomalies, voice disorders in affected subjects have gained little attention in clinical care. Related performance impairments in wind instrument players have received slightly more attention and are important not only for musicians who are instrumentalists primarily, but also because many singers play wind instruments that may affect the voice. With the expanding need of otolaryngologists to meet the vocal demands of all patients with voice disorders, learning the acoustic features and vocal traits of patients with skeletal and non-skeletal deformities has become essential. A thorough understanding of the association between dentofacial anomalies and voice and wind instrument performance is indispensable for proper patient diagnosis and counselling prior to treatment and afterward. The same is true for arts medicine physicians, teachers, and therapists who work with wind instrumentalists.

This book is unique in that sense it answers four important questions that are gaining recognition with the rise in voice health awareness in professional voice users and instrumentalists:

1. Do patients with dentofacial anomalies have distinctive voice characteristics? If so, what are these characteristics?
2. What is the impact of dentofacial anomalies on vocalists' and wind instrumentalists' performance?
3. Is the voice of affected subjects in jeopardy during and/or after treatment? If so, why, and what should the patient know?
4. Can anatomic structures (e.g., lips, palate, temporomandibular joint [TMJ]) be injured or altered by playing wind instruments, and what can be done to minimize adverse effects and optimize performance?

This book provides a concise, focused review of the anatomy and physiology of phonation in Chap. 1, the work-up of patients with voice disorders in Chaps. 2 and 3, basic techniques and evaluation of wind instrument performance and dysfunction in Chap. 4, and a comprehensive discussion of the most common skeletal and non-skeletal dentofacial anomalies, including their means of diagnosis and treatment. This includes review of literature on the vocal and acoustic features of affected patients, as well as the special considerations in wind instrumentalists. An overview of orthodontic disorders and diagnosis is provided in Chap. 5. This chapter also includes an explanation of orthodontic evaluation, cephalometric analysis, and classification of malocclusion. Chapter 6 reviews the interaction between dentofacial anomalies and morphology of the upper airway that potentially can affect sound, function, and ease of performance for vocalists and wind instrumentalists. Chapter 7 discusses common problems for professional voice users and wind instrumentalists associated with dentofacial anomalies including orofacial structure, dental and periodontal disorders, malocclusion, velopharyngeal insufficiency, and temporomandibular joint dysfunction. The relationships of fundamental frequency to dentofacial shape and growth, bodily growth, and other factors are presented in Chap. 8. The association between facial growth and embouchure development is highlighted. Chapter 9 reviews the correlation between body size/shape and performance frequencies. Acoustic implications of dentofacial anomalies on performance, and consequences for vocalists and wind instrumentalists, are presented in detail. Chapter 11 reviews the effects of orthodontic treatment (such as braces) on voice and wind instrument performance, and Chap. 12 provides an overview of orthognathic surgery (minor and extensive) and its potential effects on vocalists and wind instrumentalists. The information provided in this book should enhance awareness of the vocal characteristics and wind instrument concerns associated often with dentofacial anomalies. Teachers and players of wind instruments, at both the professional and amateur levels from elementary through adult years, have started to investigate the engagement of the vocal tract in wind performance. Despite the increased interest, the lack of relevant, scientific, and valid information has led to the development of performance pedagogy that may affect the health of the vocal tract as well as dentofacial morphology. In most chapters, and particularly in Chap. 4, information relevant to the relationship between the vocal tract and wind instruments is presented, with reference to singing and speech. The importance of these relationships and their relationships to dentofacial anomalies and treatments should be helpful to wind instrumentalists and teachers, voice professionals and their teachers, and medical and dental professionals.

This is the first book that addresses the impact of orthodontic treatment and orthognathic surgery in detail for either voice users or wind instrumentalists. Because there is not only overlap between these populations, but also cross-over risks (incorrect instrument performance can cause voice problems and vice versa), a combined discussion of both is invaluable for clinicians, teachers, and performers. The authors hope that the information in this book proves helpful, and that it inspires and focuses future research.

Beirut, Lebanon — Abdul-Latif Hamdan
Philadelphia, PA, USA — Robert Thayer Sataloff
Kutztown, PA, USA — Valerie Trollinger
Philadelphia, PA, USA — Mary J. Hawkshaw

Contents

Contributors

Anthony T. Macari, DDS, MS Orthodontics and Dentofacial Orthopedics, American University of Beirut, Beirut, Lebanon

Johnathan Brandon Sataloff, MD Department of Psychiatry, Beth Israel Deaconess Medical Center, Harvard Medical School, Boston, MA, USA

Part I

Basic Principles of Phonation and Diagnostic Work-Up

Anatomy and Physiology of the Voice

1

To treat voice patients knowledgeably and responsibly, health care providers must understand the medical aspects of voice disorders and their treatment. This requires core knowledge of the anatomy and physiology of phonation. The human voice consists of much more than simply the vocal folds, popularly known as the vocal cords. State-of-the-art voice diagnosis, nonsurgical therapy, and voice surgery depend on understanding the complex workings of the vocal tract. Physicians and dentists specializing in the care of voice patients, especially voice professionals, should be familiar with at least the basics of the latest concepts in voice function. The physiology of phonation is much more complex than this brief chapter might suggest, and readers interested in acquiring more than a clinically essential introduction are encouraged to consult other literature [1].

Anatomy

The larynx is essential to normal voice production, but the anatomy of the voice is not limited to the larynx. The vocal mechanism includes the abdominal and back musculature, rib cage, lungs, pharynx, oral cavity, and nose, among other structures. Each component performs an important function in voice production, although it is possible to produce voice even without a larynx—for example, in patients who have undergone laryngectomy. In addition, virtually all parts of the body play some role in voice production and may be responsible for voice dysfunction. Even something as remote as a sprained ankle may alter posture, thereby impairing abdominal, back, and thoracic muscle function and resulting in vocal inefficiency, weakness, and hoarseness.

The larynx is composed of four basic anatomic units: skeleton, intrinsic muscles, extrinsic muscles, and mucosa. The most important components of the laryngeal skeleton are the thyroid cartilage, cricoid cartilage, and two arytenoid cartilages (Fig. 1.1). Intrinsic muscles of the larynx are connected to these cartilages (Fig. 1.2). One of the intrinsic muscles, the *thyroarytenoid muscle* (its medial belly also is known as the vocalis muscle), extends on each side from the vocal process of the arytenoid cartilage to the inside of the thyroid cartilage just below and behind the thyroid prominence ("Adam's apple"), forming the body of the vocal folds. The vocal folds act as the *oscillator* or *voice source* of the vocal tract. The space between the vocal folds is called the *glottis* and is used as an anatomic reference point. The intrinsic muscles alter the position, shape, and tension of the vocal folds, bringing them together (adduction), moving them apart (abduction), or stretching them by increasing longitudinal tension (Fig. 1.3). They are able to do so because the laryngeal cartilages are connected by soft attachments that allow changes in their relative angles and distances, thereby permitting alteration in the shape and tension of the tissues suspended between them. The arytenoid

A.-L. Hamdan et al., *Dentofacial Anomalies*, https://doi.org/10.1007/978-3-030-69109-7_1

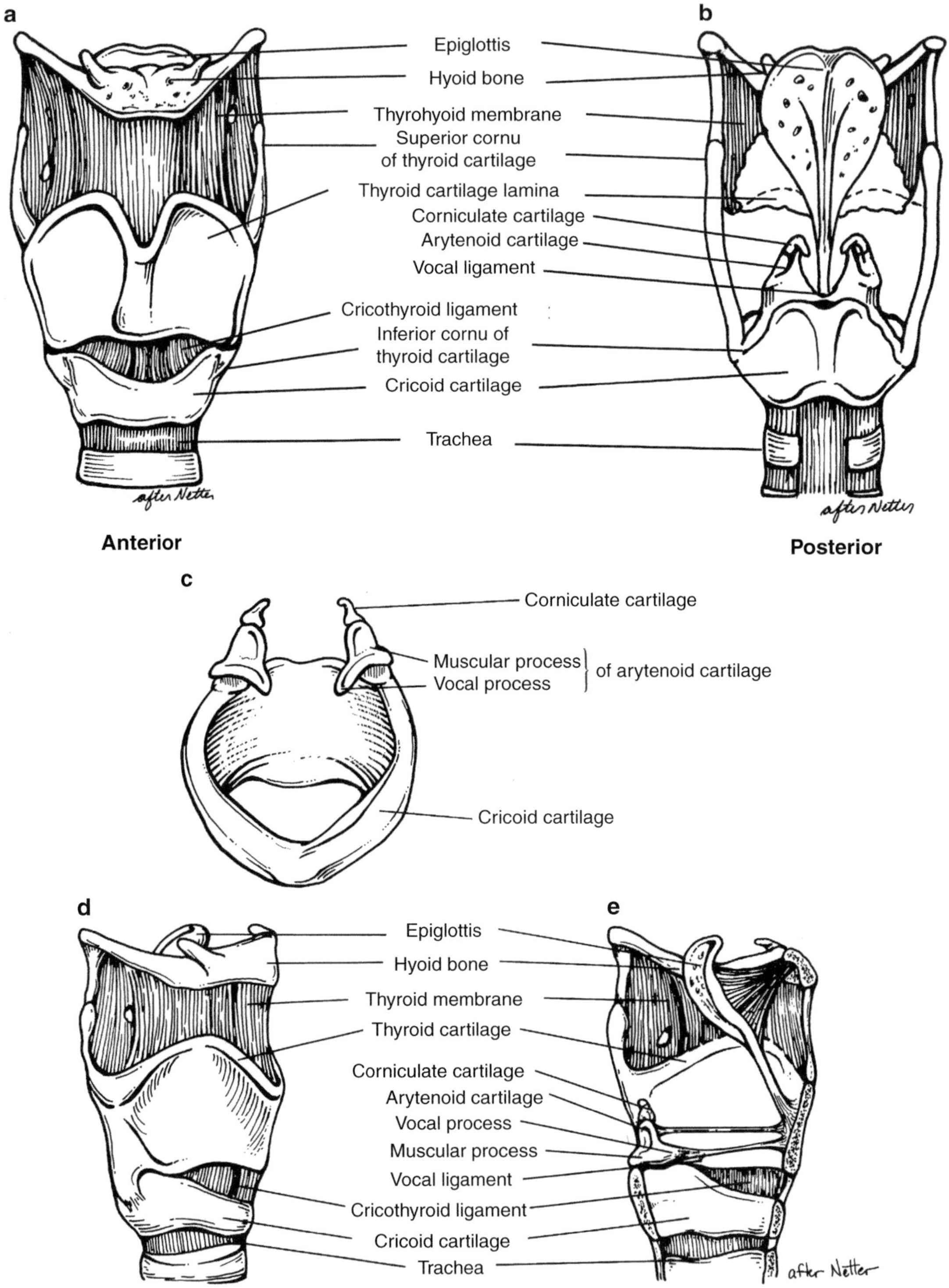

Fig. 1.1 Cartilages of the larynx

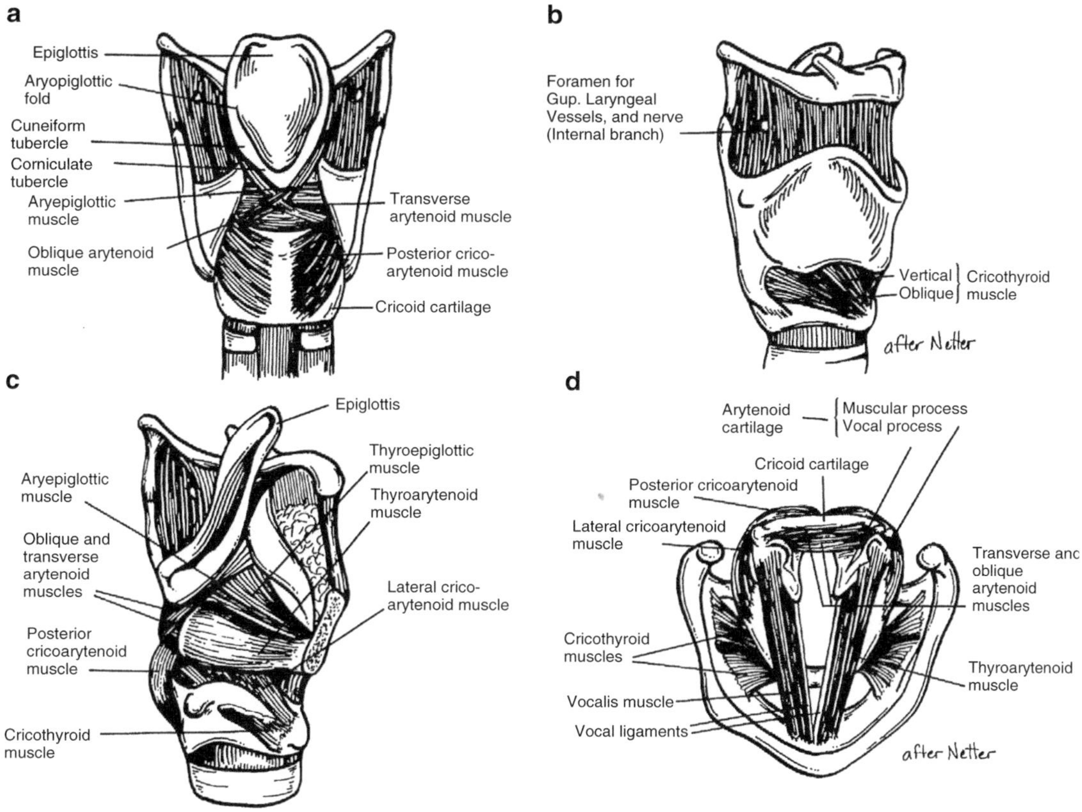

Fig. 1.2 Intrinsic muscles of the larynx

cartilages on their eliptoid cricoarytenoid joints are capable of motion in multiple planes, permitting complex vocal fold motion and alteration in the shape of the vocal fold edge associated with intrinsic muscle action (Fig. 1.4). All but one of the muscles on each side of the larynx are innervated by one of the two *recurrent laryngeal nerves*. Because this nerve runs in a long course (especially on the left) from the neck down into the chest and then back up to the larynx (hence, the name "recurrent"), it is injured easily by trauma, neck surgery, and chest surgery. Injury may result in vocal fold paresis or paralysis. The remaining muscle (*cricothyroid muscle*) is innervated by the superior laryngeal nerve on each side, which is especially susceptible to viral and traumatic injury. It causes changes in longitudinal tension that are important in voice projection and pitch control. The "false vocal folds" are located above the vocal folds, and unlike the true vocal folds, usually do not make contact during normal speaking or singing [1]. The neuroanatomy and neurophysiology of phonation are extremely complicated, and only partially understood. As the new field of neurolaryngology advances, a more thorough understanding of the subject is becoming increasingly important to clinicians. Readers interested in acquiring a deeper, scientific understanding of neurolaryngology are encouraged to consult other literature [2] and the publications cited therein.

Because the attachments of the laryngeal cartilages are flexible, the positions of the cartilages with respect to each other change when the laryngeal skeleton is elevated or lowered. Such changes in vertical height are controlled by the extrinsic laryngeal muscles, the strap muscles of the neck. When the angles and distances between cartilages change because of this accordion-like effect, the resting length of the intrinsic muscle

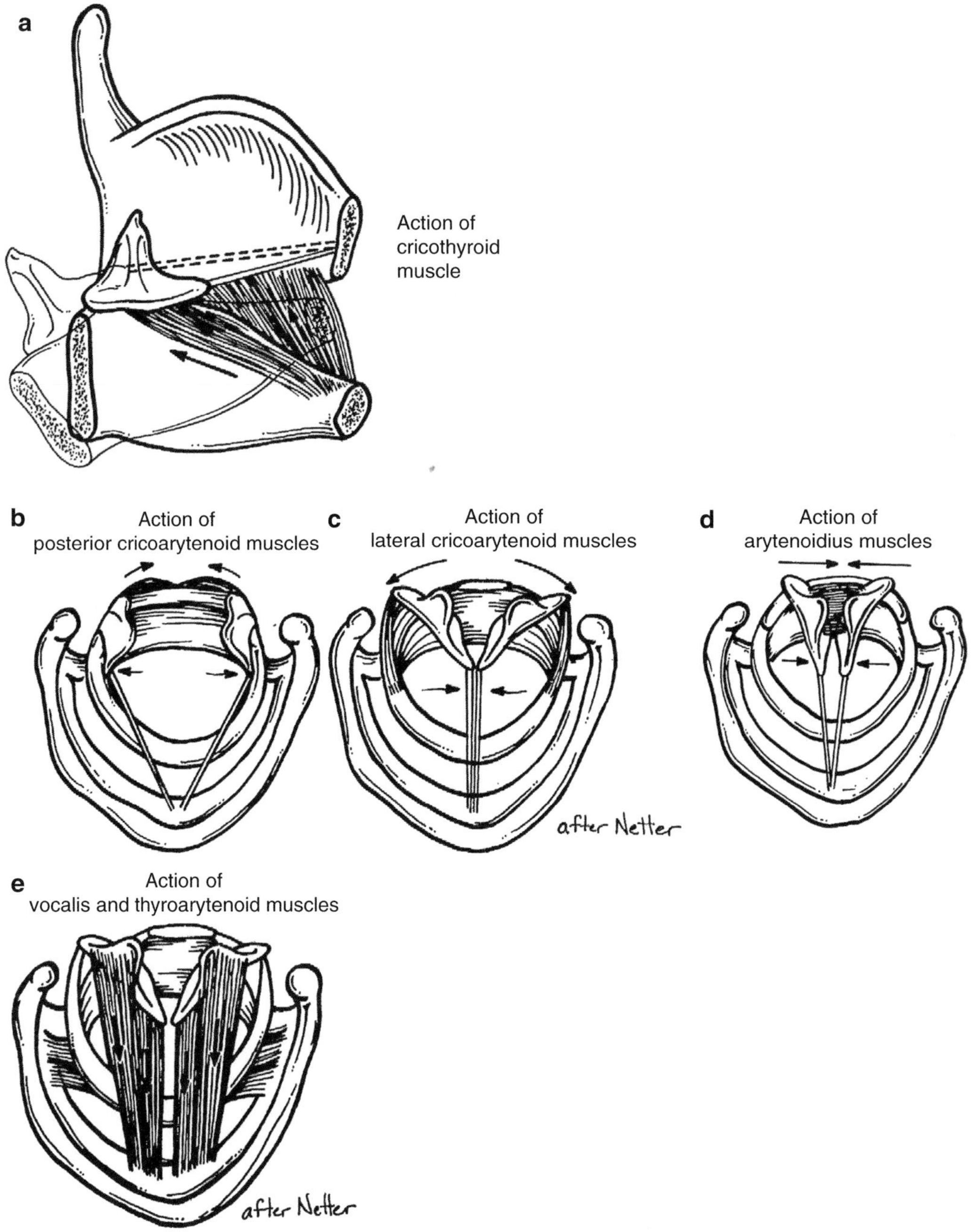

Fig. 1.3 Action of the intrinsic muscles

changes. Such large adjustments in intrinsic muscle condition interfere with fine control of smooth vocal quality. Classically trained singers generally are taught to use the extrinsic muscles to maintain the laryngeal skeleton at a relatively constant height regardless of pitch. That is, they learn to avoid the natural tendency of the larynx to rise with ascending pitch and fall with descending pitch, thereby enhancing unity of sound quality throughout the vocal range through effects on

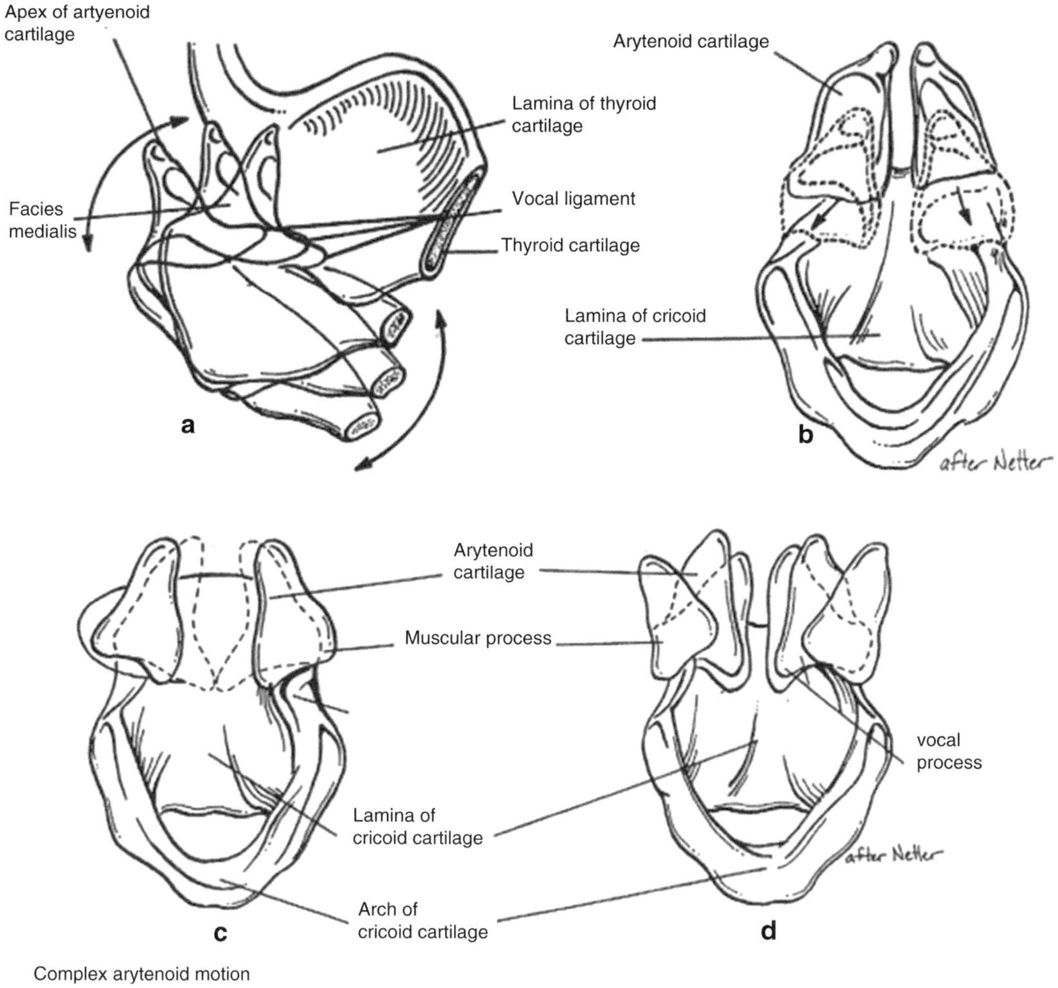

Fig. 1.4 Complex arytenoid motion

both resting muscle condition and supraglottic vocal tract posture.

The soft tissues lining the larynx are much more complex than originally thought. The mucosa forms the thin, lubricated surface of the vocal folds, which makes contact when the two vocal folds are approximated. Laryngeal mucosa might look superficially like the mucosa which lines the inside of the mouth, but it is not. Throughout most of the larynx, there are goblet cells and pseudo-stratified ciliated columnar epithelial cells designed for producing and handling mucous secretions, similar to mucosal surfaces found throughout the respiratory tract. However, the mucosa overlying the vocal folds is different. First, it is stratified squamous epithelium, which is better suited to withstand the trauma of vocal fold contact. Second, the vocal fold is not simply muscle covered with mucosa. Rather, it consists of five layers as described by Hirano [3]. Mechanically, the vocal fold structures act more like three layers consisting of the *cover* (epithelium and superficial layer of the lamina propria), *transition* (intermediate and deep layers of the lamina propria), and *body* (the vocalis muscle).

The *supraglottic vocal tract* includes the pharynx, tongue, palate, oral cavity, nose, and other structures. Together, they act as a *resonator* and are largely responsible for vocal quality or timbre and the perceived character of all phonated sounds. The vocal folds themselves produce only a "buzzing" sound. During the course of vocal training for singing, acting, or healthy speaking, changes occur not only in the larynx, but also in the muscle motion, control, and shape of the supraglottic vocal tract, and in aerobic, pulmonary, and bodily muscle function.

The *infraglottic vocal tract* (all anatomical structures below the glottis) serves as the *power source* for the voice. Singers and actors often refer to the entire power source complex as their "support" or "diaphragm." The anatomy of support for phonation is especially complicated and not completely understood. Yet, it is quite important because deficiencies in support frequently are responsible for voice dysfunction.

The purpose of the support mechanism is to generate a force that directs a controlled airstream between the vocal folds. Active respiratory muscles work in concert with passive forces. The principal muscles of inspiration are the diaphragm (a dome-shaped muscle that extends along the bottom of the rib cage) and the external intercostal muscles (located between the ribs). During quiet respiration, expiration is largely passive. The lungs and rib cage generate passive expiratory forces under many common circumstances such as after a full breath.

Many of the muscles used for active expiration also are employed in "support" for phonation. Muscles of active expiration either raise the intra-abdominal pressure, forcing the diaphragm upward, or lower the ribs or sternum to decrease the dimensions of the thorax, or both, thereby compressing air in the chest. The primary muscles of expiration are "the abdominal muscles," but internal intercostals and other chest and back muscles also are involved. Trauma or surgery that alters the structure or function of these muscles or ribs undermines the power source of the voice, as do diseases, such as asthma, that impair expiration. Deficiencies in the support mechanism often result in compensatory efforts that utilize the laryngeal muscles, which are not designed for power functions. Such behavior can result in impaired voice quality, rapid fatigue, pain, and even structural pathology such as vocal fold nodules. Current expert treatment for such vocal problems focuses on correction of the underlying malfunction rather than surgery whenever possible.

Physiology

The physiology of voice production is extremely complex. Volitional production of voice begins in the cerebral cortex (Fig. 1.5).

The command for vocalization involves complex interactions among brain centers for speech, as well as other areas. For singing, speech directives must be integrated with information from the centers for musical and artistic expression, which are discussed elsewhere [1]. The "idea" of the planned vocalization is conveyed to the precentral gyrus in the motor cortex, which transmits another set of instructions to the motor nuclei in the brainstem and the spinal cord. These areas send out the complicated messages necessary for coordinated activity of the larynx, thoracic and abdominal musculature lungs, and vocal tract articulators, among other structures. Additional refinement of motor activity is provided by the extrapyramidal and autonomic nervous systems. These impulses combine to produce a sound that is transmitted not only to the ears of the listener, but also to those of the speaker or singer. Auditory feedback is transmitted from the ear through the brainstem to the cerebral cortex, and adjustments are made within milliseconds that permit the vocalist to match the sound produced with the sound intended, integrating the acoustic properties of the performance environment. Tactile feedback from throat and other muscles involved in phonation also is believed to help in fine-tuning vocal output, although the mechanism and role of tactile feedback are not understood fully. Many trained singers and speakers cultivate the ability to use tactile feedback effectively because of expected interference with auditory feedback data from ancillary sound such as an orchestra or band.

Phonation, the production of sound, requires interaction among the power source, oscillator,

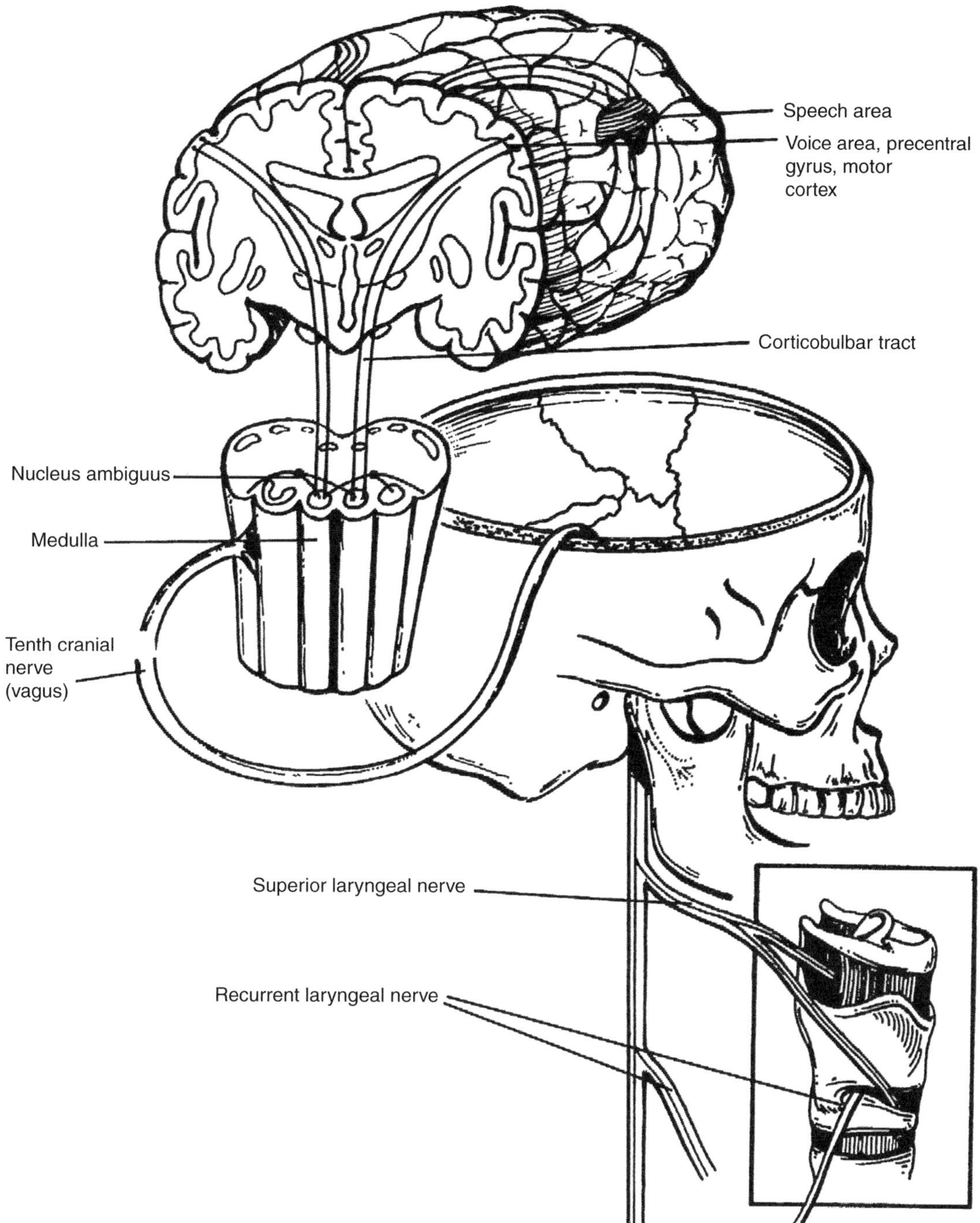

Fig. 1.5 Simplified summary of pathway for volitional phonation

and resonator. The voice may be compared to a brass instrument such as a trumpet. Power is generated by the chest, abdominal, and back musculature and a high-pressure airstream is produced. The trumpeter's lips open and close against the mouthpiece producing a "buzz" similar to the sound produced by vocal folds when they come together and move apart (oscillate) during phonation. This sound then passes through the trumpet, which has acoustic resonance characteristics that shape the sound we associate with trumpet music. If a trumpet mouthpiece is placed on a French horn, the sound we hear will sound like a French horn, not a trumpet. Quality characteristics are dependent upon the resonator more than on the oscillatory source. The non-mouthpiece portions of a brass instrument are analogous to the supraglottic vocal tract.

During phonation, the infraglottic musculature must make rapid, complex adjustments because the resistance changes almost continuously as the glottis closes, opens, and changes shape. At the beginning of each phonatory cycle, the vocal folds are approximated, and the glottis is obliterated. This permits infraglottic air pressure to build, typically to a level of about 7 cm of water for conversational speech. At that point, the vocal folds are convergent (Fig. 1.6a). Because the vocal folds are closed, there is no airflow. The subglottic pressure then pushes the vocal folds progressively farther apart from the bottom up and from the back forward (Fig. 1.6b) until a space develops (Fig. 1.6c, d) and air begins to flow. Bernoulli force created by the air passing between the vocal folds combines with the mechanical properties of the folds to begin clos-

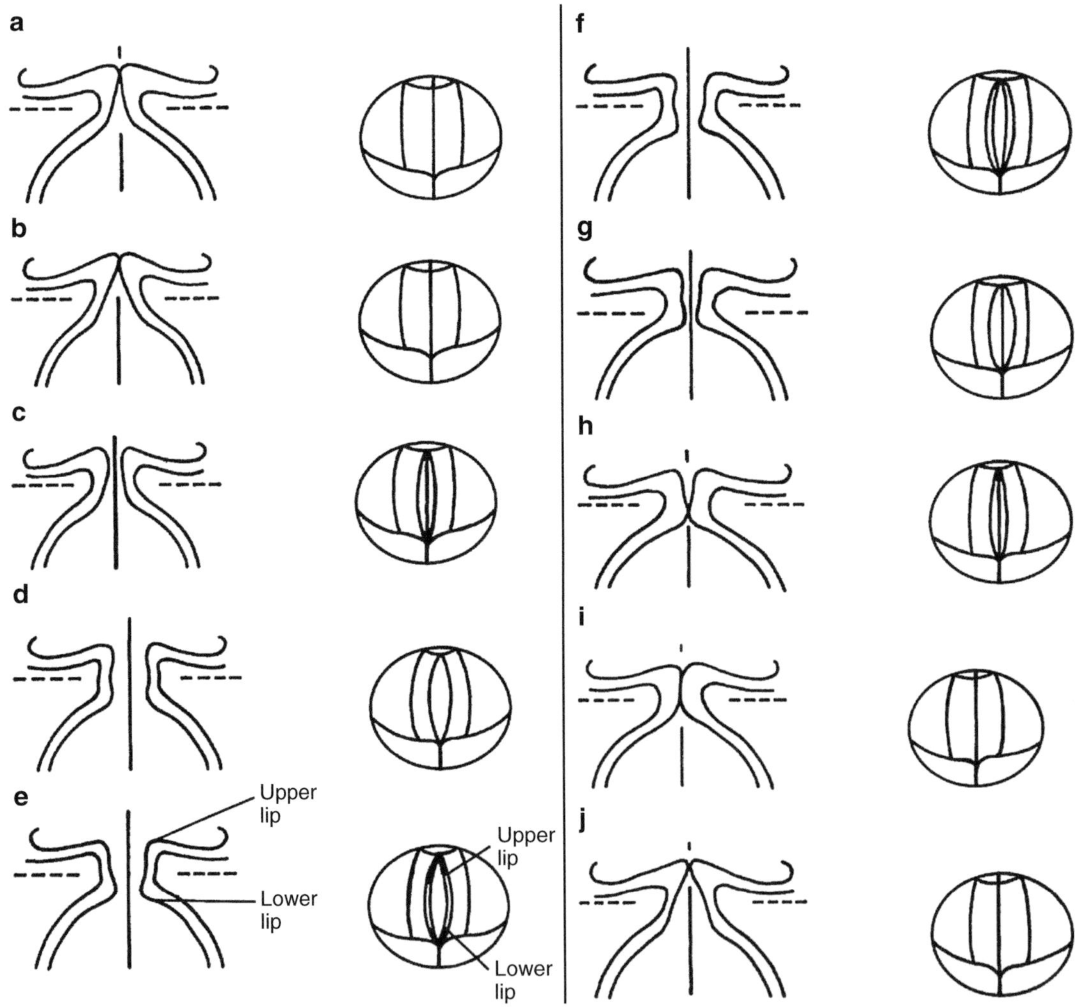

Fig. 1.6 Frontal view (left) and view from above (right) illustrating the normal pattern of vocal fold vibration. The vocal folds close and open from the inferior aspect of the vibratory margin upward, and from posterior to anterior

ing the lower portion of the vocal folds almost immediately (Fig. 1.6e–h) even while the upper edges are still separating. The principles and mathematics of Bernoulli force are complex. It is a flow effect more easily understood by familiar examples such as the sensation of pull exerted on a vehicle when passed by a truck at high speed or the inward motion of a shower curtain when the water flows past it.

The upper portion of the vocal folds has elastic properties that also tend to make the vocal folds snap back to the midline. This force becomes more dominant as the upper edges are stretched and the opposing force of the airstream diminishes because of approximation of the lower edges of the vocal folds. The upper portions of the vocal folds are then returned to the midline (Fig. 1.6i), completing the glottic cycle. Subglottal pressure then builds again (Fig. 1.6j), and the events repeat. Thus, there is a vertical phase difference. That is, the lower portion of the vocal folds begins to open and close before the upper portion. The rippling displacement of the vocal fold cover produces a mucosal wave that can be examined clinically under stroboscopic light. If this complex motion is impaired, hoarseness or other changes in voice quality may cause the patient to seek medical evaluation. The frequency of vibration (number of cycles of openings and closings per second, measured in hertz [Hz]) is dependent on the air pressure and mechanical properties of the vocal folds, which are regulated in part by the laryngeal muscles. Pitch is the perceptual correlate of frequency. Under most circumstances, as the vocal folds are thinned and stretched and air pressure is increased, the frequency of air pulse emissions increases, and pitch goes up. The myoelastic-aerodynamic mechanism of phonation reveals that the vocal folds emit pulses of air, rather than vibrating like strings.

The sound produced by the oscillating vocal folds, called the voice source signal, is a complex tone containing a fundamental frequency and many overtones, or higher harmonic partials. The amplitude of the partials decreases uniformly at approximately 12 dB per octave. Interestingly, the acoustic spectrum of the voice source is about the same in ordinary speakers as it is in trained singers and speakers. Voice quality differences in voice professionals occur as the voice source signal passes through their supraglottic vocal tract resonator system (Fig. 1.7).

The pharynx, oral cavity, and nasal cavity act as a series of infinitely variable interconnected resonators, which are more complex than that in our trumpet example or other single resonators. As with other resonators, some frequencies are attenuated, others are enhanced. Enhanced frequencies are radiated with higher relative amplitudes or intensities. Sundberg [4] showed long ago that the vocal tract has four or five important resonance frequencies called *formants* and summarized his early findings in a book that has become a classic. The presence of formants alters the uniformly sloping voice source spectrum and creates peaks at formant frequencies. These alterations of the voice source spectral envelope are responsible for distinguishable sounds of speech and song. Formant frequencies are determined by vocal tract shape, which can be altered by the laryngeal, pharyngeal, and oral cavity musculature. Overall vocal tract length and shape are individually fixed and determined by age and sex (females and children have shorter vocal tracts and formant frequencies that are higher than males). Voice training includes conscious physical mastery of the adjustment of vocal tract shape.

Although the formants differ for different vowels, one resonant frequency has received particular attention and is known as the "singer's formant." This formant occurs in the vicinity of 2300–3200 Hz for all vowel spectra and appears to be responsible for the "ring" in a singer's or trained speaker's ("speaker's formant") voice. The ability to hear a trained voice clearly even over a loud choir or orchestra is dependent primarily on the presence of the singer's formant [1]. Interestingly, there is little or no significant difference in maximum vocal intensity between trained and untrained singers. The singer's formant also contributes substantially to the differences in fach (voice classification) among voice categories, occurring in basses at about 2400 Hz, baritones at 2600 Hz, tenors at 2800 Hz, mezzo-

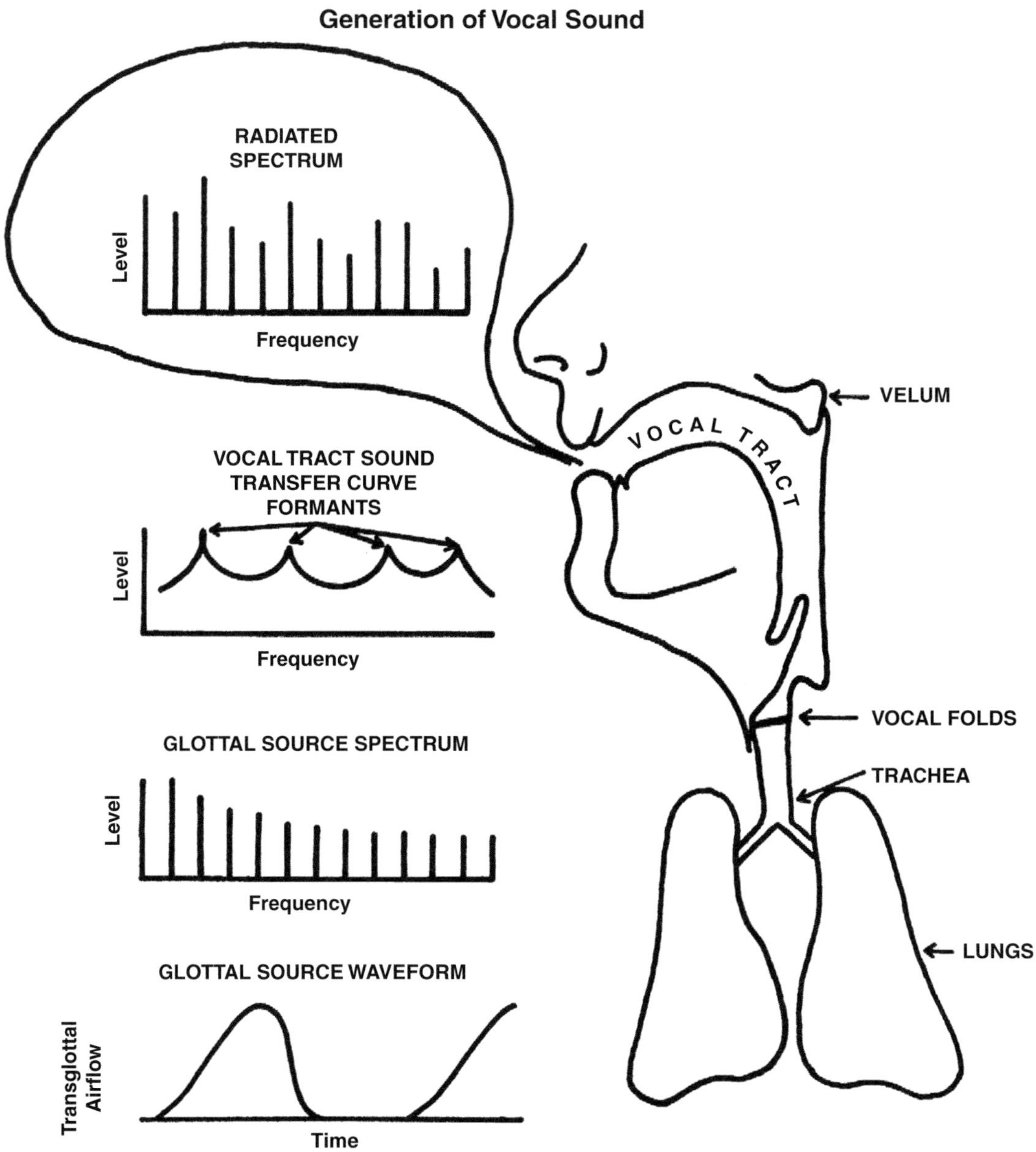

Fig. 1.7 Determinants of the spectrum of a vowel (oral-output signal)

sopranos at 2900 Hz, and sopranos at 3200 Hz. It is frequently much less prominent in high soprano singing [1].

The mechanisms that control two vocal characteristics are particularly important: fundamental frequency and intensity. Fundamental frequency, which corresponds to pitch, can be altered by changing either air pressure or the mechanical properties of the vocal folds, although the latter is more efficient under most conditions. When the cricothyroid muscle contracts, it makes the thyroid cartilage pivot on the cricothyroid joint and increases the distance between the thyroid and arytenoid cartilages, thus stretching the vocal folds. This increases the surface area exposed to subglottal pressure and makes the air pressure more effective in opening the glottis. In addition, stretching of elastic fibers of the vocal fold makes them more efficient at snapping back together. Hence, the cycles shorten and repeat more frequently, and the fundamental frequency (and pitch) rise. Other muscles, including the thyroarytenoid, also contribute [1]. Raising the pressure of the airstream also tends to increase fundamental frequency, a phenomenon for which singers must learn to compensate. Otherwise, their pitch would go up whenever they tried to sing more loudly.

Voice intensity corresponds to loudness and depends on the degree to which the glottal wave motion excites the air molecules in the vocal tract. Raising the air pressure creates greater amplitude of vocal fold oscillation and therefore increases vocal intensity. However, actually it is not the oscillation of the vocal fold, but rather the sudden cessation of airflow that is responsible for initiating an acoustic signal in the vocal tract and controlling intensity. This is similar to the mechanism of acoustic signal that results from buzzing lips. In the larynx, the sharper the cutoff of air flow, the more intense the sound [1]. In the evaluation of voice disorders, an individual's ability to optimize adjustments of air pressure and glottal resistance is assessed. When high subglottic pressure is combined with high adductory (closing) vocal fold force, glottal airflow and the amplitude of the voice source fundamental frequency are low. This is called *pressed phonation* and can be measured clinically through a technique known as flow glottography. Flow glottogram wave amplitude indicates the type of phonation being used, and the slope (closing rate) provides information about the sound pressure level or loudness. If adductory forces are so weak that the vocal folds do not make contact, the vocal folds become inefficient at resisting air leakage, and the voice source fundamental frequency is low. This is known as *breathy phonation*. *Flow phonation* is characterized by lower subglottic pressure and lower adductory force. These conditions increase the dominance of the fundamental frequency of the voice source in the perceived sound. Sundberg showed that the amplitude of the fundamental frequency can be increased by 15 dB or more when the subject changes from pressed phonation to flow phonation [4]. If a patient habitually uses pressed phonation, considerable effort will be required to achieve loud voicing. The muscle patterns and force that are used to compensate for this laryngeal inefficiency may cause vocal fold damage. Such voice behavior (i.e., pressed voice) can result from laryngeal structural problems, voice technique, psychological abnormalities, and other causes.

Acknowledgment Modified in part from Rosen DC, Sataloff JB, Sataloff RT. *Psychology of Voice Disorders*, 2nd ed. San Diego, CA: Plural Publishing, 2020; with permission.

References

1. Sataloff RT. Professional voice: the science and art of clinical care. 4th ed. San Diego, CA: Plural Publishing; 2017.
2. Sataloff RT. Neurolaryngology. San Diego, CA: Plural Publishing; 2017.
3. Hirano M. Phonosurgery: basic and clinical investigations. Otologia (Fukuoka). 1975;21:239–442.
4. Sundberg J. The science of the singing voice. DeKalb, IL: Northern Illinois University Press; 1987.

2 Patient History

A comprehensive history and physical examination usually reveal the cause of voice dysfunction. Effective history taking and physical examination depend on a practical understanding of the anatomy and physiology of voice production [1–3]. Because dysfunction in virtually any body system may affect phonation, medical inquiry must be comprehensive. The current standard of care for all voice patients evolved from advances inspired by medical problems of voice professionals such as singers and actors. Even minor problems may be particularly symptomatic in singers and actors, because of the extreme demands they place on their voices. However, a great many other patients are voice professionals. They include teachers, salespeople, attorneys, clergy, physicians, politicians, telephone receptionists, and anyone else whose ability to earn a living is impaired in the presence of voice dysfunction. Because good voice quality is so important in our society, the majority of our patients are voice professionals, and all patients should be treated as such.

The scope of inquiry and examination for most patients is similar to that required for singers and actors, except that performing voice professionals have unique needs, which require additional history and examination. Questions must be added regarding performance commitments, professional status and voice goals, the amount and nature of voice training, the performance environment, rehearsal practices, abusive habits during speech and singing, and many other matters. Such supplementary information is essential to proper treatment selection and patient counseling in singers and actors. However, analogous factors must also be taken into account for stockbrokers, factory shop foremen, elementary school teachers, homemakers with several noisy children, and many others. Physicians familiar with the management of these challenging patients are well equipped to evaluate all patients with voice complaints.

Patient History

Obtaining extensive historical background information is necessary for thorough evaluation of the voice patient, and the otolaryngologist who sees voice patients (especially singers) only occasionally cannot reasonably be expected to remember all the pertinent questions. Although some laryngologists consider a lengthy inquisition helpful in establishing rapport, many of us who see a substantial number of voice patients each day within a busy practice need a thorough but less time-consuming alternative. A history questionnaire can be extremely helpful in documenting all the necessary information, helping the patient sort out and articulate his or her problems, and saving the clinician time recording information. The author has developed a questionnaire [4] that has proven helpful. The patient is asked to complete the relevant portions of the form at home prior to his or her office visit or in

A.-L. Hamdan et al., *Dentofacial Anomalies*, https://doi.org/10.1007/978-3-030-69109-7_2

the waiting room before seeing the doctor. A similar form has been developed for voice patients who are not singers.

No history questionnaire is a substitute for direct, penetrating questioning by the physician. However, the direction of most useful inquiry can be determined from a glance at the questionnaire, obviating the need for extensive writing, which permits the physician greater eye contact with the patient and facilitates rapid establishment of the close rapport and confidence that are so important in treating voice patients. The physician is also able to supplement initial impressions and historical information from the questionnaire with seemingly leisurely conversation during the physical examination. The use of the history questionnaire has added substantially to the efficiency, consistent thoroughness, and ease of managing these delightful, but often complex, patients. A similar set of questions is also used by the speech-language pathologist with new patients and by many enlightened singing teachers when assessing new students.

How Old Are You?

Serious vocal endeavor may start in childhood and continue throughout a lifetime. As the vocal mechanism undergoes normal maturation, the voice changes. The optimal time to begin serious vocal training is controversial. For many years, most singing teachers advocated delay of vocal training and serious singing until near puberty in the female and after puberty and voice stabilization in the male. However, in a child with earnest vocal aspirations and potential, starting specialized training early in childhood is reasonable. Initial instruction should teach the child to vocalize without straining and to avoid all forms of voice abuse. It should not permit premature indulgence in operatic bravado. Most experts agree that taxing voice use and singing during puberty should be minimized or avoided altogether, particularly by the male. Voice maturation (attainment of stable adult vocal quality) may occur at any age from the early teenage years to the fourth decade of life. The dangerous tendency for young singers to attempt to sound older than their vocal years frequently causes vocal dysfunction.

All components of voice production are subject to normal aging. Abdominal and general muscular tone frequently decrease, lungs lose elasticity, the thorax loses its distensibility, the mucosa of the vocal tract atrophies, mucous secretions change character and quantity, nerve endings are reduced in number, and psychoneurologic functions change. Moreover, the larynx itself loses muscle tone and bulk and may show depletion of submucosal ground substance in the vocal folds. The laryngeal cartilages ossify, and the joints may become arthritic and stiff. Hormonal influence is altered. Vocal range, intensity, and quality all may be modified. Vocal fold atrophy may be the most striking alteration. The clinical effects of aging seem more pronounced in female singers, although vocal fold histologic changes may be more prominent in males. Excellent male singers occasionally extend their careers into their 70s or beyond [5, 6]. However, some degree of breathiness, decreased range, and other evidence of aging should be expected in elderly voices. Nevertheless, many of the changes we typically associate with elderly singers (wobble, flat pitch) are due to lack of conditioning, rather than inevitable changes of biological aging. These aesthetically undesirable concomitants of aging can often be reversed.

What Is Your Voice Problem?

Careful questioning as to the onset of vocal problems is needed to separate acute from chronic dysfunction. Often an upper respiratory tract infection will send a patient to the physician's office, but penetrating inquiry, especially in singers and actors, may reveal a chronic vocal problem that is the patient's real concern. Identifying acute and chronic problems before beginning therapy is important so that both the patient and the physician may have realistic expectations and make optimal therapeutic selections.

The specific nature of the vocal complaint can provide a great deal of information. Just as dizzy patients rarely walk into the physician's office complaining of "rotary vertigo," voice patients may be unable to articulate their symptoms without guidance. They may use the term *hoarseness* to describe a variety of conditions that the physician must separate. Hoarseness is a coarse or scratchy sound that is most often associated with abnormalities of the leading edge of the vocal folds such as laryngitis or mass lesions. Breathiness is a vocal quality characterized by excessive loss of air during vocalization. In some cases, it is due to improper technique. However, any condition that prevents full approximation of the vocal folds can be responsible. Possible causes include vocal fold paralysis, a mass lesion separating the leading edges of the vocal folds, arthritis of the cricoarytenoid joint, arytenoid dislocation, scarring of the vibratory margin, senile vocal fold atrophy (presbyphonia), psychogenic dysphonia, malingering, and other conditions.

Fatigue of the voice is inability to continue to speak or sing for extended periods without change in vocal quality and/or control. The voice may show fatigue by becoming hoarse, losing range, changing timbre, breaking into different registers, or exhibiting other uncontrolled aberrations. A well-trained singer should be able to sing for several hours without vocal fatigue.

Voice fatigue may occur through more than one mechanism. Most of the time, it is assumed to be due to muscle fatigue. This is often the case in patients who have voice fatigue associated with muscle tension dysphonia. The mechanism is most likely to be peripheral muscle fatigue and due to chemical changes (or depletion) in the muscle fibers. "Muscle fatigue" may also occur on a central (neurologic) basis. This mechanism is common in certain neuropathic disorders, such as some patients with multiple sclerosis; may occur with myasthenia gravis (actually neuromuscular junction pathology); or may be associated with paresis from various causes. However, the voice may also fatigue due to changes in the vibratory margin of the vocal fold. This phenomenon may be described as "lamina propria" fatigue (our descriptive, not universally used). It, too, may be related to chemical or fluid changes in the lamina propria or cellular damage associated with conditions such as phonotrauma and dehydration. Excessive voice use, suboptimal tissue environment (e.g., dehydration and effects of pollution), lack of sufficient time of recovery between phonatory stresses, and genetic or structural tissue weaknesses that predispose to injury or delayed recovery from trauma all may be associated with lamina propria fatigue.

Although it has not been proven, this author (RTS) suspects that fatigue may also be related to the linearity of vocal fold vibrations. However, briefly, voices have linear and nonlinear (chaotic) characteristics. As the voice becomes more trained, vibrations become more symmetrical, and the system becomes more linear. In many pathologic voices, the nonlinear components appear to become more prominent. If a voice is highly linear, slight changes in the vibratory margin may have little effect on the output of the system. However, if the system has substantial nonlinearity due to vocal fold pathology, poor tissue environment, or other causes, slight changes in the tissue (slight swelling, drying, surface cell damage) may cause substantial changes in the acoustic output of the system (the butterfly effect), causing vocal quality changes and fatigue much more quickly with much smaller changes in initial condition in more linear vocal systems.

Fatigue is often caused by misuse of abdominal and neck musculature or oversinging, singing too loudly, or too long. However, we must remember that vocal fatigue also may be a sign not only of general tiredness or vocal abuse (sometimes secondary to structural lesions or glottal closure problems) but also of serious illnesses such as myasthenia gravis. So, the importance of this complaint should not be understated.

Volume disturbance may manifest as inability to sing loudly or inability to sing softly. Each voice has its own dynamic range. Within the course of training, singers learn to sing more loudly by singing more efficiently. They also learn to sing softly, a more difficult task, through years of laborious practice. Actors and other trained speakers go through similar training. Most volume problems are secondary to intrinsic limitations of the voice or technical errors in voice use, although hormonal changes, aging, and neurologic disease are other causes. Superior laryngeal nerve paralysis impairs the ability to speak or sing loudly. This is a frequently unrecognized consequence of herpes infection (cold sores) and Lyme disease and may be precipitated by any viral upper respiratory tract infection.

Most highly trained singers require only about 10 minutes to half an hour to "warm up the voice." Prolonged warm-up time, especially in the morning, is most often caused by reflux laryngitis. Tickling or choking during singing is most often a symptom of an abnormality of the vocal fold's leading edge. The symptom of tickling or choking should contraindicate singing until the vocal folds have been examined. Pain while singing can indicate vocal fold lesions, laryngeal joint arthritis, infection, or gastric acid reflux irritation of the arytenoid region. However, pain is much more commonly caused by voice abuse with excessive muscular activity in the neck rather than an acute abnormality on the leading edge of a vocal fold. In the absence of other symptoms, these patients do not generally require immediate cessation of singing pending medical examination. However, sudden onset of pain (usually sharp pain) while singing may be associated with a mucosal tear or a vocal fold hemorrhage and warrants voice conservation pending laryngeal examination.

Do You Have Any Pressing Voice Commitments?

If a singer or a professional speaker (e.g., actor, politician) seeks treatment at the end of a busy performance season and has no pressing engagements, management of the voice problem should be relatively conservative and designed to ensure long-term protection of the larynx, the most delicate part of the vocal mechanism. However, the physician and the patient rarely have this luxury. Most often, the voice professional needs treatment within a week of an important engagement and sometimes within less than a day. Younger singers fall ill shortly before performances, not because of hypochondria or coincidence, but rather because of the immense physical and emotional stress of the preperformance period. The singer is frequently working harder and singing longer hours than usual. Moreover, he or she may be under particular pressure to learn new material and to perform well for a new audience. The singer may also be sleeping less than usual because of additional time spent rehearsing or because of the discomforts of a strange city. Seasoned professionals make their living by performing regularly, sometimes several times a week. Consequently, any time they get sick is likely to precede a performance. Caring for voice complaints in these situations requires highly skilled judgment and bold management.

Tell Me About Your Vocal Career, Long-Term Goals, and the Importance of Your Voice Quality and Upcoming Commitments

To choose a treatment program, the physician must understand the importance of the patient's voice and his or her long-term career plans, the importance of the upcoming vocal commitment, and the consequences of canceling the engagement. Injudicious prescription of voice rest can be almost as damaging to a vocal career as injudicious performance. For example, although a singer's voice is usually his or her most important commodity, other factors distinguish the few successful artists from the multitude of less successful singers with equally good voices. These include musicianship, reliability, and "professionalism." Canceling a concert at the last minute may seriously damage a performer's reputation. Reliability is especially critical early in a singer's career. Moreover, an expert singer often can modify a performance to decrease the strain on his or her voice. No singer should be allowed to perform in a manner that will permit serious injury to the vocal folds, but in the frequent borderline cases, the condition of the larynx must be weighed against other factors affecting the singer as an artist.

How Much Voice Training Have You Had?

Establishing how long a singer or actor has been performing seriously is important, especially if his or her active performance career predates the beginning of vocal training. Active untrained singers and actors frequently develop undesirable techniques that are difficult to modify. Extensive voice use without training or premature training with inappropriate repertoire may underlie persistent vocal difficulties later in life. The number of years a performer has been training his or her voice may be a fair index of vocal proficiency. A person who has studied voice for 1 or 2 years is somewhat more likely to have gross technical difficulties than is someone who has been studying for 20 years. However, if training has been intermittent or discontinued, technical problems are common, especially among singers. In addition, methods of technical voice use vary among voice teachers. Hence, a student who has had many teachers in a relatively brief period of time commonly has numerous technical insecurities or deficiencies that may be responsible for vocal dysfunction. This is especially true if the singer has changed to a new teacher within the preceding year. The physician must be careful not to criticize the patient's current voice teacher in such circumstances. It often takes years of expert instruction to correct bad habits.

All people speak more often than they sing, yet most singers report little speech training. Even if a singer uses the voice flawlessly while practicing and performing, voice abuse at other times can cause damage that affects singing.

Under What Kinds of Conditions Do You Use Your Voice?

The Lombard effect is the tendency to increase vocal intensity in response to increased background noise. A well-trained singer learns to compensate for this tendency and to avoid singing at unsafe volumes. Singers of classical music usually have such training and frequently perform with only a piano, a situation in which the balance can be controlled well. However, singers performing in large halls, with orchestras, or in operas early in their careers tend to oversing and strain their voices. Similar problems occur during outdoor concerts because of the lack of auditory feedback. This phenomenon is seen even more among "pop" singers. Pop singers are in a uniquely difficult position; often, despite little vocal training, they enjoy great artistic and financial success and endure extremely stressful demands on their time and voices. They are required to sing in large halls or outdoor arenas not designed for musical performance, amid smoke and other environmental irritants, accompanied by extremely loud background music. One frequently neglected key to survival for these singers is the proper use of monitor speakers. These direct the sound of the singer's voice toward the singer on the stage and provide auditory feedback. Determining whether the pop singer uses monitor speakers and whether they are loud enough for the singer to hear is important.

Amateur singers are often no less serious about their music than are professionals, but generally they have less ability to compensate technically for illness or other physical impairment. Rarely does an amateur suffer a great loss from postponing a performance or permitting someone to sing in his or her place. In most cases, the amateur singer's best interest is served through conservative management directed at long-term maintenance of good vocal health.

A great many of the singers who seek physicians' advice are primarily choral singers. They often are enthusiastic amateurs, untrained but dedicated to their musical recreation. They should be handled as amateur solo singers, educated specifically about the Lombard effect, and cautioned to avoid the excessive volume so common in a choral environment. One good way for a singer to monitor loudness is to cup a hand to his or her ear. This adds about 6 dB [7] to the singer's perception of his or her own voice and can be a very helpful guide in noisy surroundings. Young professional singers are often hired to augment amateur choruses. Feeling that the professional quartet has been hired to "lead" the rest of the choir, they often make the mistake of trying to accomplish that goal by singing louder than others in their sections. These singers should be advised to lead their section by singing each line as if they were soloists giving a voice lesson to the people standing next to them and as if there were a microphone in front of them recording their choral performance for their voice teacher. This approach usually not only preserves the voice but also produces a better choral sound.

How Much Do You Practice and Exercise Your Voice? How, When, and Where Do You Use Your Voice?

Vocal exercise is as essential to the vocalist as exercise and conditioning of other muscle systems is to the athlete. Proper vocal practice incorporates scales and specific exercises designed to maintain and develop the vocal apparatus. Simply acting or singing songs or giving performances without routine studious concentration on vocal technique is not adequate for the vocal performer. The physician should know whether the vocalist practices daily, whether he or she practices at the same time daily, and how long the practice lasts. Actors generally practice and warm up their voices for 10–30 minutes daily, although more time is recommended. Most serious singers practice for at least 1–2 hours per day. If a singer routinely practices in the late afternoon or evening but frequently performs in the morning (religious services, school classes, teaching voice, choir rehearsals, etc.), one should inquire into the warm-up procedures preceding such performances as well as cool-down procedures after voice use. Singing "cold," especially early in the morning, may result in the use of minor muscular alterations to compensate for vocal insecurity produced by inadequate preparation. Such crutches can result in voice dysfunction. Similar problems may result from instances of voice use other than formal singing. School teachers, telephone receptionists, salespeople, and others who speak extensively also often derive great benefit from 5 or 10 minutes of vocalization of scales first thing in the morning. Although singers rarely practice their scales too long, they frequently perform or rehearse excessively. This is especially true immediately before a major concert or audition, when physicians are most likely to see acute problems. When a singer has hoarseness and vocal fatigue and has been practicing a new role for 14 hours a day for the last 3 weeks, no simple prescription will solve the problem. However, a treatment regimen can usually be designed to carry the performer safely through his or her musical obligations.

The physician should be aware of common habits and environments that are often associated with abusive voice behavior and should ask about them routinely. Screaming at sports events and at children is among the most common. Extensive voice use in noisy environments also tends to be abusive. These include noisy rooms, cars, airplanes, sports facilities, and other locations where background noise or acoustic design impairs auditory feedback. Dry, dusty surroundings may alter vocal fold secretions through dehydration or contact irritation, altering voice function. Activities such as cheerleading, teaching, choral conducting, amateur singing, and frequent communication with hearing-impaired persons are likely to be associated with voice abuse, as is extensive professional voice use without formal training. The physician should inquire into the patient's routine voice use and should specifically ask about any activities that frequently lead to voice change such as hoarseness or discomfort in the neck or throat. Laryngologists should ask specifically about other activities that may be abusive to the vocal folds such as weight lifting, aerobics, and the playing of some wind instruments.

Are You Aware of Misusing or Abusing Your Voice During Singing?

A detailed discussion of vocal technique in singing is beyond the scope of this chapter. The most common technical errors involve excessive muscle tension in the tongue, neck, and larynx; inadequate abdominal support; and excessive volume.

Inadequate preparation can be a devastating source of voice abuse and may result from limited practice, limited rehearsal of a difficult piece, or limited vocal training for a given role. The latter error is common. In some situations, voice teachers are at fault; both the singer and the teacher must resist the impulse to "show off" the voice in works that are either too difficult for the singer's level of training or simply not suited to the singer's voice. Singers are habitually unhappy with the limitations of their voices. At some time or another, most baritones wish they were tenors and walk around proving they can sing high Cs in "Vesti la giubba." Singers with other vocal ranges have similar fantasies. Attempts to make the voice something that it is not, or at least that it is not yet, frequently are harmful.

Are You Aware of Misusing or Abusing Your Voice During Speaking?

Common patterns of voice abuse and misuse will not be discussed in detail in this chapter. Voice abuse and/ or misuse should be suspected particularly in patients who complain of voice fatigue associated with voice use, whose voices are worse at the end of a working day or week, and in any patient who is chronically hoarse. Technical errors in voice use may be the primary etiology of a voice complaint, or it may develop secondarily due to a patient's effort to compensate for voice disturbance from another cause.

Dissociation of one's speaking and singing voices is probably the most common cause of voice abuse problems in excellent singers. Too frequently, all the expert training in support, muscle control, and projection is not applied to a singers' speaking voice. Unfortunately, the resultant voice strain affects the singing voice as well as the speaking voice. Such damage is especially likely to occur in noisy rooms and in cars, where the background noise is louder than it seems. Backstage greetings after a lengthy performance can be particularly devastating. The singer usually is exhausted and distracted; the environment is often dusty and dry, and generally a noisy crowd is present. Similar conditions prevail at postperformance parties, where smoking and alcohol worsen matters. These situations should be avoided by any singer with vocal problems and should be controlled through awareness at other times.

Three particularly abusive and potentially damaging vocal activities are worthy of note. *Cheerleading* requires extensive screaming under the worst possible physical and environmental circumstances. It is a highly undesirable activity for anyone considering serious vocal endeavor. This is a common conflict in younger singers because the teenager who is the high school choir soloist often is also student council president, yearbook editor, captain of the cheerleaders, and so on.

Conducting, particularly choral conducting, can also be deleterious. An enthusiastic conductor, especially of an amateur group, frequently sings all four parts intermittently, at volumes louder than the entire choir, during lengthy rehearsals. Conducting is a common avocation among singers but must be done with expert technique and special precautions to prevent voice injury. Hoarseness or loss of soft voice control after conducting a rehearsal or concert suggests voice abuse during conducting. The patient should be instructed to record his or her voice throughout the vocal range singing long notes at dynamics from soft to loud to soft. Recordings should be made prior to rehearsal and following rehearsal. If the voice has lost range, control, or quality during the rehearsal, voice abuse has occurred. A similar test can be used for patients who sing in choirs, teach voice, or perform other potentially abusive vocal activities. Such problems in conductors can generally be managed by additional training in conducting techniques and by voice training, including warm-up and cool-down exercises.

Teaching singing may also be hazardous to vocal health. It can be done safely but requires skill and thought. Most teachers teach while seated at the piano. Late in a long, hard day, this posture is not conducive to maintenance of optimal abdominal and back support. Usually, teachers work with students continually positioned to the right or left of the keyboard. This may require the teacher to turn his or her neck at a particularly sharp angle, especially when teaching at an upright piano. Teachers also often demonstrate vocal works in their students' vocal ranges rather than their own, illustrating bad as well as good technique. If a singing teacher is hoarse or has neck discomfort, or his or her soft singing control deteriorates at the end of a teaching day (assuming that the teacher warms up before beginning to teach voice lessons), voice abuse should be suspected. Helpful modifications include teaching with a grand piano, sitting slightly sideways on the piano bench, or alternating student position to the right and left of the piano to facilitate better neck alignment. Retaining an accompanist so that the teacher can stand rather than teach from sitting behind a piano, and many other helpful modifications, are possible.

Do You Have Pain When You Talk or Sing?

Odynophonia, or pain caused by phonation, can be a disturbing symptom. It is not uncommon, but relatively little has been written or discussed on this subject. A detailed review of odynophonia is beyond the scope of this publication. However, laryngologists should be familiar with the diagnosis and treatment of at least a few of the most common causes, at least, as discussed elsewhere in this book.

What Kind of Physical Condition Are You In?

Phonation is an athletic activity that requires good conditioning and coordinated interaction of numerous physical functions. Maladies of any part of the body may be reflected in the voice. Failure to maintain good abdominal muscle tone and respiratory endurance through exercise is particularly harmful because deficiencies in these areas undermine the power source of the voice. Patients generally attempt to compensate for such weaknesses by using inappropriate muscle groups, particularly in the neck, causing vocal dysfunction. Similar problems may occur in the well-conditioned vocalist in states of fatigue. These are compounded by mucosal changes that accompany excessively long hours of hard work. Such problems may be seen even in the best singers shortly before important performances in the height of the concert season.

A popular but untrue myth holds that great opera singers must be obese. However, the vivacious, gregarious personality that often distinguishes the great performer seems to be accompanied frequently by a propensity for excess, especially culinary excess. This excess is as undesirable in the vocalist as it is in most other athletic artists, and it should be prevented from the start of one's vocal career. Appropriate and attractive body weight has always been valued in the pop music world and is becoming particularly important in the opera world as this formerly theater-based art form moves to television and film media. However, attempts at weight reduction in an established speaker or singer are a different matter. The vocal mechanism is a finely tuned, complex instrument and is exquisitely sensitive to minor changes. Substantial fluctuations in weight frequently cause deleterious alterations of the voice, although these are usually temporary. Weight reduction programs for people concerned about their voices must be monitored carefully and designed to reduce weight in small increments over long periods. A history of sudden recent weight change may be responsible for almost any vocal complaint.

How Is Your Hearing?

Hearing loss can cause substantial problems for singers and other professional voice users. This may be true especially when the voice patient is unaware that he or she has hearing loss. Consequently, not only should voice patients be asked about hearing loss, tinnitus, vertigo, and family history of hearing loss, but it is also helpful to inquire of spouses, partners, friends, or others who may have accompanied the patient to the office whether they have suspected a hearing impairment in the patient.

Have You Noted Voice or Bodily Weakness, Tremor, Fatigue, or Loss of Control?

Even minor neurologic disorders may be extremely disruptive to vocal function. Specific questions should be asked to rule out neuromuscular and neurologic diseases such as myasthenia gravis, Parkinson disease, tremors, other movement disorders, spasmodic dysphonia, multiple sclerosis, central nervous system neoplasm, and other serious maladies that may be present with voice complaints.

Do You Have Allergy or Cold Symptoms?

Acute upper respiratory tract infection causes inflammation of the mucosa, alters mucosal secretions, and makes the mucosa more vulnerable to injury. Coughing and throat clearing are particularly traumatic vocal activities and may worsen or provoke hoarseness associated with a cold. Postnasal drip and allergy may produce the same response. Infectious sinusitis is associated with discharge and diffuse mucosal inflammation, resulting in similar problems, and may actually alter the sound of a voice, especially the patient's own perception of his or her voice. Futile attempts to compensate for disease of the supraglottic vocal tract in an effort to return the sound to normal frequently result in laryngeal strain. The expert singer or speaker should compensate by monitoring technique by tactile rather than by auditory feedback, or singing "by feel" rather than "by ear."

Do You Have Breathing Problems, Especially After Exercise?

Voice patients usually volunteer information about upper respiratory tract infections and postnasal drip, but the relevance of other maladies may not be obvious to them. Consequently, the physician must seek out pertinent history.

Respiratory problems are especially important in voice patients. Even mild respiratory dysfunction may adversely affect the power source of the voice [8]. Occult asthma may be particularly troublesome [9]. A complete respiratory history should be obtained in most patients with voice complaints, and pulmonary function testing is often advisable.

Have You Been Exposed to Environmental Irritants?

Any mucosal irritant can disrupt the delicate vocal mechanism. Allergies to dust and mold are aggravated commonly during rehearsals and performances in concert halls, especially older theaters and concert halls, because of numerous curtains, backstage trappings, and dressing room facilities that are rarely cleaned thoroughly. Nasal obstruction and erythematous conjunctivae suggest generalized mucosal irritation. The drying effects of cold air and dry heat may also affect mucosal secretions, leading to decreased lubrication, a "scratchy" voice, and tickling cough. These symptoms may be minimized by nasal breathing, which allows inspired air to be filtered, warmed, and humidified. Nasal breathing, whenever possible, rather than mouth breathing, is proper vocal technique. While the performer is backstage between appearances or during rehearsals, inhalation of dust and other irritants may be controlled by wearing a protective mask, such as those used by carpenters, or a surgical mask that does not contain fiberglass. This is especially helpful when sets are being constructed in the rehearsal area.

A history of recent travel suggests other sources of mucosal irritation. The air in airplanes is extremely dry, and airplanes are noisy [10]. One must be careful to avoid talking loudly and to maintain good hydration and nasal breathing during air travel. Environmental changes can also be disruptive. Las Vegas is infamous for the mucosal irritation caused by its dry atmosphere and smoke-filled rooms. In fact, the resultant complex of hoarseness, vocal "tickle," and fatigue is referred to as "Las Vegas voice." A history of recent travel should also suggest jet lag and generalized fatigue, which may be potent detriments to good vocal function.

Environmental pollution is responsible for the presence of toxic substances and conditions encountered daily. Inhalation of toxic pollutants may affect the voice adversely by direct laryngeal injury, by causing pulmonary dysfunction that results in voice maladies, or through impairments elsewhere in the vocal tract. Ingested substances, especially those that have neurolaryngologic effects, may also adversely affect the voice. Nonchemical environmental pollutants such as noise can cause voice abnormalities, as well. Laryngologists should be familiar with the laryngologic effects of the numerous potentially irritating substances and conditions found in the environment. We must also be familiar with special pollution problems encountered by performers. Numerous materials used by artists to create sculptures, drawings, and theatrical sets are toxic and have adverse voice effects. In addition, performers are exposed routinely to chemicals encountered through stage smoke and pyrotechnic effects. Although it is clear that some of the "special effects" may result in serious laryngologic consequences, much additional study is needed to clarify the nature and scope of these occupational problems.

Do You Smoke, Live with a Smoker, or Work Around Smoke?

The effects of smoking on voice performance were reviewed recently in the *Journal of Singing* [11], and that review is recapitulated here. Smoking tobacco is the number one cause of preventable death in the United States as well as the leading cause of heart disease, stroke, emphysema, and cancer. The Centers for Disease Control and Prevention (CDC) attributes approximately 442,000 premature (shortened life expectancy) deaths annually in the United States to smoking, which is more than the combined incidence of deaths caused by highway accidents, fires, murders, illegal drugs, suicides, and AIDS [12]. Approximately 4 million deaths per year worldwide result from smoking, and if this trend continues, by 2030, this figure will increase to about 10 million deaths globally [13]. In addition to causing life-threatening diseases, smoking impairs a great many body systems, including the vocal tract. Harmful consequences of smoking or being exposed to smoke influence voice performance adversely.

Singers need good vocal health to perform well. Smoking tobacco can irritate the mucosal covering of the vocal folds, causing redness and chronic inflammation, and can have the same effect on the mucosal lining of the lungs, trachea, nasopharynx (behind the nose and throat), and mouth. In other words, the components of voice production—the generator, the oscillator, the resonator, and the articulator—all can be compromised by the harmful effects of tobacco use. The onset of effects from smoking may be immediate or delayed.

Individuals who have allergies and/or asthma are usually more sensitive to cigarette smoke with potential for an immediate adverse reaction involving the lungs, larynx, nasal cavities, and/or eyes. Chronic use of tobacco, or exposure to it, causes the toxic chemicals in tobacco to accumulate in the body, damaging the delicate linings of the vocal tract, as well as the lungs, heart, and circulatory system.

The lungs are critical components of the power source of the vocal tract. They help generate an airstream that is directed superiorly through the trachea toward the undersurface of the vocal folds. The vocal folds respond to the increase in subglottic pressure by producing sounds of variable intensities and frequencies. The number of times per second the vocal fold vibrate influences the pitch, and the amplitude of the mucosal wave influences the loudness of the sound. The sound produced by the vibration (oscillation) of the vocal folds passes upward through the oral cavity and nasopharynx where it resonates, giving the voice its richness and timbre, and eventually it is articulated by the mouth, teeth, lips, and tongue into speech or song.

Any condition that adversely affects lung function such as chronic exposure to smoke or uncontrolled asthma can contribute to dysphonia by impairing the strength, endurance, and consistency of the airstream responsible for establishing vocal fold oscillation. Any lesion that compromises vocal fold vibration and glottic closure can cause hoarseness and breathiness. Inflammation of the cover layer of the vocal folds and/or the mucosal lining of the nose, sinuses, and oral nasopharyngeal cavities can affect the quality and clarity of the voice.

Tobacco smoke can damage the lungs' parenchyma and the exchange of air through respiration. Cigarette manufacturers add hundreds of ingredients to their tobacco products to improve taste, to make smoking seem milder and easier to inhale, and to prolong burning and shelf life [14]. More than 3000 chemical compounds have been identified in tobacco smoke, and more than 60 of these compounds are carcinogens [15]. The tobacco plant, *Nicotiana tabacum*, is grown for its leaves, which can be smoked, chewed, or sniffed with various effects. The nicotine in tobacco is the addictive component and rivals crack cocaine in its ability to enslave its users. Most smokers want to stop, yet only a small percentage are successful in quitting cigarettes; the majority who quit relapse into smoking once again [16]. Tar and carbon monoxide are among the disease-causing components in tobacco products. The tar in cigarettes exposes the individual to a greater risk of bronchitis, emphysema, and lung cancer. These chemicals affect the entire vocal tract as well as the cardiovascular system (Table 2.1).

Table 2.1 Chemical additives found in tobaccos and commercial products

Tobacco chemical additives	Also found in
Acetic acid	Vinegar, hair dye
Acetone	Nail polish remover
Ammonia	Floor cleaner, toilet cleaner
Arsenic	Poison
Benzene	A leukemia-producing agent in rubber cement
Butane	Cigarette lighter fluid
Cadmium	Batteries, some oil paints
Carbon monoxide	Car exhaust
DDT	Insecticides
Ethanol	Alcohol
Formaldehyde	Embalming fluid, fabric, laboratory animals
Hexamine	Barbecue lighter
Hydrazine	Jet fuel, rocket fuel
Hydrogen cyanide	Gas chamber poison
Methane	Swamp gas
Methanol	Rocket fuel
Naphthalene	Explosives, mothballs, paints
Nickel	Electroplating
Nicotine	Insecticides
Nitrobenzene	Gasoline additive
Nitrous oxide phenols	Disinfectant
Phenol	Disinfectants, plastics
Polonium-210	A radioactive substance
Stearic acid	Candle wax
Styrene	Insulation materials
Toluene	Industrial solvent, embalmer's glue
Vinyl chloride	Plastic manufacturing, garbage bags

Cigarette smoke in the lungs can lead also to increased vascularity, edema, and excess mucous production, as well as epithelial tissue and cellular changes. The toxic agents in cigarette smoke have been associated with an increase in the number and severity of asthma attacks, chronic bronchitis, emphysema, and lung cancer, all of which can interfere with the lungs' ability to generate the stream of air needed for voice production.

Chronic bronchitis due to smoking has been associated with an increase in the number of goblet (mucous) cells, an increase in the size (hyperplasia) of the mucosal secreting glands, and a decrease in the number of ciliated cells, the cells used to clean the lungs. Chronic cough and sputum production are also seen more commonly in smokers compared with nonsmokers. Also, the heat and chemicals of unfiltered cigarette and marijuana smoke are especially irritating to the lungs and larynx.

An important component of voice quality is the symmetrical, unencumbered vibration of the true vocal folds. Anything that prevents the epithelium covering the vocal folds from vibrating or affects the loose connective tissue under the epithelium (in the superficial layer of the lamina propria known as the Reinke's space) can cause dysphonia. Cigarette smoking can cause the epithelium of the true vocal folds to become red and swollen, develop whitish discolorations (leukoplakia), undergo chronic inflammatory changes, or develop squamous metaplasia or dysplasia (tissue changes from normal to a potentially malignant state). In chronic smokers, the voice may become husky due to the accumulation of fluid in the Reinke's space (Reinke's edema). These alterations in structure can interfere with voice production by changing the biomechanics of the vocal folds and their vibratory characteristics. In severe cases, cancer can deform and paralyze the vocal folds.

Vocal misuse often follows in an attempt to compensate for dysphonia and an alerted self-perception of one's voice. The voice may feel weak, breathy, raspy, or strained. There may be a loss of range, vocal breaks, long warm-up time, and fatigue. The throat may feel raw, achy, or tight. As the voice becomes unreliable, bad habits increase as the individual struggles harder and harder to compensate vocally. As selected sound waves move upward, from the larynx toward and through the pharynx, nasopharynx, mouth, and nose (the resonators), sounds gain a unique richness and timbre. Exposing the pharynx to cigarette smoke aggravates the linings of the oropharynx, mouth, nasopharynx, sinuses, and nasal cavities. The resulting erythema, swelling, and inflammation predispose one to nasal congestion and impaired mucosal function; there may be predisposition to sinusitis and pharyngitis, in which the voice may become hyponasal, the sinus achy, and the throat painful.

Although relatively rare in the United States, cancer of the nasopharynx has been associated with cigarette smoking [17], and one of the presenting symptoms is unilateral hearing loss due to fluid in the middle ear caused by eustachian tube obstruction from the cancer. Smoking-induced cancers of the oral cavity, pharynx, larynx, and lung are common throughout the world, including in the United States.

The palate, tongue, cheeks, lips, and teeth articulate the sound modified by the resonators into speech. Cigarettes, cigar, or pipe smoking may cause a "black hairy tongue," precancerous oral lesions (leukoplakia), and/or cancer of the tongue and lips [18]. Any irritation that causes burning or inflammation of the oral mucosa can affect phonation, and all tobacco products are capable of causing these effects.

Smokeless "spit" tobacco is highly addictive, and users who dip 8–10 times a day may get the same nicotine exposure as those who smoke 1½–2 packs of cigarettes per day [19]. Smokeless tobacco has been associated with gingivitis, cheek carcinoma, and cancer of the larynx and hypopharynx.

Exposure to environmental tobacco smoke (ETS), also called secondhand smoke, side-stream smoke, or passive smoke, accounts for an estimated 3000 lung cancer deaths and approximately 35,000 deaths in the United States from heart disease in nonsmoking adults [20].

Secondhand smoke is the "passive" inhalation of tobacco smoke from environmental sources such as smoke given off by pipes, cigars, cigarettes (side-stream), or the smoke exhaled from the lungs of smokers and inhaled by other people (mainstream). This passive smoke contains a mixture of thousands of chemicals, some of which are known to cause cancer. The National Institutes of Health (NIH) lists ETS as a "known" carcinogen, and the more you are exposed to secondhand smoke, the greater your risk [21].

Infants and young children are affected particularly by secondhand smoke with increased incidences of otitis media (ear infections), bronchitis, and pneumonia. If small children are exposed to secondhand smoke, the child's resulting illness can have a stressful effect on the parent who frequently catches the child's illness. Both the illness and the stress of caring for the sick child may interfere with voice performance. People who are exposed routinely to secondhand smoke are at risk for lung cancer, heart disease, respiratory infection, and an increased number of asthma attacks [22].

There is an intricate relationship between the lungs, larynx, pharynx, nose, and mouth in the production of speech and song. Smoking can have deleterious effects on any part of the vocal tract, causing the respiratory system to lose power, damaging the vibratory margins of the vocal folds, and detracting from the richness and beauty of a voice.

The deleterious effects of tobacco smoke on mucosa are indisputable. Anyone concerned about the health of his or her voice should not smoke. Smoking causes erythema, mild edema, and generalized inflammation throughout the vocal tract. Both smoke itself and the heat of the cigarette appear to be important. Marijuana produces a particularly irritating, unfiltered smoke that is inhaled directly, causing considerable mucosal response. Voice patients who refuse to stop smoking marijuana should at least be advised to use a water pipe to cool and partially filter the smoke. Some vocalists are required to perform in smoke-filled environments and may suffer the same effects as the smokers themselves. In some theaters, it is possible to place fans upstage or direct the ventilation system so as to create a gentle draft toward the audience, clearing the smoke away from the stage. "Smoke eaters" installed in some theaters are also helpful.

Do Any Foods Seem to Affect Your Voice?

Various foods are said to affect the voice. Traditionally, singers avoid milk and ice cream before performances. In many people, these foods seem to increase the amount and viscosity of mucosal secretions. Allergy and casein have been implicated, but no satisfactory explanation has been established. In some cases, restriction of these foods from the diet before a voice performance may be helpful. Chocolate may have the same effect and should be viewed similarly. Chocolate also contains caffeine, which may aggravate reflux or cause tremor. Voice patients should be asked about eating nuts. This is important not only because some people experience effects similar to those produced by milk products and chocolate but also because they are extremely irritating if aspirated. The irritation produced by aspiration of even a small organic foreign body may be severe and impossible to correct rapidly enough to permit performance. Highly spiced foods may also cause mucosal irritation. In addition, they seem to aggravate reflux laryngitis. Coffee and other beverages containing caffeine also aggravate gastric reflux and may promote dehydration and/or alter secretions and necessitate frequent throat clearing in some people. Fad diets, especially rapid weight-reducing diets, are notorious for causing voice problems. Eating a full meal before a speaking or singing engagement may interfere with abdominal support or may aggravate upright reflux of gastric juice during abdominal muscle contraction. Lemon juice and herbal teas are considered beneficial to the voice. Both may act as demulcents, thinning secretions, and may very well be helpful.

Do You Have Morning Hoarseness, Bad Breath, Excessive Phlegm, a Lump in Your Throat, or Heartburn?

Reflux laryngitis is especially common among singers and trained speakers because of the high intraabdominal pressure associated with proper support and because of lifestyle. Singers frequently perform at night. Many vocalists refrain from eating before performances because a full stomach can compromise effective abdominal support. They typically compensate by eating heartily at postperformance gatherings late at night and then go to bed with a full stomach.

Chronic irritation of arytenoid and vocal fold mucosa by reflux of gastric secretions may occasionally be associated with dyspepsia or pyrosis. However, the key features of this malady are bitter taste and halitosis on awakening in the morning, a dry or "coated" mouth, often a scratchy sore throat or a feeling of a "lump in the throat," hoarseness, and the need for prolonged vocal warm-up. The physician must be alert to these symptoms and ask about them routinely; otherwise, the diagnosis will often be overlooked, because people who have had this problem for many years or a lifetime do not even realize it is abnormal.

Do You Have Trouble with Your Bowels or Belly?

Any condition that alters abdominal function, such as muscle spasm, constipation, or diarrhea, interferes with support and may result in a voice complaint. These symptoms may accompany infection, anxiety, various gastroenterological diseases, and other maladies.

Are You Under Particular Stress or in Therapy?

The human voice is an exquisitely sensitive messenger of emotion. Highly trained voice professionals learn to control the effects of anxiety and other emotional stress on their voices under ordinary circumstances. However, in some instances, this training may break down or a performer may be inadequately prepared to control the voice under specific stressful conditions. Preperformance anxiety is the most common example, but insecurity, depression, and other emotional disturbances are also generally reflected in the voice. Anxiety reactions are mediated in part through the autonomic nervous system and result in a dry mouth, cold clammy skin, and thick secretions. These reactions are normal, and good vocal training coupled with assurance that no abnormality or disease is present generally overcomes them. However, long-term, poorly compensated emotional stress and exogenous stress (from agents, producers, teachers, parents, etc.) may cause substantial vocal dysfunction and may result in permanent limitations of the vocal apparatus. These conditions must be diagnosed and treated expertly. Hypochondriasis is uncommon among professional singers, despite popular opinion to the contrary.

Recent publications have highlighted the complexity and importance of psychological factors associated with voice disorders [23]. A comprehensive discussion of this subject is also presented elsewhere in this book. It is important for the physician to recognize that psychological problems may not only cause voice disorders but also delay recovery from voice disorders that were entirely organic in etiology. Professional voice users, especially singers, have enormous psychological investment and personality identifications associated with their voices. A condition that causes voice loss or permanent injury often evokes the same powerful psychological responses seen following death of a loved one. This process may be initiated even when physical recovery is complete if an incident (injury or surgery) has made the vocalist realize that voice loss is possible. Such a "brush with death" can have profound emotional consequences in some patients. It is essential for laryngologists to be aware of these powerful factors and manage them properly if optimal therapeutic results are to be achieved expeditiously.

Do You Have Problems Controlling Your Weight? Are You Excessively Tired? Are You Cold When Other People Are Warm?

Endocrine problems warrant special attention. The human voice is extremely sensitive to endocrinologic changes. Many of these are reflected in alterations of fluid content of the lamina propria just beneath the laryngeal mucosa. This causes alterations in the bulk and shape of the vocal folds and results in voice change. Hypothyroidism [24–28] is a well-recognized cause of such voice disorders, although the mechanism is not fully understood. Hoarseness, vocal fatigue, muffling of the voice, loss of range, and a sensation of a lump in the throat may be present even with mild hypothyroidism. Even when thyroid function tests results are within the low normal range, this diagnosis should be entertained, especially if thyroid-stimulating hormone levels are in the high normal range or are elevated. Thyrotoxicosis may result in similar voice disturbances [25].

Do You Have Menstrual Irregularity, Cyclical Voice Changes Associated with Menses, Recent Menopause, or Other Hormonal Changes or Problems?

Voice changes associated with sex hormones are encountered commonly in clinical practice and have been investigated more thoroughly than have other hormonal changes [29, 30]. Although a correlation appears to exist between sex hormone levels and depth of male voices (higher testosterone and lower estradiol levels in basses than in tenors) [29], the most important hormonal considerations in males occur during or related to puberty [31, 32]. Voice problems related to sex hormones are more common in female singers (Carroll C, 1992, personal communication with Dr. Hans von Leden, Arizona State University at Tempe) [32–48].

Do You Have Jaw Joint or Other Dental Problems?

Dental disease, especially temporomandibular joint (TMJ) dysfunction, introduces muscle tension in the head and neck, which is transmitted to the larynx directly through the muscular attachments between the mandible and the hyoid bone and indirectly as generalized increased muscle tension. These problems often result in decreased range, vocal fatigue, and change in the quality or placement of a voice. Such tension often is accompanied by excess tongue muscle activity, especially pulling of the tongue posteriorly. This hyperfunctional behavior acts through hyoid attachments to disrupt the balance between the intrinsic and extrinsic laryngeal musculature. TMJ problems are also problematic for wind instrumentalists and some string players, including violinists. In some cases, the problems may actually be caused by instrumental technique. The history should always include information about musical activities, including instruments other than the voice.

Do You or Your Blood Relatives Have Hearing Loss?

Hearing loss is often overlooked as a source of vocal problems. Auditory feedback is fundamental to speaking and singing. Interference with this control mechanism may result in altered vocal production, particularly if the person is unaware of the hearing loss. Distortion, particularly pitch distortion (diplacusis), may also pose serious problems for the singer. This appears to be due not only to aesthetic difficulties in matching pitch but also to vocal strain that accompanies pitch shifts [49].

In addition to determining whether the patient has hearing loss, inquiry should also be made about hearing impairment occurring in family members, roommates, and other close associates. Speaking loudly to people who are hard of hearing can cause substantial, chronic vocal strain. This possibility should be investigated routinely when evaluating voice patients.

Have You Suffered Whiplash or Other Bodily Injury?

Various bodily injuries outside the confines of the vocal tract may have profound effects on the voice. Whiplash, for example, commonly causes changes in technique, with consequent voice fatigue, loss of range, difficulty singing softly, and other problems. These problems derive from the neck muscle spasm, abnormal neck posturing secondary to pain, and consequent hyperfunctional voice use. Lumbar, abdominal, head, chest, supraglottic, and extremity injuries may also affect vocal technique and be responsible for the dysphonia that prompted the voice patient to seek medical attention.

Did You Undergo Any Surgery Prior to the Onset of Your Voice Problems?

A history of laryngeal surgery in a voice patient is a matter of great concern. It is important to establish exactly why the surgery was done, by whom it was done, whether intubation was necessary, and whether voice therapy was instituted pre-or postoperatively if the lesion was associated with voice abuse (vocal nodules). If the vocal dysfunction that sent the patient to the physician's office dates from the immediate postoperative period, surgical trauma must be suspected.

Otolaryngologists frequently are asked about the effects of tonsillectomy on the voice. Singers especially may consult the physician after tonsillectomy and complain of vocal dysfunction. Certainly removal of tonsils can alter the voice [50, 51]. Tonsillectomy changes the configuration of the supraglottic vocal tract. In addition, scarring alters pharyngeal muscle function, which is trained meticulously in the professional singer. Singers must be warned that they may have permanent voice changes after tonsillectomy; however, these can be minimized by dissecting in the proper plane to lessen scarring. The singer's voice generally requires 3–6 months to stabilize or return to normal after surgery, although it is generally safe to begin limited singing within 2–4 weeks following surgery. As with any procedure for which general anesthesia may be needed, the anesthesiologist should be advised preoperatively that the patient is a professional singer. Intubation and extubation should be performed with great care, and the use of nonirritating plastic rather than rubber or ribbed metal endotracheal tubes is preferred. Use of a laryngeal mask may be advisable for selected procedures for mechanical reasons, but this device is often not ideal for tonsillectomy, and it can cause laryngeal injury such as arytenoid dislocation.

Surgery of the neck, such as thyroidectomy, may result in permanent alterations in the vocal mechanism through scarring of the extrinsic laryngeal musculature. The cervical (strap) muscles are important in maintaining laryngeal position and stability of the laryngeal skeleton, and they should be retracted rather than divided whenever possible. A history of recurrent or superior laryngeal nerve injury may explain a hoarse, breathy, or weak voice. However, in rare cases, even a singer can compensate for recurrent laryngeal nerve paralysis and have a nearly normal voice.

Thoracic and abdominal surgery interferes with respiratory and abdominal support. After these procedures, singing and projected speaking should be prohibited until pain has subsided and healing has occurred sufficiently to allow normal support. Abdominal exercises should be instituted before resumption of vocalizing. Singing and speaking without proper support are often worse for the voice than not using the voice for performance at all.

Other surgical procedures may be important factors if they necessitate intubation or if they affect the musculoskeletal system so that the person has to change stance or balance. For example, balancing on one foot after leg surgery may decrease the effectiveness of the support mechanism.

What Medications and Other Substances Do You Use?

A history of alcohol abuse suggests the probability of poor vocal technique. Intoxication results in incoordination and decreased awareness, which undermine vocal discipline designed to optimize and protect the voice. The effect of small amounts of alcohol is controversial. Although many experts oppose its use because of its vasodilatory effect and consequent mucosal alteration, many people do not seem to be adversely affected by small amounts of alcohol such as a glass of wine with a meal. However, some people have mild sensitivities to certain wines or beers. Patients who develop nasal congestion and rhinorrhea after drinking beer, for example, should be made aware that they probably have a mild allergy to that particular beverage and should avoid it before voice commitments.

Patients frequently acquire antihistamines to help control "postnasal drip" or other symptoms. The drying effect of antihistamines may result in decreased vocal fold lubrication, increased throat clearing, and irritability leading to frequent coughing. Antihistamines may be helpful to some voice patients, but they must be used with caution.

When a voice patient seeking the attention of a physician is already taking antibiotics, it is important to find out the dose and the prescribing physician, if any, as well as whether the patient frequently treats himself or herself with inadequate courses of antibiotics often supplied by colleagues. Singers, actors, and other speakers sometimes have a "sore throat" shortly before important vocal presentations and start themselves on inappropriate antibiotic therapy, which they generally discontinue after their performance.

Diuretics are also popular among some performers. They are often prescribed by gynecologists at the vocalist's request to help deplete excess water in the premenstrual period. They are not effective in this scenario, because they cannot diurese the protein-bound water in the laryngeal ground substance. Unsupervised use of these drugs may cause dehydration and consequent mucosal dryness.

Hormone use, especially use of oral contraceptives, must be mentioned specifically during the physician's inquiry. Women frequently do not mention them routinely when asked whether they are taking any medication. Vitamins are also frequently not mentioned. Most vitamin therapy seems to have little effect on the voice. However, high-dose vitamin C (5–6 g/d), which some people use to prevent upper respiratory tract infections, seems to act as a mild diuretic and may lead to dehydration and xerophonia [52].

Cocaine use is common, especially among pop musicians. This drug can be extremely irritating to the nasal mucosa, causes marked vasoconstriction, and may alter the sensorium, resulting in decreased voice control and a tendency toward vocal abuse.

Many pain medications (including aspirin and ibuprofen), psychotropic medications, and others may be responsible for a voice complaint. So far, no adverse vocal effects have been reported with selective COX-2 inhibiting anti-inflammatory medications (which do not promote bleeding, as do other nonsteroidal anti-inflammatory medicines and aspirin) such as celecoxib (Celebrex; Pfizer, Inc., New York, New York) and valecoxib (Bextra; Pharmacia Corp, New York, New York). However this group of drugs has been demonstrated to have other side effects, and should in our view only be taken under the care of a physician [53]. The effects of other new medications such as sildenafil citrate (Viagra; Pfizer, Inc.) and medications used to induce abortion remain unstudied and unknown, but it seems plausible that such medication may affect voice function, at least temporarily. Laryngologists should be familiar with the laryngologic effects of the many substances ingested medically and recreationally.

Acknowledgment Modified in part from Rubin J, Sataloff R, Korovin G. *Diagnosis and Treatment of Voice Disorders*, 4th ed. San Diego, CA: Plural Publishing; 2014; with permission.

References

1. Sataloff RT. Professional singers: the science and art of clinical care. Am J Otolaryngol. 1981;2:251–66.
2. Sataloff RT. The human voice. Sci Am. 1992;267:108–15.
3. Sundberg J. The science of the singing voice. DeKalb: Northern Illinois University Press; 1987.
4. Sataloff RT. Efficient history taking in professional singers. Laryngoscope. 1984;94:1111–4.
5. Ackerman R, Pfan W. Gerontology studies on the susceptibility to voice disorders in professional speakers. Folia Phoniatr (Basel). 1974;26:95–9.
6. von Leden H. Speech and hearing problems in the geriatric patient. J Am Geriatr Soc. 1977;25:422–6.
7. Schiff M. Comment. Presented at: seventh symposium on care of the professional voice; June 15–16, 1978; The Juilliard School, New York.
8. Spiegel JR, Cohn JR, Sataloff RT, et al. Respiratory function in singers: medical assessment, diagnoses, treatments. J Voice. 1988;2:40–50.
9. Cohn JR, Sataloff RT, Spiegel JR, et al. Airway reactivity-induced asthma in singers (ARIAS). J Voice. 1991;5:332–7.
10. Feder RJ. The professional voice and airline flight. Otolaryngol Head Neck Surg. 1984;92:251–4.

11. Anticaglia A, Hawkshaw M, Sataloff RT. The effects of smoking on voice performance. J Singing. 2004;60:161–7.
12. Centers for Disease Control and Prevention (CDC). Annual smoking-attributable, mortality, years of potential life lost, and economic costs, United States—1995–1999. MMWR Morb Mortal Wkly Rep. 2002;51(14):300–3.
13. World Health Organization. World health report 1999. Geneva: World Health Organization; 1999.
14. United States Department of Health Services (USDHHS). Tobacco products fact sheet. Washington, DC: Government Printing Office; 2000.
15. National Cancer Institute. Environmental tobacco smoke. Fact sheet 3.9; 1999. http://cis.nci.nih.gov/fact/3_9htm.
16. Centers for Disease Control and Prevention. Cigarette smoking among adults—United States, 1993. MMWR Morb Mortal Wkly Rep. 1994;3:925–9.
17. Chow WH, McLaughlin JK, Hrubec Z, et al. Tobacco use and nasopharyngeal carcinoma in a cohort of US veterans. Int J Cancer. 1993;55(4):538–40.
18. Casiglia J, Woo SB. A comprehensive view of oral cancer. Gen Dent. 2001;49(1):72–82.
19. Centers for Disease Control and Prevention. Determination of nicotine pH and moisture content of six U.S. commercial moist snuff products. MMWR Morb Mortal Wkly Rep. 1999;48(19):398.
20. American Cancer Society. Cancer facts and figures 2002. Atlanta: American Cancer Society; 2002.
21. National Toxicology Program (NTP). Report on carcinogens. 10th ed. Research Triangle Park: U.S. Department Health and Human Services, Public Health Service, National Toxicology Program; 2002. http://ehp.niehs.nih.gov/roc/toc10.html
22. Academy of Pediatrics, Committee on Environmental Health. Environmental tobacco smoke; a hazard to children. Pediatrics. 1997;99(4):639–42.
23. Rosen DC, Sataloff RT. Psychology of voice disorders. 2nd ed. San Diego: Plural Publishing, Inc.; 2020.
24. Gupta OP, Bhatia PL, Agarwal MK, et al. Nasal pharyngeal and laryngeal manifestations of hypothyroidism. Ear Nose Throat J. 1997;56:10–21.
25. Malinsky M, Muller C, Cerceau N. Etude clinique et electrophysiologique des alterations de la voix au cours des thyrotoxioses. Ann Endocrinol (Paris). 1997;38:171–2.
26. Michelsson K, Sirvio P. Cry analysis in congenital hypothyroidism. Folia Phoniatr (Basel). 1976;28:40–7.
27. Ritter FN. The effect of hypothyroidism on the larynx of the rat. Ann Otol Rhinol Laryngol. 1964;67:404–16.
28. Ritter FN. Endocrinology. In: Paparella M, Shumrick D, editors. Otolaryngology, vol. I. Philadelphia: Saunders; 1973. p. 727–34.
29. Meuser W, Nieschlag E. Sex hormones and depth of voice in the male [in German]. Dtsch Med Wochenschr. 1977;102:261–4.
30. Schiff M. The influence of estrogens on connective tissue. In: Asboe-Hansen G, editor. Hormones and connective tissue. Copenhagen: Munksgaard Press; 1967. p. 282–341.
31. Brodnitz F. The age of the castrato voice. J Speech Hear Disord. 1975;40:291–5.
32. Brodnitz F. Hormones and the human voice. Bull NY Acad Med. 1971;47:183–91.
33. von Gelder L. Psychosomatic aspects of endocrine disorders of the voice. J Commun Disord. 1974;7:257–62.
34. Lacina O. Der Einfluss der Menstruation auf die Stimme der Sangerinnen. Folia Phoniatr (Basel). 1968;20:13–24.
35. Wendler J. The influence of menstruation on the voice of the female singer. Folia Phoniatr (Basel). 1972;24:259–77.
36. Brodnitz F. Medical care preventive therapy (panel). In: Lawrence VL, editor. Transcripts of the seventh annual symposium, care of the professional Voice, vol. 3. New York: The Voice Foundation; 1978. p. 86.
37. Dordain M. Etude Statistique de l'influence des contraceptifs hormonaux sur la voix. Folia Phoniatr (Basel). 1972;24:86–96.
38. Pahn J, Goretzlehner G. Voice changes following the use of oral contraceptives [in German]. Zentralbl Gynakol. 1978;100:341–6.
39. Schiff M. "The pill" in otolaryngology. Trans Am Acad Ophthalmol Otolaryngol. 1968;72:76–84.
40. von Deuster CV. Irreversible vocal changes in pregnancy [in German]. HNO. 1977;25:430–2.
41. Flach M, Schwickardi H, Simen R. Welchen Einfluss haben Menstruation and Schwangerschaft auf die augsgebildete Gesangsstimme? Folia Phoniatr (Basel). 1968;21:199–210.
42. Arndt HJ. Stimmstorungen nach Behandlung mit Androgenen und anabolen Hormonen. Munch Med Wochenschr. 1974;116:1715–20.
43. Bourdial J. Les troubles de la voix provoques par la therapeutique hormonale androgene. Ann Otolaryngol Chir Cervicofac. 1970;87:725–34.
44. Damste PH. Virilization of the voice due to anabolic steroids [in Dutch]. Ned Tijdschr Geneeskd. 1963;107:891–2.
45. Damste PH. Voice changes in adult women caused by virilizing agents. J Speech Hear Disord. 1967;32:126–32.
46. Saez S, Francoise S. Recepteurs d'androgenes: mise en evidence dans la fraction cytosolique de muqueuse normale et d'epitheliomas phryngolaryngеs humains. C R Acad Sci Hebd Seances Acad Sci D. 1975;280:935–8.
47. Vuorenkoski V, Lenko HL, Tjernlund P, et al. Fundamental voice frequency during normal and abnormal growth, and after androgen treatment. Arch Dis Child. 1978;53:201–9.
48. Imre V. Hormonell bedingte Stimmstorungen. Folia Phoniatr (Basel). 1968;20:394–404.

49. Sundberg J, Prame E, Iwarsson J. Replicability and accuracy of pitch patterns in professional singers. In: Davis PJ, Fletcher NH, editors. Vocal fold physiology: controlling chaos and complexity. San Diego: Singular Publishing Group; 1996. p. 291–306.
50. Gould WJ, Alberti PW, Brodnitz F, Hirano M. Medical care preventive therapy [Panel]. In: Lawrence VL, editor. Transcripts of the seventh annual symposium, care of the professional voice, vol. 3. New York: The Voice Foundation; 1978. p. 74–6.
51. Wallner LJ, Hill BJ, Waldrop W, Monroe C. Voice changes following adenotonsillectomy. Laryngoscope. 1968;78:1410–8.
52. Lawrence VL. Medical care for professional voice (panel). In: Lawrence VL, editor. Transcripts from the annual symposium, care of the professional voice, vol. 3. New York: The Voice Foundation; 1978. p. 17–8.
53. Cannon CP. COX-2 inhibitors and cardiovascular risk. Science. 2012;336(6087):1386–7.

3 Physical Examination

A detailed history frequently reveals the cause of a voice problem even before a physical examination is performed. However, a comprehensive physical examination, often including objective assessment of voice function, also is essential [1–3].

Physical examination must include a thorough ear, nose, and throat evaluation and assessment of general physical condition. A patient who is extremely obese or appears fatigued, agitated, emotionally stressed, or otherwise generally ill has increased potential for voice dysfunction. This could be due to any number of factors: altered abdominal support, loss of fine motor control of laryngeal muscles, decreased bulk of the submucosal vocal fold ground substance, change in the character of mucosal secretions, or other similar mechanisms. Any physical condition that impairs the normal function of the abdominal musculature is suspect as cause for dysphonia. Some conditions, such as pregnancy, are obvious; however, a sprained ankle or broken leg that requires the singer to balance in an unaccustomed posture may distract him or her from maintaining good abdominal support and thereby result in voice dysfunction. A tremorous neurologic disorder, endocrine disturbances such as thyroid dysfunction or menopause, the aging process, and other systemic conditions also may alter the voice. The physician must remember that maladies of almost any body system may result in voice dysfunction, and the doctor must remain alert for conditions outside the head and neck. If the patient uses his or her voice professionally for singing, acting, or other vocally demanding professions, physical examination should also include assessment of the patient during typical professional vocal tasks. For example, a singer should be asked to sing. Evaluation techniques for assessing performance are described in greater detail elsewhere in this book.

Complete Ear, Nose, and Throat Examination

Examination of the ears must include assessment of hearing acuity. Even a relatively slight hearing loss may result in voice strain as a singer tries to balance his or her vocal intensity with that of associate performers. Similar effects are encountered among speakers, but they are less prominent in the early stages of hearing loss. This is especially true of hearing losses acquired after vocal training has been completed. The effect is most pronounced with sensorineural hearing loss. Diplacusis, distortion of pitch perception, makes vocal strain even worse. With conductive hearing loss, singers tend to sing more softly than appropriate rather than too loudly, and this is less harmful.

During an ear, nose, and throat examination, the conjunctivae and sclerae should be observed routinely for erythema that suggests allergy or irritation, for pallor that suggests anemia, and for other abnormalities such as jaundice. These

A.-L. Hamdan et al., *Dentofacial Anomalies*, https://doi.org/10.1007/978-3-030-69109-7_3

observations may reveal the problem reflected in the vocal tract even before the larynx is visualized. Hearing loss in a spouse may be problematic as well if the voice professional strains vocally to communicate.

The nose should be assessed for patency of the nasal airway, character of the nasal mucosa, and nature of secretions, if any. A patient who is unable to breathe through the nose because of anatomic obstruction is forced to breathe unfiltered, unhumidified air through the mouth. Pale gray allergic mucosa or swollen infected mucosa in the nose suggests abnormal mucosa elsewhere in the respiratory tract.

Examination of the oral cavity should include careful attention to the tonsils and lymphoid tissue in the posterior pharyngeal wall, as well as to the mucosa. Diffuse lymphoid hypertrophy associated with a complaint of "scratchy" voice and irritative cough may indicate infection. The amount and viscosity of mucosal and salivary secretions also should be noted. Xerostomia is particularly important. The presence of scalloping of the lateral aspects of the tongue should be noted. This finding is caused commonly by tongue thrust and may be associated with inappropriate tongue tension and muscle tension dysphonia. Dental examination should focus not only on oral hygiene but also on the presence of wear facets suggestive of bruxism. Bruxism is a clue to excessive tension and may be associated with dysfunction of the temporomandibular joints, which should also be assessed routinely. Thinning of the enamel of the central incisors in a normal or underweight patient may be a clue to bulimia. However, it may also result from excessive ingestion of lemons, which some singers eat to help thin their secretions.

The neck should be examined for masses, restriction of movement, excess muscle tension and/or spasm, and scars from prior neck surgery or trauma. Laryngeal vertical mobility is also important. For example, tilting of the larynx produced by partial fixation of cervical muscles cut during previous surgery may produce voice dysfunction, as may fixation of the trachea to overlying neck skin. Particular attention should be paid to the thyroid gland. Examination of posterior neck muscles and range of motion should not be neglected. The cranial nerves should also be examined. Diminished fifth nerve sensation, diminished gag reflex, palatal deviation, or other mild cranial nerve deficits may indicate cranial polyneuropathy. Postviral, infectious neuropathies may involve the superior laryngeal nerve(s) and cause weakness of the vocal fold muscle secondary to decreased neural input, fatigability, and loss of range and projection in the voice. The recurrent laryngeal nerve is also affected in some cases. More serious neurologic disease may also be associated with such symptoms and signs.

Laryngeal Examination

Examination of the larynx begins when the singer or other voice patient enters the physician's office. The range, ease, volume, and quality of the speaking voice should be noted. If the examination is not being conducted in the patient's native language, the physician should be sure to listen to a sample of the patient's mother tongue, as well. Voice use is often different under the strain or habits of foreign language use. Rating scales of the speaking voice may be helpful [4, 5]. The classification proposed by the Japanese Society of Logopedics and Phoniatrics is one of the most widely used. It is known commonly as the GRBAS Voice Rating Scale and is discussed in the section on psychoacoustic evaluation [6].

Physicians are not usually experts in voice classification. However, the physicians should at least be able to discriminate substantial differences in range and timbre, such as between bass and tenor, or alto and soprano. Although the correlation between speaking and singing voices is not perfect, a speaker with a low, comfortable bass voice who reports that he is a tenor may be misclassified and singing inappropriate roles with consequent voice strain. This judgment should be deferred to an expert, but the observation should lead the physician to make the appropriate referral. Excessive volume or obvious strain during speaking clearly indicates that voice abuse is present and may be contributing to the patient's singing complaint. The speaking voice can be evaluated more consistently and accurately using standardized reading passages, and such assessments are performed routinely by speech-language pathologists, by phoniatricians, and sometimes by laryngologists.

The definition of "register" or "registration" is controversial, and many different terms are used by musicians and scientists. Often, the definitions are unclear. Terms to describe register include chest, creek, falsetto, head, heavy, light, little, low, middle, modal, normal, pulse, upper, vocal fry, voce di petto, voce di mista, voce di testa, and whistle (also called flageolet and flute register). A register is a range of frequencies that has a consistent quality or timbre. The break between registers is an area of instability called the passaggio. During vocal training, singers are taught to integrate qualities of their various registers and to smooth and obscure the transition between registers. Registers occur not only in voices but also in some instruments, notably the organ. Vocal register changes are associated with changes in laryngeal musculature and in vocal fold shape. For example, in chest register, contraction of the thyroarytenoid muscles causes thickening of the vocal folds, with a square-shaped glottis and large vibratory margin contact area. In falsetto in men and head voice in women, cricothyroid muscle contraction is dominant, vocal folds are elongated, and the contact area is much thinner and more triangular than in chest voice. Vertical phase differences are diminished in head voice in comparison with chest voice. Controversy remains on the use of traditional terms in males such as chest, middle, head and falsetto register, or chest and head register in females. Voice scientists commonly prefer terms such as modal register. In any case, health care professionals should understand that there is a difference between the terms *register* and *range*. For example, if a singer complains of inability to sing high notes, this should be described as a loss of upper range, not a loss of upper register. Register and range difficulties should be noted.

Vibrato is a fluctuation of the fundamental frequency of a note. It is produced by the vocal mechanism under neural control and is present naturally in adult voices. The primary components of vibrato include rate (the number of frequency fluctuations per second), extent (number of Hertz of fluctuation above and below the center frequency), regularity (consistency of frequency variations from one cycle to the next), and wave form. Rate and extent have been studied most extensively and are arguably the most important components in determining how the vibrato is perceived. Natural vibrato generally is about 6 Hz. Vibrato rate is slower in males than in females, and vocal pitch and effort do not have a substantial influence on vibrato. However, singers are able to alter vibrato rate and pitch oscillation voluntarily for stylistic purposes. The athletic choice of vibrato rate varies over time. For example, vibrato rates of 6–7 Hz were popular in classical Western (operatic) singing in the early twentieth century, but a vibrato rate of 5.5–6 Hz was considered more attractive by the end of the twentieth century. In general, pitch fluctuation covers about 1 semitone (half a semitone above and half a semitone below the center frequency) at present. A prominent wobble, as may be heard in some elderly singers who are not in ideal physical and vocal condition generally, is referred to as a tremolo. The excessive pitch (and sometimes intensity) fluctuations are caused by muscle activity, sometimes with a respiratory component, and are superimposed on the individual's vibrato in most cases, rather than actually being a widened, distorted vibrato. The true source of natural vibrato is uncertain, although the larynx, pharynx, tongue, and other components of the vocal tract may move in concert with vibrato, as well as with tremolo. Vibrato is thought not to be due primarily to phonatory structural activity rather than to respiratory source. The pressure of vibrato abnormalities or tremolo should be documented.

Any patient with a voice complaint should be examined by indirect laryngoscopy at least. It is not possible to judge voice range, quality, or other vocal attributes by inspection of the vocal folds. However, the presence or absence of nodules, mass lesions, contact ulcers, hemorrhage, erythema, paralysis, arytenoid erythema (reflux), and other anatomic abnormalities must be established. Erythema and edema of the laryngeal

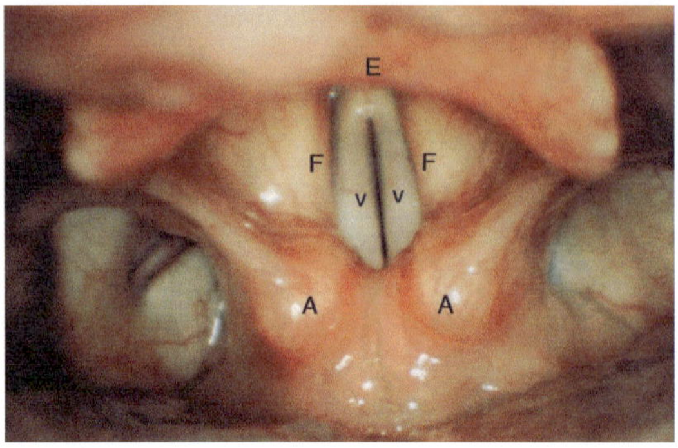

Fig. 3.1 Normal larynx showing the true vocal folds (V), false vocal folds (F), arytenoids (A), and epiglottis (E)

surface of the epiglottis are seen often in association with muscle tension dysphonia and with frequent coughing or clearing of the throat. It is caused by direct trauma from the arytenoids during these maneuvers. The mirror or a laryngeal telescope often provides a better view of the posterior portion of the endolarynx than is obtained with flexible endoscopy. Stroboscopic examination adds substantially to diagnostic abilities (Fig. 3.1), as discussed below. Another occasionally helpful adjunct is the operating microscope. Magnification allows visualization of small mucosal disruptions and hemorrhages that may be significant but overlooked otherwise. This technique also allows photography of the larynx with a microscope camera. Magnification may also be achieved through magnifying laryngeal mirrors or by wearing loupes. Loupes usually provide a clearer image than do most of the magnifying mirrors available.

A laryngeal telescope may be combined with a stroboscope to provide excellent visualization of the vocal folds and related structures. The author usually uses a 70° laryngeal telescope, although 90° telescopes are required for some patients. The combination of a telescope and stroboscope provides optimal magnification and optical quality for assessment of vocal fold vibration. However, it is generally performed with the tongue in a fixed position, and the nature of the examination does not permit assessment of the larynx during normal phonatory gestures.

Flexible fiberoptic laryngoscopy can be performed as an office procedure and allows inspection of the vocal folds in patients whose vocal folds are difficult to visualize indirectly. In addition, it permits observation of the vocal mechanism in a more natural posture than does indirect laryngoscopy, permitting sophisticated dynamic voice assessment. In the hands of an experienced endoscopist, this method may provide a great deal of information about both speaking and singing techniques. The combination of a fiberoptic laryngoscope with a laryngeal stroboscope may be especially useful. This system permits magnification, photography, and detailed inspection of vocal fold motion. Sophisticated systems that permit flexible or rigid fiberoptic strobovideolaryngoscopy are currently available commercially. They are invaluable assets for routine clinical use. The video system also provides a permanent record, permitting reassessment, comparison over time, and easy consultation. A refinement not currently available commercially is stereoscopic fiberoptic laryngoscopy, accomplished by placing a laryngoscope through each nostril, fastening the two together in the pharynx, and observing the larynx through the eyepieces [7]. This method allows visualization of laryngeal motion in three dimensions. However, it is used primarily in a research setting.

Rigid endoscopy under general anesthesia may be reserved for the rare patient whose vocal folds cannot be assessed adequately by other means or for patients who need surgical procedures to remove or biopsy laryngeal lesions. In some cases, this may be done with local anesthesia, avoiding the need for intubation and the traumatic coughing and vomiting that may occur even after general anesthesia administered by mask. Coughing after general anesthesia may be minimized by using topical anesthesia in the larynx and the trachea. However, topical anesthetics may act as severe mucosal irritants in a small number of patients. They may also predispose the patient to aspiration in the postoperative period. If a patient has had difficulty with a topical anesthetic administered in the office, it should not be used in the operating room. When used in general anesthesia cases, topical anesthetics should usually be applied at the end of the procedure. Thus, if inflammation occurs, it will not interfere with performance of microsurgery. Postoperative duration of anesthesia is also optimized. The author has had the least difficulty with 4% Xylocaine.

Objective Tests

Reliable, valid, objective analysis of the voice is extremely important and is an essential part of a comprehensive physical examination [2]. It is as valuable to the laryngologist as audiometry is to the otologist [8, 9]. Familiarity with some of the measures and technological advances currently available is helpful. This information is covered in greater detail elsewhere in this book but is included here as a brief overview for the convenience of the reader.

Strobovideolaryngoscopy

Integrity of the vibratory margin of the vocal fold is essential for the complex motion required to produce good vocal quality. Under continuous light, the vocal folds vibrate approximately 250 times per second while phonating at middle C. Naturally, the human eye cannot discern the necessary details during such rapid motion. The vibratory margin may be assessed through high-speed photography, strobovideolaryngoscopy, high-speed video, videokymography, electroglottography (EEG), or photoglottography. Strobovideolaryngoscopy provides the necessary clinical information in a practical fashion. Stroboscopic light allows routine slow-motion evaluation of the mucosal cover layer of the leading edge of the vocal fold. This state-of-the-art physical examination permits detection of vibratory asymmetries, structural abnormalities, small masses, submucosal scars, and other conditions that are invisible under ordinary light [10, 11]. Documentation of the procedure by coupling stroboscopic light with the video camera allows later reevaluation by the laryngologist or other health care providers.

Stroboscopy does not provide a true slow-motion image, as obtained through high-speed photography (Fig. 3.2). The stroboscope actually illuminates different points on consecutive vocal fold waves, each of which is retained on the retina for 0.2 s. The stroboscopically lighted portions of the successive waves are fused visually, and thus the examiner is actually evaluating simulated cycles of phonation. The slow-motion effect is created by having the stroboscopic light desynchronized with the frequency of vocal fold vibration by approximately 2 Hz. When vocal fold vibration and the stroboscope are synchronized exactly, the vocal folds appear to stand still, rather than move in slow motion (Fig. 3.3). In most instances, this approximation of slow motion provides all the clinical information necessary. Our routine stroboscopy protocol is described elsewhere [11]. We use a modification of the standardized method of subjective assessment of strobovideolaryngoscopic images, as proposed by Bless et al. [12] and Hirano [13]. Characteristics evaluated include the fundamental frequency, the symmetry of movements, periodicity, glottic closure, the amplitude of vibration, the mucosal wave, the presence of nonvibrating portions of the vocal fold, and other unusual findings. With practice, perceptual judgments of stroboscopic images provide a great deal of information. However, it is easy for the inexperienced observer to draw unwarranted conclusions because of normal variations in vibration. Vibrations depend on fundamental frequency, intensity, and vocal register. For example, failure of glottic closure occurs normally in falsetto phonation. Consequently, it is important to note these characteristics and to examine each voice under a variety of conditions.

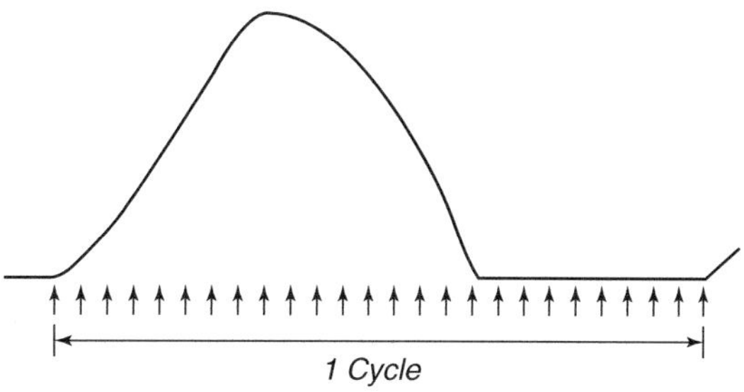

Fig. 3.2 The principle of ultrahigh-speed photography. Numerous images are taken during each vibratory cycle. This technique is a true slow-motion representation of each vocal fold vibration

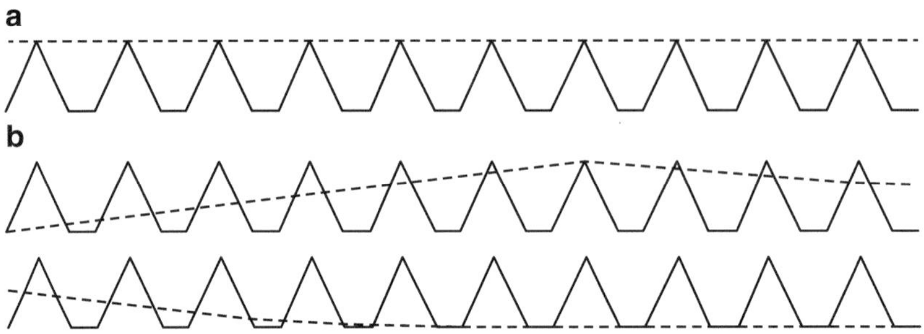

Fig. 3.3 The principle of stroboscopy. The stroboscopic light illuminates portions of successive cycles. The eye fuses the illuminated points into an illusion of slow motion. (**a**) If the stroboscope is synchronized with vocal fold vibration, a similar point is illuminated on each successive cycle and the vocal fold appears to stand still. (**b**) If the stroboscope is slightly desynchronized, each cycle is illuminated at a slightly different point, and the slow-motion effect is created

Other Techniques to Examine Vocal Fold Vibration

Other techniques to examine vocal fold vibration include ultrahigh-speed photography, electroglottography (EGG), photoelectroglottography, ultrasound glottography, and most recently videokymography [14] and high-speed video (digital or analog). Ultrahigh-speed photography provides images that are in true slow motion, rather than simulated. High-speed video offers similar advantages without most of the disadvantages of high-speed motion pictures. Videokymography offers high-speed imaging of a single line along the vocal fold. EGG uses two electrodes placed on the skin of the neck above the thyroid laminae. It traces the opening and closing of the glottis and can be compared with stroboscopic images [15]. EGG allows objective determination of the presence or absence of glottal vibrations and easy determination of the fundamental period of vibration and is reproducible. It reflects the glottal condition more accurately during its closed phase. Photo electroglottography and ultrasound glottography are less useful clinically [16].

Measures of Phonatory Ability

Objective measures of phonatory ability are easy to use, readily available to the laryngologist, helpful in the treatment of professional vocalists with specific voice disorders, and quite useful in assessing the results of surgical therapies. Maximum phonation time is measured with a stopwatch. The patient is instructed to sustain the vowel /a/ for as long as possible after deep inspiration, vocalizing at a comfortable frequency and intensity. The frequency and intensity may be determined and controlled by an inexpensive frequency analyzer and sound level meter. The test is repeated three times, and the greatest value is recorded. Normal values have been determined [16]. Frequency range of phonation is recorded in semitones and documents the vocal range from the lowest note in the modal register (excluding vocal fry) to the highest falsetto note. This is the physiologic frequency range of phonation and disregards quality. The musical frequency range of phonation measures lowest to highest notes of musically acceptable quality. Tests for maximum phonation time, frequency ranges, and many of the other parameters discussed later (including spectrographic analysis) may be preserved on a tape recorder or digitized and stored for analysis at a convenient future time and used for pre- and post-treatment comparisons. Recordings should be made in a standardized, consistent fashion.

Frequency limits of vocal register also may be measured. The registers are (from low to high) vocal fry, chest, mid, head, and falsetto. However, classification of registers is controversial, and many other classifications are used. Although the classification listed above is common among musicians, at present, most voice scientists prefer to classify registers as pulse, modal, and loft. Overlap of frequency among registers occurs routinely.

Testing the speaking fundamental frequency often reveals excessively low pitch, an abnormality associated with chronic voice abuse and development of vocal nodules. This parameter may be followed objectively throughout a course of voice therapy. Intensity range of phonation (IRP) has proven a less useful measure than frequency range. It varies with fundamental frequency (which should be recorded) and is greatest in the middle frequency range. It is recorded in sound pressure level (SPL) (re 0.0002 microbar). For healthy adults who are not professional vocalists, measuring at a single fundamental frequency, IRP averages 54.8 dB for males and 51 dB for females [17]. Alterations of intensity are common in voice disorders, although IRP is not the most sensitive test to detect them. Information from these tests may be combined in a fundamental frequency-intensity profile [16], also called a *phonetogram*.

Glottal efficiency (ratio of the acoustic power at the level of the glottis to subglottal power) provides useful information but is not clinically practical because measuring acoustic power at the level of the glottis is difficult. Subglottic power is the product of subglottal pressure and airflow rate. These can be determined clinically. Various alternative measures of glottic efficiency have been proposed, including the ratio of radiated acoustic power to subglottal power [18], airflow intensity profile [19], and ratio of the root mean square value of the AC component to the mean volume velocity (DC component) [20]. Although glottal efficiency is of great interest, none of these tests are particularly helpful under routine clinical circumstances.

Aerodynamic Measures

Traditional pulmonary function testing provides the most readily accessible measure of respiratory function. The most common parameters measured include (1) tidal volume, the volume of air that enters the lungs during inspiration and leaves during expiration in normal breathing; (2) functional residual capacity, the volume of air remaining in the lungs at the end of inspiration during normal breathing, which can be divided into expiratory reserve volume (maximal additional volume that can be exhaled) and residual volume (the volume of air remaining in the lungs at the end of maximal exhalation); (3) inspiratory capacity, the maximal volume of air that can be inhaled starting at the functional residual capacity; (4) total lung capacity, the volume of air in the lungs following maximal inspiration; (5) vital capacity, the maximal volume of air that can be exhaled from the lungs following maximal inspiration; (6) forced vital capacity, the rate of air flow with rapid, forceful expiration from total lung capacity to residual volume; (7) FEV_1, the forced expiratory volume in 1 s; (8) FEV_3, the forced expiratory volume in 3 s; and (9) maximal mid-expiratory flow, the mean rate of airflow over the middle half of the forced vital capacity (between 25% and 75% of the forced vital capacity). For singers and professional speakers with an abnormality caused by voice abuse, abnormal pulmonary function tests may confirm deficiencies in aerobic conditioning or reveal previously unrecognized asthma [21]. Flow glottography with computer inverse filtering is also a practical and valuable diagnostic for assessing flow at the vocal fold level, evaluating the voice source, and imaging the results of the balance between adductory forces and subglottal pressure [22]. It also has therapeutic value as a biofeedback tool.

The spirometer, readily available for pulmonary function testing, can also be used for measuring airflow during phonation. However, the spirometer does not allow simultaneous display of acoustic signals, and its frequency response is poor. A pneumotachograph consists of a laminar air resistor, a differential pressure transducer, and an amplifying and recording system. It allows measurement of airflow and simultaneous recording of other signals when coupled with a polygraph. A hot-wire anemometer allows determination of airflow velocity by measuring the electrical drop across the hot wire. Modern hot-wire anemometers containing electrical feedback circuitry that maintains the temperature of the hot wire provide a flat response up to 1 kHz and are useful clinically.

The four parameters traditionally measured in the aerodynamic performance of a voice are subglottal pressure (P_{sub}), supraglottal pressure (P_{sup}), glottal impedance, and the volume velocity of airflow at the glottis. These parameters and their rapid variations can be measured under laboratory circumstances. However, clinically their mean value is usually determined as follows:

$$P_{sub} - P_{sup} = \mathrm{MFR} \times \mathrm{GR}$$

where MFR is the mean (root mean square) flow rate and GR is the mean (root mean square) glottal resistance. When vocalizing the open vowel /*a*/, the supraglottic pressure equals the atmospheric pressure, reducing the equation to

$$P_{sub} = \mathrm{MFR} \times \mathrm{GR}$$

The mean flow rate is a useful clinical measure. While the patient vocalizes the vowel /*a*/, the mean flow rate is calculated by dividing the total volume of air used during phonation by the duration of phonation. The subject phonates at a comfortable pitch and loudness either over a determined period of time or for a maximum sustained period of phonation.

Air volume is measured by the use of a mask fitted tightly over the face or by phonating into a mouthpiece while wearing a nose clamp. Measurements may be made using a spirometer, pneumotachograph, or hot-wire anemometer. The normal values for mean flow rate under habitual phonation, with changes in intensity or register, and under various pathologic circumstances, were determined in the 1970s [16]. Normal values are available for both adults and children. Mean flow rate also can be measured and is a clinically useful parameter to follow during treatment for vocal nodules, recurrent laryngeal nerve paralysis, spasmodic dysphonia, and other conditions.

Glottal resistance cannot be measured directly, but it may be calculated from the mean flow rate and mean subglottal pressure. Normal glottal resistance is 20–100 dyne seconds/cm^5 at low and medium pitches and 150 dyne seconds/cm^5 at high pitches [18]. The normal values for subglottal pressure under various healthy and pathologic voice conditions have also been determined by numerous investigators [16]. The phonation quotient is the vital capacity divided by the maximum phonation time. It has been shown to correlate closely with maximum flow rate [23] and is a more convenient measure. Normative data determined by various authors have been published [16]. The phonation quotient provides an objective measure of the effects of treatment and is particularly useful in cases of recurrent laryngeal nerve paralysis and mass lesions of the vocal folds, including nodules.

Acoustic Analysis

Acoustic analysis equipment can determine frequency, intensity, harmonic spectrum, cycle-to-cycle perturbations in frequency (jitter), cycle-to-cycle perturbations in amplitude (shimmer), harmonics/noise ratios, breathiness index, and many other parameters. The DSP Sona-Graph Sound Analyzer Model 5500 (Kay Elemetrics, Lincoln Park, New Jersey) is an integrated voice analysis system. It is equipped for sound spectrography capabilities. Spectrography provides a visual record of the voice. The acoustic signal is depicted using time (*x*-axis), frequency (*y*-axis), and intensity (*z*-axis), shading of light versus dark. Using the bandpass filters, generalizations about quality, pitch, and loudness can be made. These observations are used in formulating the voice therapy treatment plan. Formant structure and strength can be determined using the narrow-band filters, of which a variety of configurations are possible. In clinical settings in which singers and other professional voice users are evaluated and treated routinely, this feature is extremely valuable. A sophisticated voice analysis program (an optional program) may be combined with the Sona-Graph and is an especially valuable addition to the clinical laboratory. The voice analysis program (Computer Speech Lab; Kay Elemetrics) measures speaking fundamental frequency, frequency perturbation (jitter), amplitude perturbation (shimmer), and harmonics-to-noise ratio and provides many other useful values. An electroglottograph may be used in conjunction with the Sona-Graph to provide some of these voicing parameters. Examining the EGG waveform alone is possible with this setup, but its clinical usefulness has not yet been established. An important feature of the Sona-Graph is the long-term average (LTA) spectral capability, which permits analysis of longer voice samples (30–90 s). The LTA analyzes only voiced speech segments and may be useful in screening for hoarse or breathy voices. In addition, computer interface capabilities (also an optional program) have solved many data storage and file maintenance problems.

In analyzing acoustic signals, the microphone may be placed at the level of the mouth or positioned in or over the trachea, although intratracheal recordings are used for research purposes only. The position should be standardized in each office or laboratory [24]. Various techniques are being developed to improve the usefulness of acoustic analysis. Because of the enormous amount of information carried in the acoustic signal, further refinements in objective acoustic analysis should prove particularly valuable to the clinician.

Laryngeal Electromyography

Electromyography (EMG) requires an electrode system, an amplifier, an oscilloscope, a loudspeaker, and a recording system [25]. Electrodes are placed transcutaneously into laryngeal muscles. EMG can be extremely valuable in confirming cases of vocal fold paresis, in differentiating paralysis from arytenoid dislocation, distinguishing recurrent laryngeal nerve paralysis from combined recurrent and superior nerve paralysis, diagnosing other more subtle neurolaryngologic pathology, and documenting functional voice disorders and malingering. It is also recommended for needle localization when using botulinum toxin for treatment of spasmodic dysphonia and other conditions.

Psychoacoustic Evaluation

Because the human ear and brain are the most sensitive and complex analyzers of sound currently available, many researchers have tried to standardize and quantify psychoacoustic evaluation. Unfortunately, even definitions of basic terms such as hoarseness and breathiness are still controversial. Psychoacoustic evaluation protocols and interpretations are not standardized. Consequently, although subjective psychoacoustic analysis of voice is of great value to the individual skilled clinician, it remains generally unsatisfactory for comparing research among laboratories or for reporting clinical results.

The GRBAS scale [6] helps standardize perceptual analysis for clinical purposes. It rates the voice from a scale from 0 to 3, with regrading to grade, roughness, breathiness, asthenia, and strain. Grade 0 is normal, 1 is slightly abnormal, 2 is moderately abnormal, and 3 is extremely abnormal. Grade refers to the degree of hoarseness or voice abnormality. Roughness refers to the acoustic/auditory impression of irregularity of vibration and corresponds with gear and shimmer. Breathiness refers to the acoustic/auditory impression of air leakage and corresponds to turbulence. Asthenic evaluation assesses weakness or lack of power and corresponds to vocal intensity and energy in higher harmonics. Strain refers to the acoustic/auditory impression of hyperfunction and may be related to fundamental frequency, noise in the high-frequency range, and energy in higher harmonics. For example, a patient's voice might be graded as G2, R2, B1, A1, S2.

Outcomes Assessment

Measuring the impact of a voice disorder has always been challenging. However, recent advances have begun to address this problem. Validated instruments such as the Voice Handicap Index (VHI) [26] are currently in clinical use and are likely to be used widely in future years.

Voice Impairment and Disability

Quantifying voice impairment and assigning a disability rating (percentage of whole person) remain controversial. This subject is still not addressed comprehensively even in the most recent editions (2008, 6th edition) of the American Medical Association's *Guidelines for the Evaluation of Impairment and Disability* (The Guides). The Guides still do not take into account the person's profession when calculating disability. Alternative approaches have been proposed [27], and advances in this complex arena are anticipated over the next few years.

Evaluation of the Singing Voice

The physician must be careful not to exceed the limits of his or her expertise, especially in caring for singers. However, if voice abuse or technical error is suspected, or if a difficult judgment must be reached on whether to allow a sick singer to perform, a brief observation of the patient's singing may provide invaluable information. This is accomplished best by asking the singer to stand and sing scales either in the examining room or in the soundproof audiology booth. Similar maneuvers may be used for professional speakers, including actors (who can vocalize and recite lines), clergy and politicians (who can deliver sermons and speeches), and virtually all other voice patients. The singer's stance should be balanced, with the weight slightly forward. The knees should be bent slightly, and the shoulders, torso, and neck should be relaxed. The singer should inhale through the nose whenever possible allowing filtration, warming, and humidification of inspired air. In general, the chest should be expanded, but most of the active breathing is abdominal. The chest should not rise substantially with each inspiration, and the supraclavicular musculature should not be involved obviously in inspiration. Shoulders and neck muscles should not be tensed even with deep inspiration. Abdominal musculature should be contracted shortly before the initiation of the tone. This may be evaluated visually or by palpation (Fig. 3.4).

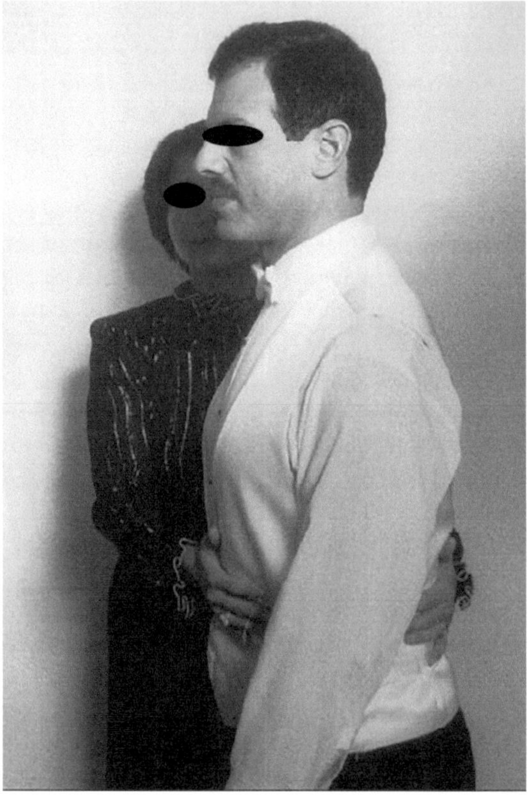

Fig. 3.4 Bimanual palpation of the support mechanism. The singer should expand posteriorly and anteriorly with inspiration. Muscles should tighten prior to onset of sung tone

Muscles of the neck and face should be relaxed. Economy is a basic principle of all art forms. Wasted energy and motion and muscle tension are incorrect and usually deleterious.

The singer should be instructed to sing a scale (a 5-note scale is usually sufficient) on the vowel /a/, beginning on any comfortable note. Technical errors are usually most obvious as contraction of muscles in the neck and chin, retraction of the lower lip, retraction of the tongue, or tightening of the muscles of mastication. The singer's mouth should be open widely but comfortably. When singing /a/, the singer's tongue should rest in a neutral position with the tip of the tongue lying against the back of the singer's mandibular incisors. If the tongue pulls back or demonstrates obvious muscular activity as the singer performs the scales, improper voice use can be confirmed on the basis of posi-

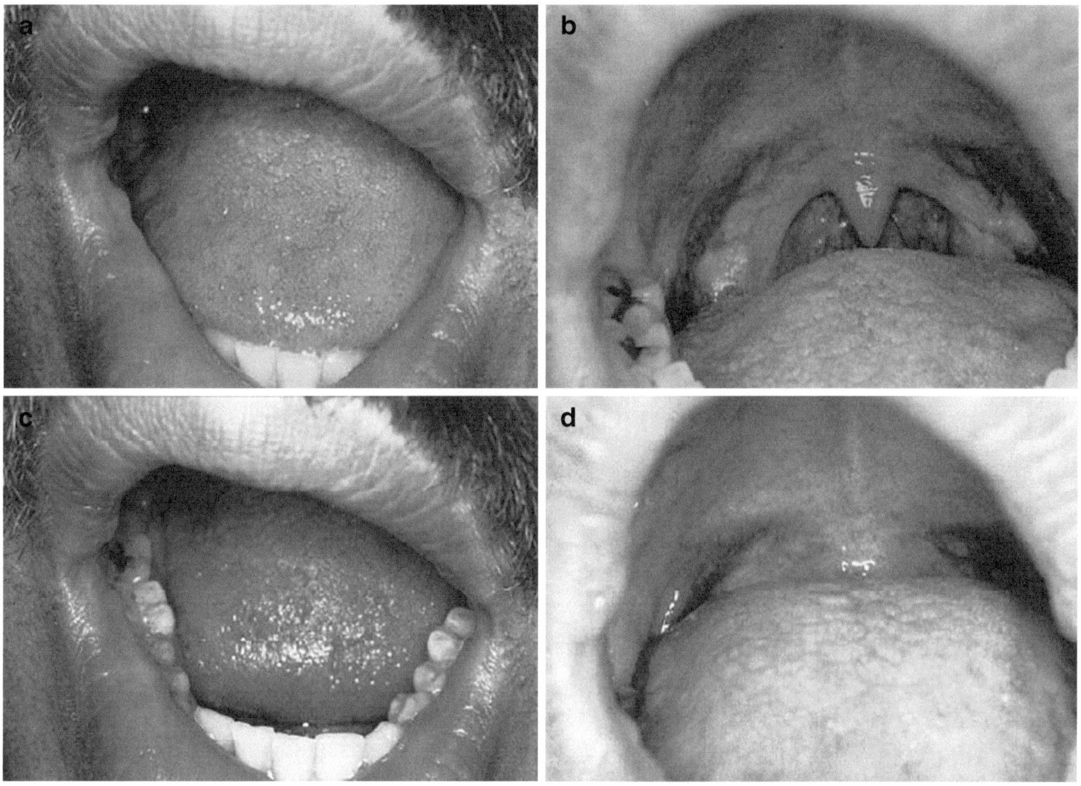

Fig. 3.5 Proper relaxed position of the anterior (**a**) and posterior (**b**) portions of the tongue. Common improper use of the tongue pulled back from the teeth (**c**) and raised posteriorly (**d**)

tive evidence (Fig. 3.5). The position of the larynx should not vary substantially with pitch changes. Rising of the larynx with ascending pitch is evidence of technical dysfunction. This examination also gives the physician an opportunity to observe any dramatic differences between the qualities and ranges of the patient's speaking voice and the singing voice. A physical examination summary form has proven helpful in organization and documentation [3].

Remembering the admonition not to exceed his or her expertise, the physician who examines many singers can often glean valuable information from a brief attempt to modify an obvious technical error. For example, deciding whether to allow a singer with mild or moderate laryngitis to perform is often difficult. On the one hand, an expert singer has technical skills that allow him or her to compensate safely. On the other hand, if a singer does not sing with correct technique and does not have the discipline to modify volume, technique, and repertoire as necessary, the risk of vocal injury may be increased substantially even by mild inflammation of the vocal folds. In borderline circumstances, observation of the singer's technique may greatly help the physician in making a judgment.

If the singer's technique appears flawless, the physician may feel somewhat more secure in allowing the singer to proceed with performance commitments. More commonly, even good singers demonstrate technical errors when experiencing voice difficulties. In a vain effort to compensate for dysfunction at the vocal fold level, singers often modify their technique in the neck and supraglottic vocal tract. In the good singer, this usually means going from good technique to bad technique. The most common error involves pulling back the tongue and tightening the cervical muscles. Although this increased muscular activity gives the singer the illusion of making the voice more secure, this technical maladjustment undermines vocal efficiency and increases vocal strain. The physician may ask the singer to hold the top note of a 5-note scale; while the note is being held, the singer may simply be told, "Relax your tongue." At the same time, the physician points to the singer's abdominal musculature. Most good singers immediately correct to good technique. If they do, and if upcoming performances are particularly important, the singer may be able to perform with a reminder that meticulous technique is essential. The singer should be advised to "sing by feel rather than by ear," consult his or her voice teacher, and conserve the voice except when it is absolutely necessary to use it. If a singer is unable to correct from bad technique to good technique promptly, especially if he or she uses excessive muscle tension in the neck and ineffective abdominal support, it is generally safer not to perform with even a mild vocal fold abnormality. With increased experience and training, the laryngologist may make other observations that aid in providing appropriate treatment recommendations for singer patients. Once these skills have been mastered for the care of singers, applying them to other patients is relatively easy, so long as the laryngologist takes the time to understand the demands of the individual's professional, avocational, and recreational vocal activities.

If treatment is to be instituted, making at least a tape recording of the voice is advisable in most cases and essential before any surgical intervention. The author routinely uses strobovideolaryngoscopy for diagnosis and documentation in virtually all cases as well as many of the objective measures discussed. Pretreatment testing is extremely helpful clinically and medicolegally.

Additional Examinations

A general physical examination should be performed whenever the patient's systemic health is questionable. Debilitating conditions such as mononucleosis may be noticed first by the singer as vocal fatigue. A neurologic assessment may be particularly revealing. The physician must be careful not to overlook dysarthrias and dysphonias, which are characteristic of movement disorders and of serious neurologic disease. Dysarthria is a defect in rhythm, enunciation, and articulation that usually results from neuromuscular impairment or weakness such as may occur after a stroke. It may be seen with oral deformities or illness, as well. Dysphonia is an abnormality of vocalization usually caused by problems at the laryngeal level.

Physicians should be familiar with the six types of dysarthria, their symptoms, and their importance [28, 29]. Flaccid dysarthria occurs in lower motor neuron or primary muscle disorders such as myasthenia gravis and tumors or strokes involving the brainstem nuclei. Spastic dysarthria occurs in upper motor neuron disorders (pseudobulbar palsy) such as multiple strokes and cerebral palsy. Ataxic dysarthria is seen with cerebellar disease, alcohol intoxication, and multiple sclerosis. Hypokinetic dysarthria accompanies Parkinson disease. Hyperkinetic dysarthria may be spasmodic, as in the Gilles de la Tourette disease, or dystonic, as in chorea and cerebral palsy. Mixed dysarthria occurs in amyotrophic lateral sclerosis (ALS) or Lou Gehrig disease. The preceding classification actually combines dysphonic and dysarthric characteristics but is very useful clinically. The value of a comprehensive neurolaryngologic evaluation [30] cannot be overstated. More specific details of voice changes associated with neurologic dysfunction and their localizing value are available elsewhere [2, 31].

It is extremely valuable for the laryngologist to assemble an arts-medicine team that includes not only a speech-language pathologist, singing voice specialist, acting voice specialist, and voice scientist but also medical colleagues in other disciplines. Collaboration with an expert neurologist, pulmonologist, endocrinologist, psychologist, psychiatrist, internist, physiatrist, and others with special knowledge of, and interest in, voice disorders is invaluable in caring for patients with voice disorders. Such interdisciplinary teams have not only changed the standard of care in voice evaluation and treatment but are also largely responsible for the rapid and productive growth of voice as a subspecialty.

Acknowledgment Modified in part from Rubin J, Sataloff R, Korovin G. *Diagnosis and Treatment of Voice Disorders*, 4th ed. San Diego, CA: Plural Publishing; 2014; with permission.

References

1. Sataloff RT. Professional singers: the science and art of clinical care. Am J Otolaryngol. 1981;2:251–66.
2. Rubin J, Sataloff R, Korovin G. Diagnosis and treatment of voice disorders. 4th ed. San Diego: Plural Publishing; 2014.
3. Sataloff RT. The professional voice: part II, physical examination. J Voice. 1987;1:91–201.
4. Fuazawa T, Blaugrund SM, El-Assuooty A, Gould WJ. Acoustic analysis of hoarse voice: a preliminary report. J Voice. 1988;2(2):127–31.
5. Gelfer M. Perceptual attributes of voice: development and use of rating scales. J Voice. 1988;2(4):320–6.
6. Hirano M. Clinical examination of the voice. New York: Springer-Verlag; 1981. p. 83–4.
7. Fujimura O. Stereo-fiberoptic laryngeal observation. J Acoust Soc Am. 1979;65:70–2.
8. Sataloff RT, Spiegel JR, Carroll LM, Darby KS, Hawkshaw MJ, Rulnick RK. The clinical voice laboratory: practical design and clinical application. J Voice. 1990;4:264–79.
9. Sataloff RT, Heuer RH, Hoover C, Baroody MM. Laboratory assessment of voice. In: Gould WJ, Sataloff RT, Spiegel JR. Voice surgery. St. Louis: Mosby; 1993. p. 203–16.
10. Sataloff RT, Spiegel JR, Carroll LM, Schiebel BR, Darby KS, Rulnick RK. Strobovideolaryngoscopy in professional voice users: results and clinical value. J Voice. 1986;1:359–64.
11. Sataloff RT, Spiegel JR, Hawkshaw MJ. Strobovideolaryngoscopy: results and clinical value. Ann Otol Rhinol Laryngol. 1991;100:725–7.
12. Bless D, Hirano M, Feder RJ. Video stroboscopic evaluation of the larynx. Ear Nose Throat J. 1987;66:289–96.
13. Hirano M. Phonosurgery: basic and clinical investigations. Otologia (Fukuoka). 1975;21:239–442.
14. Svec J, Shutte H. Videokymography: high-speed line scanning of vocal fold vibration. J Voice. 1996;10:201–5.
15. Leclure FLE, Brocaar ME, Verscheeure J. Electroglottography and its relation to glottal activity. Folia Phoniatr (Basel). 1975;27:215–24.
16. Hirano M. Clinical examination of the voice, vol. 25–27. New York: Springer-Verlag; 1981. p. 85–98.
17. Coleman RJ, Mabis JH, Hinson JK. Fundamental frequency sound pressure level profiles of adult male and female voices. J Speech Hear Res. 1977;20:197–204.
18. Isshiki N. Regulatory mechanism of voice intensity variation. J Speech Hear Res. 1964;7:17–29.
19. Saito S. Phonosurgery: basic study on the mechanisms of phonation and endolaryngeal microsurgery. Otologia (Fukuoka). 1977;23:171–384.
20. Isshiki N. Functional surgery of the larynx. In: Report of the 78th annual convention of the oto-rhino-laryngological society of Japan. Fukuoka: Kyoto University; 1977.
21. Cohn JR, Sataloff RT, Spiegel JR, Fish JE, Kennedy K. Airway reactivity-induced asthma in singers (ARIAS). J Voice. 1991;5:332–7.
22. Sundberg J. The science of the singing voice. Dekalb: Northern Illinois University Press; 1987. p. 11, 66, 77–89.
23. Hirano M, Koike Y, von Leden H. Maximum phonation time and air usage during phonation. Folia Phoniatr (Basel). 1968;20:185–201.
24. Price DB, Sataloff RT. A simple technique for consistent microphone placement in voice recording. J Voice. 1988;2:206–7.
25. Sataloff RT, Mandel S, Heman-Ackah YD, Abaza M. Laryngeal electromyography. 3rd ed. San Diego: Plural Publishing, Inc; 2017.
26. Benninger MS, Syamal MN, Gardner GM, Jacobson BH. New dimensions in measuring voice treatment outcomes and quality of life. In: Sataloff RT. Professional voice: the science and art of clinical care. 4th ed. San Diego: Plural Publishing, Inc; 2017. p. 547–58.
27. Sataloff RT. Voice impairment, disability, handicap, and medical-legal evaluation. In: Sataloff RT, editor. Professional voice: the science and art of clinical care. 4th ed. San Diego: Plural Publishing, Inc; 2017. p. 1741–54.
28. Darley FL, Aronson AE, Brown JR. Differential diagnostic of patterns of dysarthria. J Speech Hear Res. 1969;12(2):246–9.
29. Darley FL, Aronson AE, Brown JR. Clusters of deviant speech dimensions in the dysarthrias. J Speech Hear Res. 1969;12(3):462–96.
30. Rosenfield DB. Neurolaryngology. Ear Nose Throat J. 1987;66:323–6.
31. Raphael BN, Sataloff RT. Increasing vocal effectiveness. In: Sataloff RT. Professional voice: the science and art of clinical care. 4th ed. San Diego: Plural Publishing, Inc; 2017. p. 1201–12.

4 Wind Instrument Technique, Function, and Evaluation: An Overview

Introduction

The interaction of the larynx, pharynx, jaws, tongue, teeth, and lip behaviors and the consequences of those behaviors have been studied by researchers in medical, voice science, and wind instrumentalist communities. The research has been somewhat limited, and research foci have varied. The purpose of this chapter is to connect the practical pedagogical approaches used by wind instrument teachers with medical, dental, orthodontic, and voice science research and to identify unresolved issues and misinformation, summarize what has been done in research, and to suggest areas of further investigation that might be beneficial to the medical and dental community, as well as to wind instrumentalists. *Wind instrumentalists* (including brass and woodwind players) have been identified through research as professional voice users in that laryngeal and pharyngeal activity are involved in playing instruments, and through that wind instrumentalists can develop voice discomfort and damage as a result of performing on their instruments [1–4].

Pedagogical and Practical Considerations of Teaching and Learning Wind Instruments

Students who wish to play wind instruments often begin at the age when they start to deal with growth spurts and for many, the possibility of getting braces or other orthodontic treatments. This poses the potential for a multitude of orthodontic problems to develop: medical and musical. So, understanding how children and novices start learning to play instruments is critical for any dental or voice care professional.

Historically, children (and any musical instrument novice) started instrument lessons with a teacher who was well-trained on the instrument. Unfortunately, since the 1990s, that is no longer the case. Most children begin lessons in their public school programs in group lessons (if they attend a school that is based on the traditional western music education curriculum) with a teacher who has been trained minimally to play the instruments (with the exception of his/her major instrument, if there was one). In many schools in the USA, it is becoming more common for choral directors, who may have no wind instrument playing background at all, to teach beginning band instruments. The focus of school band programs is to teach fingerings and have the beginners be able to play well enough so that they can perform in an ensemble. Detailed attention to embouchure, breathing, and especially the larynx and oral cavity are addressed either

A.-L. Hamdan et al., *Dentofacial Anomalies*, https://doi.org/10.1007/978-3-030-69109-7_4

later or not at all. The focus is on making sound; and *how* that is done beyond learning correct fingerings and basic embouchure usually is not a major concern. The late Chicago Symphony Principal Tuba player Arnold Jacobs likely summed up the approach best through his exhortations to his own students to focus on the sound they wanted, and the body would then figure out a way to produce it [5].

Students who decide that they are serious about the instrument will sometimes (but not usually) try to find a teacher who specializes and continue instruction with someone who has expertise. However, most professional wind musicians and music teachers are not trained on the anatomy of the vocal tract; and consequently, a number of strategies are promoted that might help a student create a desired sound but might compromise the health of the vocal tract. Indeed, recent research has shown that wind instrumentalists, from amateur to professional including college level, can experience a number of discomforting consequences such as throat pain, dry throat, and hoarseness after playing their instruments over a period of time, such as in a rehearsal or extended recording or practice session [3, 4, 6].

The revelation that the entire vocal tract can suffer damage or discomfort has gained more focus as a central topic of investigation, as opposed to an anecdotal observation, over approximately the past 70 years [7]. However, most current research focuses more on observations and measurements of small groups of instrumentalists or on self-reports, including most of the research reviewed later in this chapter. Pedagogical information presented comes from published books and materials. However, most of it is quite subjective, with the idea that instrumentalists focus on getting a particular sound and will manipulate themselves as needed to do so. So, there is tremendous variability in approaches and almost no evidence-based confirmation of their efficacy or risks. Subjective terminology commonly used by musicians will be used to help the medical specialist understand their viewpoints. Comparing and contrasting objective evaluations with subjective behaviors, observations, and terminology may seem confusing. However, it is hoped that sharing the information will better inform dentists, orthodontists, and voice specialists as they work with this population, and that this information will improve their ability to interpret the language their patients use to describe their performance concerns. Analogous strategies and information were central to the development of medical care for professional voice users [1, 8].

Issues with Beginning Woodwind Musicians

The instrument that most beginners end up playing is based upon accessibility (e.g., a parent has an old clarinet in the house, or an instrument is particularly cheap at a big-box store) and what the school will offer. Most young students start on clarinet, saxophone, or flute. The oboe and bassoon typically are saved for older students. Other considerations include the band director's assessment of over- and under-bite, ease of playing the instrument, and finally the child's preference. It is not unusual for a child to prefer to play a more difficult instrument, such as the oboe or bassoon or a larger sax, but due to the size of the child and the size of the instrument, in addition to the myriad of problems with double-reed instruments, most children will be urged to start on one of the instruments mentioned above and then eventually transition to a double-reed, which in itself can lead to more problems as discussed later in this section and throughout this book.

A unique characteristic of woodwind instruments is that every instrument requires a different embouchure (the manner in which the lips, jaw, and teeth are configured to blow into the instrument efficiently). Most instrument teachers depend upon basic explanations and heuristic imagery to describe the embouchures to students. This non-clinical terminology often references using "smile muscles" or "pucker muscles." Additionally, embouchures can be either a double-lipped or single-lipped type when reeds are considered (the flute does not have a reed). The "lipped" term refers to the amount of lip covering the teeth. Figure 4.1 provides illustrations and brief descriptions of each embouchure for each

Instrument	Embouchure	Description
Flute	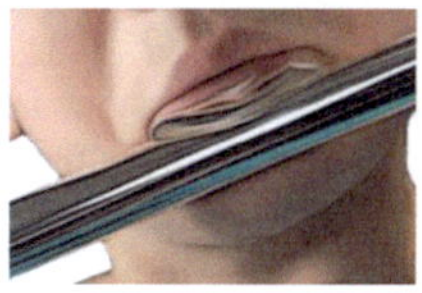	The example shows a traditional flute embouchure that demonstrates the focused central airstream. However, players with a tear-drop shaped upper lip will usually offset the embouchure a bit to the left to accommodate. Flute players will roll the mouthpiece aperture toward themselves and away to adjust for higher and lower notes.
Oboe	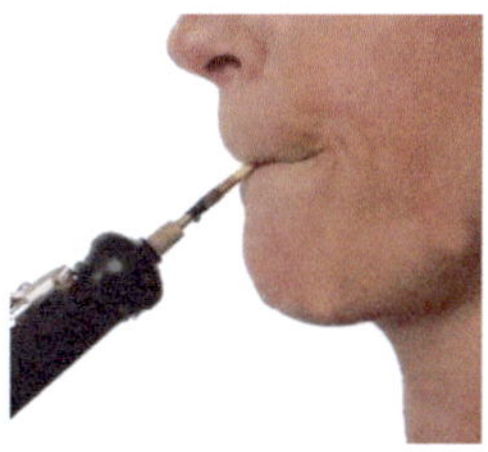	Traditional double-lipped oboe embouchure. Note the chin is rounded and not flat. The instrument is held close to a 45-degree angle to the mouth, and the player can actually play the instrument straight out horizontally from the mouth as well, for certain pieces.
Clarinet	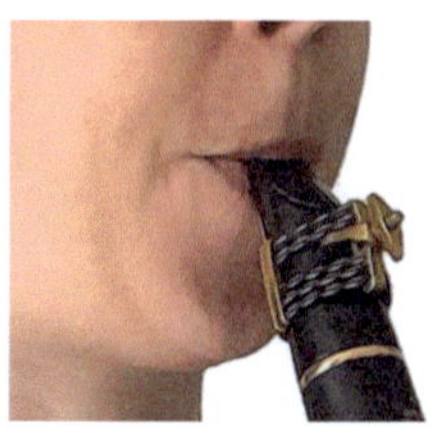	Traditional clarinet embouchure. Note the flattened & pointed chin and that the red parts of both lips is observable. The clarinet embouchure is unique in that it does not move while playing. Squeaks indicate that the mouthpiece is not fully supported by the embouchure. Also, note the angle of the mouthpiece as it enters the mouth: It is closer into the body than the oboe and saxophone. The player cannot play this instrument straight out horizontally from the mouth.
Saxophone	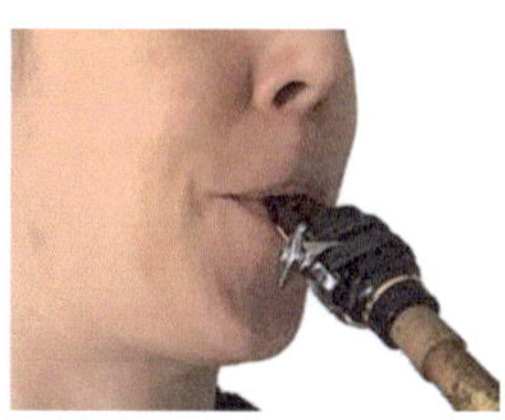	The saxophone embouchure is similar to the clarinet. However, the chin is much less pointed. Alto, tenor, baritone and bass saxophones also enter the mouth at a wider angle than the clarinet. Musicians who play soprano sax often hold the instrument out more horizontally, but that is due to personal preference.
Bassoon – high note embouchure	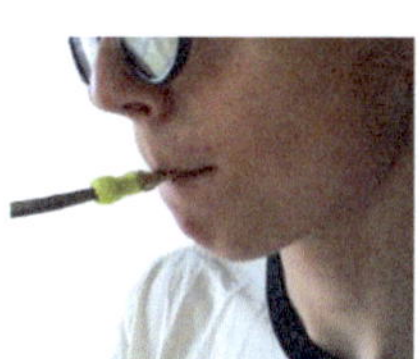	The bassoon is the only wind instrument that allows and encourages the player to move the reed in and out of the mouth to assist with playing in certain ranges. The embouchure at the left demonstrates a currently -taught modified overbite, double-lipped embouchure with much of the reed in the mouth to take advantage of the more resistant parts of the reed to aid in playing in the extreme high range of the instrument. Please note: students who switch to bassoon from clarinet often try to play the bassoon with a

Fig. 4.1 Annotated embouchures. (Photos provided by: MaryBeth Kern, John Flohr, and Dayne Kishbaugh.)

		clarinet embouchure, which includes a flattened and pointed chin, which is not seen here.
Bassoon – low note embouchure	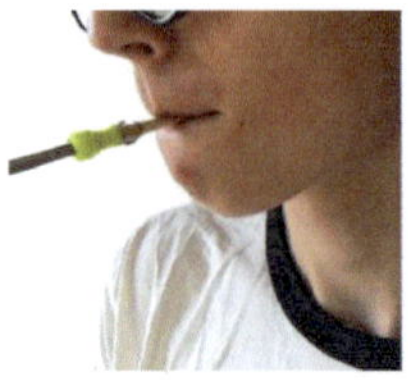	This embouchure demonstrates the double-lipped one used to aid in playing very low notes, to take advantage of the less resistant parts of the reed. Please also note that the student demonstrating the embouchures wears braces. 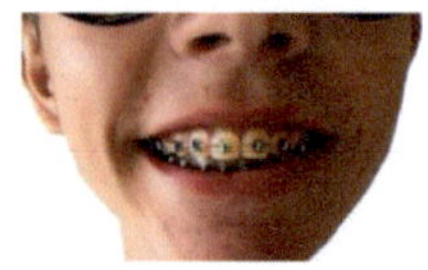
Bassoon – extreme overbite embouchure	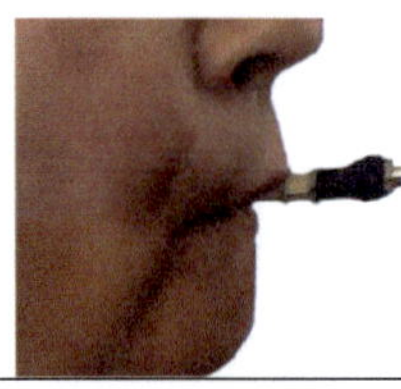	This photo shows the older traditional bassoon embouchure with a pronounced overbite, which is still taught by some teachers and school instrumental teachers.
Trumpet- high note embouchure	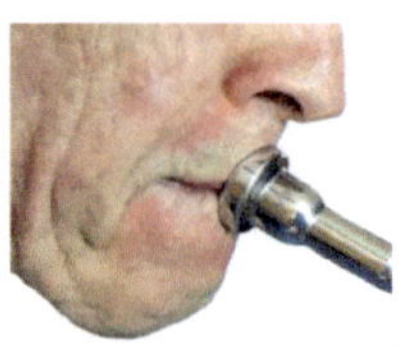	Brass players change the tightness of their lips to aid in playing in the higher and lower ranges of the instruments. This photo of a trumpet player shows how the lips are tightened, with less red showing, to play high notes.
Trumpet- low note embouchure	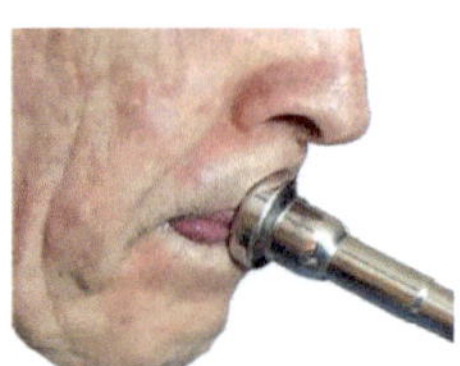	Low notes require more relaxed lips with more of the body of each lip showing.

Fig. 4.1 (continued)

woodwind instrument. Dental and medical professionals are encouraged strongly to ask their patients of any age to describe or demonstrate the embouchure they use on their instrument. The assumption that the embouchure used is the correct one should not be made without seeing it. Although Fig. 4.1 focuses on muscle use and unique characteristics of each embouchure, it is important to know that both smile and pucker muscles are used, but differently, on each instrument.

Objective research and classification of embouchure types were investigated initially in 1939 with the first work of Edward Strayer, a Philadelphia orthodontist and performing bassoonist, whose work was updated in 2019 by Clemente, Mendes, Moreira et al. (2019) [9]. While instrument teachers generally are not familiar with dental classifications, it has long been thought (and anecdotally applied) that band directors should look for certain mouth qualities when having students play woodwind instruments, such as having a pronounced overbite to play the bassoon; and past research seemed to suggest that this advice was not unwarranted [10, 11]. For more information concerning the interface of the embouchure with orthodontic considerations, please refer to Chap. 9 of this book.

While woodwind instrument embouchures seem to be developed clearly for each instrument, there is a plethora of problems that emerge commonly if a student who started on one instrument with a very prescribed embouchure, such as the clarinet, decides after several years to play another woodwind instrument, such as the bassoon, which has a completely different embouchure. The reason these lateral moves are difficult is because the embouchures have already been shaped on the previous instrument, and trying to change to a completely different one can be extremely difficult to nearly impossible, especially if the musician was self-taught. It is not uncommon for college-level bassoon and oboe teachers to struggle with students who insist on playing these instruments with clarinet embouchures, which means that they will be likely to bite hard on the reeds (as they will use smile muscles, not the pucker ones as needed) and constrict their air flow. The resultant tension could be damaging to the larynx, including the vocal folds. Additionally, it is not uncommon for students to decide that they will not study with a teacher and instead will teach themselves how to play other wind instruments, as it is commonly and anecdotally communicated to younger woodwind instrumentalists that basic concepts such as fingerings, support, air flow, and other skills are similar and can be transferred easily (but usually no detailed attention to developing the correct embouchure shape is advised).

Brass Instrument Embouchures

Unlike woodwind instruments, brass instrument embouchures are essentially identical and function the same. However, that does not mean a trumpet player can easily play a tuba. The higher instruments, such as all of the trumpets and French horn, require a tighter embouchure formation, while low brass instruments typically require a more relaxed embouchure formation. Beginning students are started on cornet (and then move to trumpet), trombone, and euphonium. French horn is saved for older and more serious students, and those young students who wish to play tuba start first on euphonium due to the size of the instrument. In younger players, as well as professional players, these embouchures can collapse, which can end a career. Focal dystonia and other embouchure problems in brass musicians are discussed later in this chapter.

Mouthpieces and Their Characteristics

Woodwind instruments use either a single reed, a double reed, or no reed at all. Brass instruments use cupped mouthpieces, while the French horn has a V-shaped mouthpiece. All reeds and mouthpieces come in varying sizes and resistance levels. This section provides basic foundations of reeds and mouthpieces so that dental and laryngological specialists can ask detailed questions of patients if and when needed during evaluations.

Single Reeds

Clarinet and saxophone players use single reeds which are shaped, gouged, and profiled to specific thickness from the tip to the collar (where the bark starts). The reed is made of a particular type of bamboo cane called *Arundo donax sativa*, that is grown in Southern France but has recently been grown successfully in China. The reed is attached to a rubber, wood, plastic, or even glass or metal mouthpiece by a ligature mechanism so that the reed can vibrate against the window opening of the mouthpiece. The mouthpiece is then attached to the instrument. A unique quality of these mouthpieces is that they can be pushed in or pulled out as needed to make sure that the instrument plays in tune. For clarinetists, mouthpieces can range from mass-molded factory-made plastic kinds (which means they may not be very reliable) to specifically made, professional-level ones that will be matched to specific clarinets based on the needs of the performer. Saxophone mouthpieces are more often plastic or rubber, with the same considerations of playing level and need, and jazz saxophonists also have been known to play on metal mouthpieces.

The reed itself can be a source of consternation and grief for young players, especially dentally, because a reed that is too soft (meaning that it vibrates too freely) will not have enough rigidity to support high notes. Many young players believe that the first reed that they get is the one that they will play for their first year of instruction, or longer, no matter how moldy it may become. Most band directors order single reeds in massive quantities and hand them out when a student needs one, but therein lies more problems. Single reeds come in 5 strengths: 1 = very soft to 5 = very hard. Beginners often are started on a reed that is 2.5 or so, and then as their strength and support and range increase, they use more rigid reeds. It is not known why a level 1 strength even exists. However, there are several major caveats: Reeds may come in boxes marked as a 2-strength, but they may actually be closer to a 4-strength. This is because after reeds are cut, shaped, and dried, they tend to do what reed musicians refer to euphemistically as "healing," because they harden between the time they are made and the time they are taken out of the box and played, therefore requiring time to break in. Second, not all reeds will break in, and the majority of band directors do not have the necessary equipment or know how to use it to adjust the reed and make it playable. Finally, not all reeds will play, even if there are attempts at adjusting them. For professional single-reed players, it is not unusual to test 3 boxes of 10 Vandoren [12] 5-strength clarinet reeds and find out that out of those 30 reeds that after adjustment, only about 10 will play to meet the needs of the clarinetist.

For younger players, those who do not play seriously, those who do not study with a professional single-reed musician, and for adults who just want to play clarinet by figuring it out on their own (e.g., as a doubler or tripler [someone who plays multiple instruments] in a community band), a number of tension-producing behaviors attributable to the wrong reed can develop that can cause dental, oropharyngeal, and laryngeal damage. For example, a person playing on a reed that is too soft will bite on the mouthpiece and the reed to play high sounds. Biting may result in a tongue that is raised in the back of the throat (again, as an attempt to squeeze out high notes) which will add additional constriction to the vocal tract. Essentially, where one system of sound production is not optimal, other systems attempt to compensate. In this case, the suboptimal component is a weak reed. This biting problem is very common in young and inexperienced players; and as evidence, it is normal to see teeth marks gouged into the top of the mouthpiece. When a child is playing on a reed that is too hard and has not been adjusted, there will be excessive fatigue when playing because instead of excessive biting, she or he will blow too hard and too often, and usually they will start the air from the throat by opening and closing the glottis (using a hard "huh" sound to start and slapping the tongue hard on the reed), which may result in throat pain. For young players who do not play seriously or study with a professional single-reed musician, and for adults who play clarinet by "figuring it out" on their own (e.g., as a doubler or tripler [someone who plays multiple instruments] in a community band), a number of tension-producing behaviors can cause dental, oropharyngeal, and laryngeal damage that is attributable to the wrong reed. There really is no rough time range of how long a reed will last, being that length of time practicing, acidity of the mouth saliva, kind of music played, and general hygiene of reed care will all affect if the reed lasts for a week or if it lasts longer, but generally, harder reeds last longer than softer ones.

For any dental or medical professional working with young or amateur clarinetists or saxophonists with dental or voice issues, asking to see the reed and mouthpiece may provide evidence of how the issues developed. Additional questions medical professionals should ask are whether the student is studying with a professional on the instrument, when the reed was changed last, what the strength of the reed is, if the reed was adjusted in any way, and the kind of music the player is working on. These would be in addition to any other questions concerning voice use, singing, and voice health.

Double Reeds

Whereas single reed players can order their reeds by the boxful, double-reed players do not have that option. Students who decide to study seriously a double-reed instrument often scare their school band directors, as most of them do not learn double reeds as part of their training. However, there are band directors, especially at the high school level, who will encourage a particularly talented student on sax or clarinet or flute to consider trying the bassoon or oboe that is stored in the basement of the school; and often these students try these instruments and then decide they will teach themselves. The reason that many students go this route is because the band director will supply the reed and the instrument, and there are few professional teachers available; so, they are expensive.

Younger and beginning double-reed players of any age often come from a different instrument, meaning that the correct embouchure may not be used. Also, double reeds are the entire mouthpiece of the oboe and bassoon (not attached to a rubber or plastic mouthpiece as with a clarinet or sax), and as such, can deteriorate quickly, are often in need of adjustment, and also need to be made to work with each individual instrument. An oboe reed that works on one oboe will not necessarily work on another oboe. Bassoons and oboes are very expensive, and those owned by schools are usually very old, not maintained, and will leak a lot of air, making the instruments much harder to play than an instrument that is in good condition.

Double-reeds need to be hand-crafted specifically to work with instruments. It is common for band directors to give their bassoon and oboe players plastic reeds instead of those made out of cane, because the plastic reeds will blow easily and allow the student to create a sound right away, but they will sound like either an annoyed cow or angry sheep instead of the traditional beautiful bassoon or oboe sound. Factory-made cane reeds are available and come in the same kinds of strengths that single reeds do. However, there is much more variability in the strengths in that a double reed that is labelled as medium-soft may actually be very hard. Band directors generally do not know that these reeds will not play right out of the box and often require adjustment, either making them less or more resistant by either sanding the reed or clipping it, and they will not know how to adjust them. Therefore, it is critical that any person who wishes to play a double-reed instrument study with a professional on the instrument, which can help the young musician develop playing behaviors that will not be damaging to the teeth, oropharynx, and larynx. However, most double-reed professionals are not educated in anatomy. So, while they may encourage the development of some healthy behaviors, they will not consistently prevent unhealthy techniques until better music teacher and musician education is available.

It is important for voice and medical professionals to know that attempts have been made to develop plastic reeds for professionals that are considered "perfect" and will never need to be replaced. These reeds cost about $125.00 USD, and reviews on their success are very mixed. While unlikely, it is possible that a wind instrument patient may be using one of these.

Double-reed instruments require specific embouchures, and the lips serve more as cushions and should never be overly tense for any length of time. As with the clarinet and saxophone, the reed goes into the mouth, which will require the tongue to arch further in the back of the mouth (research discussed later in this chapter will review this in more detail); but because the reed goes further into the mouth than a single-reed mouthpiece, a number of tension-creating issues can develop easily including biting on the reeds, constricting the airway with the arched tongue, and excessive jaw tension.

As with single reeds, dental and voice professionals working with double-reed musicians from beginner to professional level should ask about reed strengths, age of the reed, who makes the reed; and if the player makes it, then the kind of reed that the player prefers to make. When working with accomplished players, finding out whether the player prefers a harder/darker sound or lighter/flexible sound will provide information on the thickness and openness of the reed, and on the forces applied during playing. Some players use a particular style of reed regularly, while others craft particular reeds for particular pieces. Observing how the player blows the reed will allow the medical or dental specialist to observe tension in the body through watching inhalation, exhalation, neck and body muscle tension, and how the mouth is set.

Lifetime of All Reeds

The lifetime of a single or double reed is variable. Some will play well for several months, some for several weeks, and even some for only a few days. The lifetime of the reed depends upon a number of variables, such as how long the reed is played regularly, the acidity of the player's saliva, the basic hygiene care of the reed and mouthpiece, and the kind of music that is being performed with the reed. However, assigning a standard ball-park figure of lifetimes is very difficult because of so much variability, but it can be helpful to think that as soon as a reed is played, it then begins the process of wearing out, which reed players refer to "dying." Depending upon the player and the reed, the reed may die quickly or it may take a long time. While this terminology may seem a bit trite, it is the most common term used with reeds and reed life and death among woodwind players. Clarinet and sax reeds can play well for up to several weeks, while oboe reeds traditionally play well for only a few days. Bassoon reeds tend to last the longest, although if one is crafted for a particular performance, it may not work for any other pieces beyond that performance.

Flute Head Joints

The part of the flute into which the player blows is called the head joint. Blowing into the hole is like blowing across the top of a bottle. Young and beginner flute players usually start on flutes with head joints that come with the instrument; and when they begin, they often overblow and get dizzy, as it takes time to learn to focus the airstream correctly. Professional and advanced players regularly use different head joints on their flutes, finding one that helps them create the sound and flexibility of expressiveness that they want. Often, these joints are made of silver, platinum, or gold. Fortunately, there are no documented research publications concerning vocal tract problems with flute players, likely because the mouthpiece is outside of the body; and developing incorrect embouchures is unlikely, and there is little-to-no pressure on the teeth. However, anecdotal evidence suggests that orthognathic surgery can compromise one's ability to play flute. Orthognathic surgery is discussed in Chap. 12 of this book.

Brass Instrument Mouthpieces

While it might seem that brass instrument mouthpieces are less fussy than reeds, unfortunately that is not the case. There is a variety of mouthpieces available for all of these instruments and additionally, philosophical playing approaches of teachers and professionals differ concerning preference and how they should be used.

Mouthpieces come primarily in two shapes: c-cup and v-cup, with variations for each shape. While most trumpets, trombones, and tubas traditionally use c-cup mouthpiece, and French horn uses a v-cup mouthpiece, it is not unusual to have the opposite occur as well. The thickness of the mouthpiece, the material from which it is made, the size of the rim, and the depth of the c-cup or v-cup all contribute to the sound the instrument will make.

The mouthpiece size and style can cause problems for young players. If the student trumpet player is using an old, 1920's style silver cornet with an old mouthpiece that is too shallow, the student will have difficulty playing lower notes and due to inexperience will likely push hard against the teeth when trying to produce high notes. Beginners on trumpet often start on a B-flat cornet when young (ages 9–10 years) because the instrument is smaller and fits more easily in the hands, and they change to trumpet when a little older. The traditional cup size of the mouthpieces for beginners is modelled after the Bach 7C [13]. This is generally copied across the industry for beginners. However, it is not unusual to have serious students exchange the 7C for other mouthpieces as they improve. The purpose of the mouthpiece is to provide evenness of tone and pitch stability throughout the range of the instrument, especially for beginners. If the size is a higher number, that indicates the cup is shallow and made for high notes specifically (as in lead trumpet for jazz ensembles). A number smaller than Bach 3 or 7 would be unlikely to be found in a young student's instrument case.

French horn students often start on a Conn No. 2 [14, 15] or similar sizes. Trombone, euphonium, and tuba players have much larger cup-sized mouthpieces. Less detail is provided in this chapter concerning those mouthpieces because research indicates that musicians who play these lower brass instruments suffer fewer vocal tract issues than trumpet and French horn players [11]. There are numerous websites devoted to brass instrument mouthpieces, and the reader is encouraged to explore those via a simple search.

Traditionally, brass players are taught to buzz their lips either with or without a mouthpiece. Some players can actually buzz tunes with their lips alone, without the mouthpiece. However. there are other players who do not think that that is a necessary skill. Additionally, most young players play on one mouthpiece only, while more advanced and professional players may have an entire collection of mouthpieces that are switched out for various performance venues and repertoire; however, there are those who believe that one mouthpiece should be used for all performances. Decisions on mouthpieces used is purely personal and due to preferences of the performer and/or teacher. The advantage that brass players have over wind instrumentalists is that their mouthpieces do not wear out in a few weeks, nor do they regularly make their own. However, they can be custom made and some players currently are working on creating new types and styles of mouthpieces. The materials commonly used are brass, and older mouthpieces may be made from nickel silver. An excellent guide to varieties, sizes, and foundations of mouthpieces is available through Yamaha [16]. Additional well-known models currently used are those developed by and named after Vincent Bach [13], Robert Giardinelli [17], and Renold Schilke [18].

Dental, orthodontic, and voice specialists who work with young brass players should be aware of some issues that may affect the teeth and jaw, as well as the vocal tract. The most common issues concern embouchure. The first major issue is that young trumpet players often push the rim of the mouthpiece against their teeth when first learning to play notes higher than C5 (C above middle C). This would be analogous to biting on a wind instrument. While band instrument instructors are aware of this common problem and address it, the success may be minimal because they will not be able to remind the musician every day. The problem is overcome through learning better support, and it also has been suggested that raising and arching the tongue toward the back of the mouth will also help. Anecdotally, it has been shared that braces help younger trumpet players avoid developing the habit of excessive pressure, because they will shred their lips.

Another bad habit that can be developed by young trumpet and trombone players is holding the instrument at an angle that will change the embouchure. While holding these instruments at 90 degrees is usually required for marching band, it is better to hold the instruments at a comfortable angle that is less than 90 degrees. However, some students may hold the instrument far more vertically, which for trumpet players may let them develop something more like a woodwind instrument embouchure if they are not monitored and corrected quickly. The vertical position is usually a result of arm fatigue. For trombonists, the problem is less common but is due to difficulty in reaching seventh position as the arm may not be long enough. However, some players can become lazy and have the slide nearly touch the floor or ground when extended, resulting in the "farmer plowing the field" style of playing. Fortunately, this is usually just a bad habit and the young players correct it immediately once they are called out on it, so it should not affect dental or voice health.

Other Considerations for All Wind Instruments

Much has been written about the desire for young instrumentalists to play instruments that will not interfere with the jaws and teeth (see Chap. 11 in this book for more discussion). For many young people, this would limit the options available to them; and, in fact, they would not be able to play the instrument of their dreams. The selection of the instrument a young musician wishes to play well is rarely determined by his or her teeth; moreover, music psychology research has investigated why children choose the instruments that they do, with the final question being "does the child choose the instrument or the instrument choose the child?" [19–21]. Therefore, the relationship between the instrument and the human who plays it, especially for committed musicians, is personal and should not be considered lightly when working with instrumentalists who present with any dental or vocal tract problems. Many musicians feel that the instrument is an extension of and part of themselves, and anything that may jeopardize that relationship may seem threatening.

Use of Vowels in Assisting with Pitch, Tone, and Resonance, Also Known As "Voicing" Technique

A common pedagogical application in wind instrument playing, called "voicing," is promoted by many teachers to aid with pitch, tone, and resonance for all wind instruments [22–25]. The approach claims to get the idea from singers, and as such, promotes the idea that forming the vowel shape in the throat will help with the notes. However, a few issues, most unknown to the wind players, must be recognized with this approach. First, the wind players who have promoted this approach think of pure vowels, not modified vowels that would be used by singers, especially when singing in a high range. For example, a student may be encouraged to make an /i/ vowel shape in the throat while playing a high B on the bassoon. Second, manipulating the vocal tract to create these vowels is likely to add more tension and therefore inhibit the breath support needed to play the instrument. This approach has not been investigated scientifically in relationship to dental implications or vocal health, but it is possible that it may contribute to overall tension and vocal tract problems.

Contemporary Performance Practice Concerns

In contemporary pieces, it is not unusual for an instrument to be played in a different way from which it was intended traditionally. A current trend of composers require differing tonguing/articulation techniques (e.g., double and triple tonguing, flutter-tonguing, slap tonguing), vocal productions of sounds while playing the instrument (e.g., singing while playing, either in tune or in harmony, or creating shrieks; and also creating unvoiced sounds that are more percussive-like) and in some works, taking the mouthpiece from one instrument and using it to make sounds on another (e.g., the bassoon reed and bocal [the metal tube of the bassoon on which the reed is placed] are placed into the mouthpiece of a trombone, making a new instrument called the "tromboon.") and playing the mouthpiece differently than usual (such as playing the clarinet mouthpiece upside down), playing only a piece of the instrument, and playing with something inserted into the instrument to make a different kind of sound. As composers look for more ways to add new sounds to music, it is likely that these kinds of performance skills will be required more often. It is not unlikely that a wind musician may experience discomfort, pain, and soreness after practicing and perfecting these kinds of sounds or modified embouchures.

The Value of Warming Up

Most wind instrumentalists think of warming up as in (1) warming up the instrument so it will respond correctly and (2) warming up the hands and fingers to work with technical passages. It would be rare that a wind instrumentalist would be thinking of warming up the voice as part of this process. Additionally, cooling-down the instrument after playing is generally not done in woodwind performance; however, it is becoming a more common practice with high-brass musicians, especially trumpet players, to do so after a long practice session or performance. While a number of trumpet pedagogy websites provide information on cooling-down, there is no research concerning the value of this process to the vocal tract. Another reason why warming-down is not a common behavior among wind instrumentalists after performing is that most venues want the players to leave the premises as soon as possible.

The value of wind instrument and voice warm-up and cool-down exercises has not been studied. Neither has the efficacy of singing training for wind instrumentalists. However, anecdotally, the authors (VLT and RTS) have found singing training and voice therapy very helpful in addressing such possibilities in wind instrumentalists.

Questions to Ask Wind Instrument Musicians as Part of an Evaluation

While at this time there are no published protocols in place to evaluate the vocal tract in relationship to wind instrument playing, there is documented evidence of particular orofacial and vocal tract issues that could be exacerbated by playing a wind instrument [26]. These issues are addressed later in this chapter. However, understanding whether there is a connection between the instrument and how it is played, and the possible diagnosis requires the medical and dental specialist to collect other information from the patient. Suggested questions include the following:

1. How long have you played your instrument?
   - 2a. *For woodwind instrumentalists*:
     - a. For young players: "Tell me about your instrument. Why did you pick it, or did it pick you? How long have you been playing? Is the instrument owned by you, is it borrowed from school, or is it rented (important for instrument maintenance, as the instrument may leak or have cracks that make playing it more difficult)? Are you studying with a professional on this instrument? Did you play another wind instrument before this one and are you playing more than one kind of wind instrument now?"
     - b. What strength of reed are you using? How old is it?
     - c. For young musicians or beginners: "Can you show me the embouchure you use while playing the instrument?" (If the instrument is present, then the musician can demonstrate. The medical and dental specialist should look for indication of tension in the body, and if the musician has a sax or clarinet, if teeth indentations are seen on the mouthpiece that will indicate the musician is biting too hard).
     - d. Professionals and accomplished players can be asked simply "What is your set-up?" and they will share the make, model, age of the instrument, and all of its parts, what everything is made of, usually including kinds of reeds and strengths.
   - 2b. *For brass instrumentalists:*
     - a. For young players: "Tell me about your instrument. Why did you pick it, or did it pick you? How long have you been playing? Is the instrument owned

by you, or borrowed from the school, or is it rented (important for instrument maintenance, as the instrument may leak, which makes playing it more difficult)? Are you studying with a professional on this instrument?"

   b. Professionals and accomplished players can be asked simply "What is your set-up?" and they will share the make, model, age of the instrument, and all of its parts, kinds of mouthpieces used for what circumstances, if they double or triple on other brass instruments, and so forth.
   c. If the instrument is available, the musician should play it and the medical or dental specialist look for signs of tension.

3. Have you had any bodily (musculoskeletal) injuries that have caused pain or changes that might have affected your instrument performance?

Laryngoscopic Examination Suggestions

At this time, validated protocols are not available to assist laryngoscopic evaluation while playing a wind instrument. However, several observations can be made during laryngoscopic examination while playing the instrument:

- If the larynx is rising while playing.
- If the vocal folds are touching, or approximating tensely.
- If there is evidence of swelling.
- If there is evidence of excessive vocal fold rigidity in position relative to the midline that seems more pronounced on one side than the other.
- When the musician is playing with vibrato, if the vocal folds move differently – or not at all – on either side.

These behaviors can be observed readily by (1) having the musician play a scale from low to high and back down several times, at a fast speed, (2) having the musician play sustained notes (low, middle, and high parts of the instrument range) with vibrato (professional and accomplished) or without vibrato (professional, accomplished, and beginners), and (3) having the person play a piece or excerpt of a piece of music in which she or he notices throat discomfort with (if they have that problem) or not, and as a contrast, one piece/excerpt in with the discomfort does not occur.

Research Focus in Medicine Concerning Laryngeal and Vocal Tract Behaviors

Most research conducted by medical professionals has used small numbers of professional wind instrumentalists as subjects. The foci generally have been on *oromandibular* issues concerning embouchure (the formation of the lips around the reed or mouthpiece), *focal dystonias* in some wind instrumentalists, and intraocular and intraoral pressure in individuals while playing high-pressure instruments. Other areas of medical research have looked at *pneumoparotitis*, in which air forced through the parotid ducts from the mouth during performance causes swelling in the face [27]. *Palate paresis* was found to be common in woodwind players, and it can lead to *velopharyngeal insufficiency* (VPI) [28, 29]. Evans et al. reported that the highest prevalence of VPI was reported in musicians who played the following instruments in this order: (1) clarinet, (2) oboe, (3)saxophone, (4), bassoon, (5) French Horn, (6) trumpet [30]. Males reported a higher incidence of VPI than females, and the degree of occurrence of VPI was attributed by the musicians in the study in descending order to: (1) muscular fatigue, (2) performance-related stress, (3) other kinds of stress, (4) prolonged and intense periods of music-making, and (5) returning to practice after a significant vacation from the instrument. The primary and most obvious symptom of VPI was a grunting sound in the back of the throat (reported by 83%). In a later study, the researchers concluded further that fatigue and stress, along with specific anatomical features of the musicians who were investigated, may affect velopharyngeal closure in musicians diagnosed with stress VPI [31]. The occurrence is not painful, but it is annoying and uncomfortable physically as well as audibly to the performer and to the musicians sitting nearby. Most musicians who suffer regularly from VPI do not know that the problem can be remediated medically or surgically or that it can be addressed through speech and voice therapy. It is not known whether musicians with high incidence of VPI suffer from other vocal health issues. These medical and surgical problems are addressed in more detail in Chap. 7 of this book.

Laryngocele, an abnormal air-filled laryngeal sac, has been found primarily in brass musicians [27, 32, 33]. *Pharyngocele*, which is an expansion of the pharynx that involves the common air and food passageway presents commonly as expansion in the neck. Wind musicians who experience this often leave the top of their shirts open at the neck or buy shirts a neck size larger than their usual size to accommodate the expansion. A recent case study highlights the susceptibility to laryngoceles and pharyngoceles, particularly in young brass musicians who may engage in improper performance techniques, poor practice habits, experience performance anxiety more readily, and may not have had enough instruction on injury prevention [34], although these conditions may develop in musicians with good technique, as well. The researchers add that the research literature available is confusing in that there are multiple names for similar problems, and that physicians need to be aware that confusing the terminology may lead to misdiagnosis. Additional concern has been expressed about the development of *laryngopharyngeal diverticulae* in wind instrumentalists, designating a musician-acquired diverticulum as an "occupational overuse syndrome" [35].

Embouchure, when addressed, has been identified by the medical community primarily as being the strongest contributor in controlling instrumental tone color. This is very different from how wind musicians view the importance of embouchure. They consider the lips and mouth muscles as cushions or conduits rather than as a primary source of manipulation to change tone color, and excessive tension in the lip and mouth area is viewed as a negative behavior in wind instrument performance. Some research has identified the pharynx as responsible for tone color [36].

Overall, instrument pedagogy or teaching methodology that influenced the musician research subjects has not been a strong consideration when conducting medical research. Although some studies cite older books written by musicians concerning pedagogy, the information may not have been applied with complete understanding. Additionally, wind musicians also learn through oral traditions, similar to the way singers learn to sing from voice teachers who pass down legend and lore associated with performance that may not be supported through scientific research.

Eckley's research concerning glottis configuration in wind players during performance was unique in that not only did she report what was seen in the laryngeal behaviors of the instrumentalists in the study, but she also offered medical observations, which had not been offered in previous or subsequent research [2]. The study looked at (1) the position of the vocal and ventricular folds during sound production, (2) anteroposterior and lateral laryngeal dimensions during the sound production, (3) tongue base and pharyngeal position and behavior while blowing into the instrument, and (4) the presence or absence of vibrato and the apparent location of the vibrato source in the vocal tract. Ten wind instrumentalists participated as subjects. Eckley reported the following: (1) musical tones were performed with partially adducted vocal folds; (2) the greater the technical difficulty of the passage, the greater the lateral tension in the larynx and the constriction in the entire vocal tract; and (3) instrumentalists reported dysphonia after intense instrumental playing (5 out of 10) and increased throat secretions after intense playing (8 out of 10), and in difficult passages (4 out of 10) which were not identified by the researcher. It was observed in all participants that musical tones were played with partially adducted vocal folds and that the greater the technical difficulty reported by the player, more the playing was associated with increased lateral tension in the larynx as well as constriction in the vocal tract. Medically, Eckley noted arytenoid and interarytenoid edema and hyperemia in eight of the ten participants at a moderate intensity (5 on a scale of 1–10), and one subject presented with mild edema (3 on a scale of 1–10) [2]. The findings of this study could potentially have important implications for wind instrument musicians. However, follow-up research has not been done, nor have any other medical professionals addressed these issues.

Research Conducted by Wind Instrumentalists with Voice Scientists

The major area of research interest, as well as contention, of wind instrumentalists concerns laryngeal behavior as it relates to vibrato production, primarily with regard to the intrinsic muscles of the larynx. However, how the vocal tract contributes to the creation of instrumental sounds and tone colors has often been misunderstood or misapplied. In wind instrument pedagogy, musicians are encouraged to keep an "open throat" while playing. However, there often is confusion as to what an "open throat" actually means. Common imagery used asks the musician to imagine that there is an orange or a tennis ball in the back of the throat that keeps the throat open. Applying these pedagogical approaches in research by wind instrumentalists (often in collaboration with voice scientists at local universities, who are not always musically trained) can lead to well-intentioned research studies with baffling results. This problem highlights the need for expert, collaborative research.

Generally, most wind instrumentalists who have conducted research do not have a strong background in vocal tract anatomy, speech science, or in singing (many have not studied voice professionally), leading to some misunderstandings on how the vocal tract behaves in singing and in instrument playing, occasionally leading to some humorous assumptions and conclusions, particularly when arguing that vibrato in reed instruments should be like vibrato in the human voice. One phenomenon in recent research or opinion articles cited often concerns the "goat's trill" which was a performance practice, and not necessarily pleasant, in early Baroque opera [37], which required glottal articulations, and which has been referred to as an "Elmer Fudd" voice [38, 39]. Many woodwind instrumentalist researchers believe firmly that the intrinsic muscles of the larynx control vibrato, despite the absence of convincing evidence to support that notion. Brass instrument researchers have shown that vibrato is controlled primarily by the embouchure or with the slide for trombonists. Their research interests focus more on investigations into issues with embouchures and air pressure. Both kinds of researchers have valid concerns, and both areas will be addressed separately here.

Woodwind Research

Internal laryngeal behaviors in five professional bassoonists were evaluated using a nasopharyngeal fiberoptic endoscope as they performed part of the second movement of the Mozart *Bassoon Concerto, K.191* and the second movement final solo in Tchaikovsky's *4th Symphony*, played both with straight tone and with vibrato [40]. The results of the study indicated clearly that the glottal opening and the arytenoid cartilages were engaged during vibrato, and the conclusion of the study was that the larynx contributes directly to the creation of vibrato. Additionally, the researcher proposed that the manner in which the vibrato was created was the same way it was created in singers. His conclusions have been perpetuated by many woodwind instrumentalists for years in that students frequently are encouraged to create vibrato the same way they do when they sing. Teachers refer to research that shows that laryngeal engagement also causes the movements of the tongue and pharynx during performance, and that the vocal folds serve primarily to assist in controlling airflow, but also are used to assist in the production of vibrato in the flute [39, 41–44]. In investigating all woodwind instrument laryngeal behaviors, Scott et al. stated "Vibrato activity for flute, oboe and bassoon varied greatly between individuals, but there was no doubt that the vibrato originated in the throat, not the diaphragm" [41]. Kahane et al. reported vocal fold and soft palate motion during bassoon playing in vibrato, but added that it was not known if these were active or passive behaviors [45]. Watson noted that manipulating the glottis and the degree of closure affected airflow into the instrument [46]. In a more recent study, Adduci investigated the amount of intraoral and sound pressure in oboists, and observed that the arytenoids were more closed during performance of lower intensity sounds and were more open during higher intensity sounds [47]. With the exception of Kahane (a voice scientist) et al., the musicians proposed that the larynx was actively creating the vibrato, as it does in singing (in part), but did not consider the possibility that the behaviors were instead passive. They also assumed that because laryngeal movement was observed, it was causally related to vibrato; but no causal relationship has been established. In nearly all cases, the researchers also revealed a lack of understanding of the complex issues and controversies regarding vibrato production in singers.

The frequent conclusions in this research that woodwind vibrato is like voice vibrato also are problematic and illustrate the lack of understanding among woodwind musicians of how the vocal tract works. One primary difference between wind instrument sound production and the voice is that in singing the vocal folds touch longitudinally and separate to create sound. In wind instrument playing, the vocal folds usually are held fairly rigidly while they are adducted partially, and they do not touch in the same way that they do in singing. The degree of rigidity is unknown.

Brass Instrument Research

Research conducted by or with brass musicians has focused primarily on issues of embouchure and air pressure. Both are areas of great concern, with the primary foci being the embouchure and the pressure of the mouthpiece against the mouth. The most worrisome problem is referred to by wind musicians as "embouchure collapse," but it also includes the condition known as focal dystonia. The former term also encompasses a temporary loss of embouchure formation due to overuse and fatigue, as well as permanent loss attributable to focal dystonia, which is reported to happen more frequently in men than women, possibly because of sex hormones [48]. Many brass musicians have anecdotally attributed the phenomenon to mouthpiece pressure, but there is no research to support that speculation. The cause is not known, and the problem still ends careers of very promising musicians, particularly brass instrumentalists. Excellent and comprehensive reviews of orofacial problems in brass musicians can be accessed in many studies found in the journal *Medical Problems of Performing Artists* [49], including a review by Rodriguez-Lozano [49].

The physical effects of performance anxiety on brass musicians also have been studied. The physical manifestations of performance anxiety, particularly in brass instrumentalists, can lead to termination of professional careers [50], and "dry mouth" in brass musicians can be especially troublesome in performance [51]. Physical manifestations displayed most commonly by brass musicians include breathing, pain, and tension issues, all of which can affect performance; and they often are associated with added jaw tension [51]. Unfortunately, the internet is full of recordings of notable brass performance "fails," and anecdotal stories abound about how conductors have used mistakes in rehearsal and unedited live performance recordings, particularly in professional unionized orchestras, to encourage brass musicians to consider early retirement [52]. While an overall discussion of performance anxiety is not part of this chapter, the physical manifestations of it, particularly in brass instruments, might engage the vocal tract in ways that could be damaging. Similar issues occur in voice, particularly in singers and other professional voice users [53].

Laryngeal Activity and Positioning in Wind Instrument Performance

Laryngeal activity researched broadly in the medical and musical fields has included the role of the glottis in air control and laryngeal positioning in performance [2, 27, 33, 54–58]. Glottal concerns have included controlling the air for vibrato and glottis formation, especially in controlling exhalation into an instrument. Students often first learn to play wind instruments during compulsory education using soprano recorder that is taught in general music classes, often in the fourth grade in the USA. The most popular method used in the classroom (in which students master songs and some basic note-reading skills to earn colored belts that are tied on to their recorders) does not address healthy articulation. While many music educators have argued over the articulation sound that should be used (either "doo" or "thoo"), most teachers do not address how air is initiated into the instrument. Many very young instrumentalists instinctively inhale and slam the glottis shut to keep the air from coming out until they open the glottis and the air rushes out; and they often continue that behavior through their playing careers unless they are taught otherwise. Forceful, habitual, high-pressure glottis closure can lead to vocal fold injury in speakers and singers, and it is almost certainly similarly hazardous in wind instrumentalists. Many researchers refer to this behavior as a Valsalva maneuver, although not all researchers agree with the application of the term. According to Dr. Peter Iltis, a French Horn player who also earned a PhD in kinesthesiology, the "true Valsalva maneuver involves closing the vocal apparatus (otherwise known as the glottis) and forcefully bearing down with the abdominal muscles and the internal intercostal muscles, and suddenly releasing the pressure by reopening the glottis in wind players, when the problem of starting notes due to a "locking" (sic) of the tongue and closing of the throat occurs, they are utilizing the same mechanism of glottal closure, and they can indeed build up pressure to some extent in the thorax, but they are not performing a true Valsalva maneuver" [59]. The recommended remediation for this behavior (described but not named by Dr. Iltis) is to use the same breathing technique that is used in singing – to inhale, suspend the breath but not close the glottis, and release the breath, using the tongue to articulate the sound on the instrument. It is not known how many wind instrument teachers apply this knowledge, nor whether the repeated, forceful adduction of the vocal folds in the instinctive approach contributes to vocal fold damage in instrumentalists, but the author (RTS) has treated patients in whom these instrumental performance misuses appear to have been the only causes of voice pathology. In such patients, voice function improves with excellent teaching of less traumatic instrument-playing technique. This is an area that needs more research in both young beginners and professional players.

Researchers have reported that the larynx is lowered in flute, saxophone, and oboe playing [44, 60]. However, it is not clear whether the researchers were referring to the larynx at a resting position or actively forced lower during playing, not unlike the vocal pedagogy approaches used in Germany in the late 1800s to 1900s [61]. It was reported that when musicians played higher notes, the larynx rose in single-reed instrument players, but stayed in a lower position for double-reed players [36, 62]. Additionally, researchers pointed out that every woodwind instrument requires a different laryngeal position [44], and that tone quality can be modified by changes in embouchure, reed, breath support, and throat configuration [63]. The date range of the earlier studies is from 1964 to 1998, and there have been many changes in the ways instruments are engineered since then, with the exception of the bassoon which has remained the least successfully modernized. Current instrument developers have sought to design and develop instruments and plastic reeds that require less work (both physical and respiratory) from the performer, particularly plastic instruments sold inexpensively by big-box retail stores for beginner and amateur musicians. The implications of learning to play on a plastic instrument or with a plastic reed, and how that will affect a student transferring to a wooden or brass instrument are not known.

When playing an instrument causes dysphonia, that usually indicates that the musician's technique is faulty and involves excess tension. Optimizing all aspects of technique and elimination hyperfunction usually leads to resolution of the dysphonia. This process may be facilitated by voice therapy and singing lessons which may teach players muscle control or relaxation through a process that provokes less anxiety than trying to change or abandon performance habits in their primary instrument. However, since most voice therapy and singing lessons do not involve a reed or mouthpiece intruding into the mouth, the effect of the tongue tension release strategies still needs investigation as to how wind players modify those strategies while playing the instrument.

Another area not addressed in research concerning the larynx and vocal tract in instrumentalists is the effect of overall body muscle tension while the wind instrumentalist performs [64]. This may be of particular concern for instrumentalists who need to hold the instrument in an uncomfortable or physically compromising position for long periods of time. For example, a baritone saxophonist using a neckstrap to hold about 25 pounds of instrument around the neck, particularly in a marching band, often experiences muscle tension in the shoulders that may translate to tension in the laryngeal area. Clarinetists and oboists who do not use neckstraps balance their instruments on their thumbs, creating tension and eventually pain in the thumb joint and the arms, which also can translate to tension in the arm, shoulder, neck, and possibly the larynx. Amateur and self-taught musicians, and students still in training, often engage in tension-producing habits while performing: hands are shaped as tensed claws, fingers are pressed down too hard to cover keys or holes (evidenced by the finger tips becoming white), arms are held in awkward positions, shoulders are raised and lowered in the misguided belief that such movement adds to musicality, and so forth. The adverse effects of bodily tension upon voice performance are well recognized and may occur whether the tension has been caused by singing, speaking, playing an instrument, or other factors, including trauma [65].

Interestingly, the question of whether a "natural larynx" is even needed for wind instrument performance has been raised, as demonstrated by a case study concerning a professional trombonist who underwent a total laryngectomy and had a Blom-Singer voice prosthesis with a tracheoesophageal shunt inserted. The researchers reported that the prosthesis created enough of a regulated, strong airflow to play a brass instrument. However, the air pressure required to play trombone was too high for the prosthesis. Thus, the musician changed to a valved tenor horn and was successful in playing and teaching the instrument [66].

Other Vocal Tract Behaviors

Several other behaviors in addition to velopharyngeal insufficiency should be considered, including acoustical coupling behaviors between the lip valves and vocal folds, vocal tract resonance in wind instrument performance, and the role of the tongue. A fairly exhaustive group of studies has shown that there is disagreement on how the vocal tract engages or manipulates sounds in wind instruments. Musicians generally believe that the shape of the mouth affects the sound, but there are some scientists who disagree [56, 67–74]. Scientists have investigated vocal tract behaviors two ways: (1) by working with professional musicians, primarily trombonists, clarinetist, saxophonists, and digeridoo performers, and (2) by creating artificial players with latex lips [67]. All of the studies indicate that the vocal tract can be engaged in controlling pitch, and to some degree tone color, via vocal tract tuning. However, the degree of involvement is unknown. Additionally, the studies have been conducted using primarily professional players (when humans are used) playing long tones in various ranges of the instrument or engaging in an extended pitch-producing technique, such as pitch-bending. Tongue position has been investigated and reported as in a high position for high notes and a low position for low notes [67]. Additionally, some instruments may require more vocal tract engagement than others. For example, hypothetically, instruments that have the mouthpieces outside of the mouth (e.g., brass instruments and flute) may require a different degree of engagement from those that have the mouthpiece inserted into the mouth (e.g., clarinet, oboe, bassoon, and saxophone), but there is no research in this area. Moreover, vocal tract behavior may be affected by the degree of mouthpiece insertion into the mouth (the bassoon requires changes in this factor, such as putting more reed in when playing higher notes, and less reed when playing lower notes, while the same strategy on a clarinet would result in a series of squeaks). Unfortunately, there are no studies that investigate vocal tract behaviors in these areas from a health standpoint, and it is not clear whether these behaviors are learned or created in response to the instrument.

Studies that investigate tongue position and movement in a number of techniques used regularly by professionals, such as *flutter-tonguing*, and *double* and *triple* tonguing, have not been undertaken. These techniques are physically difficult and time-consuming to learn, and they require a great amount of muscle effort to do well, depending upon the instrument. Flutter-tonguing is used commonly in performances of jazz music, but it is also a standard part of classical music repertoire. Flutter-tonguing would be akin to a steady vocally rolled /r/ sound but without the phonation. Air pressure must be very strong and steady, since it cannot waiver as it progresses through the instrument. Double tonguing can be taught several ways, with the two most common being a /tɑ/—/kɑ/ approach in which /tɑ/ is one articulation and /kɑ/ is the other articulation. For double reeds, particularly the bassoon and contrabassoon, the approach is different, using a "good-dog" approach that moves the articulations further to the back of the mouth to accommodate the intrusion of the reed into the oral cavity. Students learn to double-tongue by gradually increasing the speed of the articulation using a metronome. There is no established desired speed; however, generally it is believed that the faster, the better. Triple tonguing can be performed either as "ta-ka-ta ta-ka-ta" or "duh-gah-duh duh-gah-duh," again depending upon the position of the mouthpiece. This technique is often required for marches, and for a great variety of symphonic music. Double, triple, and flutter-tonguing are exhausting techniques, especially when they need to be done over extended periods of time, and can result in temporary tongue and throat pain, even in expert professional wind instrumentalists. Of particular concern are students who are just learning these techniques and may experience pain, fatigue, and soreness more readily. The effect of extended vocal tract techniques, such as these tonguing techniques, should be investigated to see if they impact to vocal health over time.

Many other issues worthy of consideration are beyond the scope of this chapter but include other commonalities and potential commonalities among singers and wind instrumentalists. For example, reflux is a well-recognized problem found very commonly in singers. Interestingly, Cammarota et al. showed in a study of 1083 musicians that reflux is also an issue for instrumentalists and is more common in wind instrumentalists (especially flute and double-reed players) than in other instrumentalists [75]. Since reflux is known to affect the vocal tract, reflux is likely to have consequences not only for singers but also for wind instrumentalists. The same study revealed that the incidence of overweight (36.75%) and obesity (11%) was significantly higher in wind players than in other instrumentalists (22.31% and 4.78%, respectively.). It is not known whether obesity has an adverse effect on wind instrumentalists, but obesity decreases the area of the vocal tract and has adverse effects on voice [76]. Obesity seems likely to affect wind instrument performance but studies are needed. Interestingly, although obesity is associated with obstructive sleep apnea (OSA), the prevalence of OSA is lower in double-reed players than in non-wind instrumentalists; and the more hours they played, the lower their risk of OSA [77]. The study surveyed 906 musicians, and other wind instrumentalists did not differ from non-wind players. Respiratory and vocal tract muscle training is the likely cause of lower prevalence of OSA in double-reed players. However, in a study of 340 professional orchestra musicians, no difference in snoring or daytime fatigue was found when comparing wind instrumentalists with other professional musicians [78]. These issues would benefit from further investigation, as would many other questions regarding the vocal tract in wind instrumentalists.

Concurrent Studies of Wind Instruments and Singing

The primary study that looks at the interrelationship between singing and playing a wind instrument was undertaken in 1989 and the issue to be revisited and investigated further. In an electromyographic study investigating concurrent relationships among oboists studying voice, the researcher concluded that concurrent study introduced several problems that the oboists displayed that affected their singing including (1) greater supra- versus sub-glottal air pressure, (2) greater jaw tension, (3) greater lip tension, (4) and less tongue flexibility [79]. It was recommended that vocalists not study wind instrument performance due to these findings. More recently, a study looked at the effect of a vocal polyp on a female singer/saxophonist/French hornist and found that the polyp affected singing, but did not affect performance on the other instruments [27]. Updated and relevant research addressing the interaction of voice instruction and wind instrument instruction is needed.

Conclusion

Controversies remain regarding concurrent study and / or performance of singing and wind instruments. Both involve pharyngeal and laryngeal activity, possibly in different degrees from novice to expert wind instrument players. It appears likely that, if excellent technique is employed, playing wind instruments and singing concurrently should be safe and possibly even complementary. It also is likely that if either activity is performed with excessive laryngeal and pharyngeal tension, fatigue, and more serious consequences of one musical activity could affect the other. Further research is needed to determine whether this association is confirmed. Clearly, there is important anatomic and physiologic overlap between vocal and instrumental performance techniques, but many of the interactions and consequences remain unknown. Additional clinical observation, pedagogical investigation, and evidenced-based research should be encouraged.

Acknowledgment Modified in part from Sataloff RT. *Professional Voice: The Science and Art of Clinical Care*, 4th ed. San Diego, CA: Plural Publishing; 2017; with permission.

References

1. Sataloff RT. Professional voice: science and art of clinical care. 4th ed. San Diego: Plural Publishing; 2017.
2. Eckley CA. Glottic configuration in wind instrument players. Braz J Otorhinolaryngol (Brazil). 2006;72:45–7.
3. Trollinger V. Relationships among self-reported vocal and laryngeal health and performance career success in professional wind instrumentalists. Invited research poster presentation presented at 48th annual symposium: Care of the Professional Voice; May 29-June 2, 2019; Philadelphia, PA.
4. Cappellaro J, Beber BC. Vocal tract discomfort and voice-related quality of life in wind instrumentalists. J Voice. 2018;32(3):314–8.
5. Campos FG. Trumpet technique. New York: Oxford University Press; 2005.
6. Trollinger V, Sataloff RT. Laryngeal and vocal health issues for double reed players. Double Reed. 2017;40(2):145–50.
7. Ghirardi A, Goulart I, Riberio S. Voice and vocal tract of wind instrumentalists: integrative literature review. Disturb Comun. 2020;32(1):64–72.
8. Sataloff R. Professional singers: the science and art of clinical care. Am J Otolaryngol. 1981;2(3):251–66.
9. Clemente M, Mendes J, Moreira A, et al. A new classification of wind instruments: orofacial considerations. J Oral Biol Craniofac Res. 2019;9(3):268–76.
10. Porter M. Dental aspects of orchestral wind instrument playing with special reference to the embouchure. Br Dent J. 1952;93:66–73.
11. Engelman JA. Measurement of perioral pressures during playing of musical wind instruments. Am J Orthod. 1965;51(11):856–64.

12. Vandoren France. https://vandoren.fr/en/. Accessed June 24, 2020, 2020.
13. Vincent Bach Mouthpieces. https://www.bachbrass.com/instruments/mouthpieces. Published 2020. Accessed June 17, 2020.
14. Farkas P. Art of French horn playing. Los Angeles: Summy-Birchard; 1956.
15. Conn-Selmer Corporation. https://www.conn-selmer.com/en-us/instruments/band-instruments/french-horns. Published 2020. Accessed June 24, 2020, 2020.
16. Yamaha Corporation. Mouthpieces for Brass & Woodwind Instruments. https://usa.yamaha.com/files/download/brochure/6/1267056/WA-37R.pdf. Published 2017. Accessed June 24 2020. Hamamatsu, Shizuoka, Japan.
17. Giardinelli. http://giardinelli.com/. Accessed June 17, 2020.
18. Schilke – Selecting a Brass Mouthpiece. https://www.schilkemusic.com/products/mouthpieces/. Published 2014. Accessed June 17, 2020.
19. Millican JS. Band instrument selection and assignment:a review of the literature. Update Appl Res Music Educ. 2017;35(2):46–53.
20. Coffman DD, Sehmann KH. Musical instrument preference: implications for music educators. Update Appl Res Music Educ. 1989;7(2):32–4.
21. Geringer JM. An assessment of children's musical instrument preferences. J Music Ther. 1977;14:172–9.
22. Heyne M, Derrick D, Al-Tamimi J. Native language influence on Brass instrument performance: an application of Generalized Additive Mixed Models (GAMMs) to midsagittal ultrasound images of the tongue. Front Psychol. 2019;10:2597.
23. Walker K. Spirited wind playing. Bloomington: Indiana University Press; 2016.
24. González D, Payri B. A vowel-based method for vocal tract control in clarinet pedagogy. Int J Music Educ. 2017;35(3):435–45.
25. Nowak JaN H. The art of expressing playing. Carl Fischer: New York; 2004.
26. Yeo DKL, Pham TP, Baker J, Porters SAT. Specific orofacial problems experienced by musicians. Aust Dent J. 2002;47(1):2–11.
27. Gallivan GJ, Eitnier CM. Vocal fold polyp in a professional brass/wind instrumentalist and singer. J Voice (United States). 2006;20:157–64.
28. Levine HL. Functional disorders of the upper airway associated with playing wind instruments. Cleve Clin Q. 1986;53(1):11–3.
29. Evans A, Ackermann B, Driscoll T. Functional anatomy of the soft palate applied to wind playing. Med Probl Perform Art. 2010;25(4):183–9.
30. Stone R, Cuper PH. Best practices for teacher leadership : what award-winning teachers do for their professional learning communities. Thousand Oaks: Corwin Press; 2006.
31. Evans A, Driscoll T, Livesey J, Fitzsimons D, Ackermann B. Nasendoscopic evaluation of stress velopharyngeal insufficiency in wind musicians: a pilot study. Med Probl Perform Art. 2015;30(1):47–53.
32. Isaacson G, Sataloff RT. Bilateral laryngoceles in a young trumpet player: case report. Ear Nose Throat J. 2000;79(4):272–4.
33. Gallivan KH, Gallivan GJ. Bilateral mixed laryngoceles: simultaneous strobovideolaryngoscopy and external video examination. J Voice. 2002;16(2):258–66.
34. Flores-Franco RA, Limas-Frescas NE. The overused airway: lessons from a young trumpet player. Med Probl Perform Art. 2010;25(1):35–8.
35. Costa MM, Alvite FL. Lateral laryngopharyngeal diverticula: a videofluoroscopic study of laryngopharyngeal wall in wind instrumentalists. Arq Gastroenterol. 2012;49(2):99–106.
36. Fritz C, Wolfe J. How do clarinet players adjust the resonances of their vocal tracts for different playing effects? J Acoust Soc Am. 2005;118(5):3306–15.
37. Sadie JA. Companion to baroque music. Los Angeles: University of California Press; 1998.
38. Burns M. Thoughts and strategies for bassoon vibrato. Double Reed. 2005;28(2):121–4.
39. Weait C, Shea J. Vibrato: an audio-videofluorographic investigation of a bassoonist. Appl Radiol. 1977;6:89.
40. Pool CS. Observations of the larynx during vibrato production among professional bassoonists as indicated in experiments utilizing fiberoptic laryngoscopy. [Doctoral dissertation.]. Phoenix, University of Arizona; 2004.
41. Scott J, Weait C, Veazey C, Clardy M. Functions of the throat in wind playing: new views. Flutist Quarter. 1988;13(2):44–8.
42. Brown A. A cineflourographic study of the throat while vibrato tones are played on flute and oboe. [Doctoral dissertation], Iowa City, IA University of Iowa; 1973.
43. Carr W. A videoflurographic investigation of tongue and throat positions in playing flute, oboe, clarinet, bassoon and saxophone. [Doctoral dissertation]. Los Angeles: University of Southern California; 1978.
44. King AI, Ashby J, Nelson C. Laryngeal function in wind instrumentalists: the woodwinds. J Voice. 1988;1(4):365–7.
45. Kahane JC, Beckford NS, Chorna LB, Teachey JC, McClelland DK. Videofluoroscopic and Laryngoscopic evaluation of the upper airway and larynx of professional bassoon players. J Voice. 2006;20:297–307.
46. Watson A. The biology of musical performance and performance-related injury. New York: Scarecrow Press; 2009.
47. Adduci M. Dynamic measurement of intraoral pressure and sound pressure with laryngoscopic characterization during oboe performance. [Doctoral dissertation]. Denton; University of North Texas; 2011.
48. Rosset-Llobet J, Pascual-Leone A, Fàbregas-Molas S. Role of female reproductive hormones in musicians' dystonia. Med Probl Perform Art. 2012;27(3):156–8.
49. Rodríguez-Lozano FJ, Sáez-Yuguero MR, Bermejo-Fenoll A. Orofacial problems in musicians: a

review of the literature. Med Probl Perform Art. 2011;26(3):150–6.
50. van Kemenade JF, van Son MJ, van Heesch NC. Performance anxiety among professional musicians in symphonic orchestras: a self-report study. Psychol Rep. 1995;77(2):555–62.
51. Slocumb BS. Causes, effects and solutions to performance-related anxiety: suggestions for the teaching of brass instruments. [Doctoral dissertation] Greensboro, NC; University of North Carolina at Greensboro; 2009.
52. Dallas-Fort Worth Musicians Master Agreement. 72–147 D-FWPMAL. Master Agreement. http://musiciansdfw.org/files/2014/02/DO_12_16.pdf. Published 2012. Accessed July 4, 2015.
53. Rosen DC, Sataloff JB, Sataloff RT. Psychology of voice disorders. 2nd ed. San Diego: Plural Publishing; 2021.
54. Cavalot AL, Schindler A, Juliani E, Schindler O, Cortesina G. Playing a brass instrument after total laryngectomy: a case report. Head Neck. 2009;31(8):1102–6.
55. Chapman R. A strategy for proper utilization of the glottis and implications of improper use in trumpet performance. [Doctoral dissertation]. Miami: University of Miami; 2014.
56. Tarnopolsky A, Fletcher N, Hollenberg L, Lange B, Smith J, Acoustics WJ. The vocal tract and the sound of a didgeridoo. Nature. 2005;436(7047):39.
57. King AI, Ashby J, Nelson C. Laryngeal function in wind instruments: the brass. J Voice. 1989;3(1):65–7.
58. Miethe E. Video-endoscopic findings in playing various wind instruments. HNO. 1991;39(11):445–7.
59. Iltis P. Medical and scientific issues: the physiology of breathing: setting the record straight. Horn Call. 2013;43(2):35–8.
60. Rydell R, Karlsson M, Milesson A, Schalén L. Laryngeal activity during wind instrument playing: video endoscopic documentation. Logoped Phoniatr Vocol. 1996;21(1):43–8.
61. Miller R. Historical overview of vocal pedagogy. In: Sataloff RT, editor. Professional voice: the science and art of clinical care, vol. 2. 4th ed. San Diego: Plural Publishing; 2017. p. 1217–29.
62. Sommerfeldt SD, Strong WJ. Simulation of a player-clariinet system. J Acoust Soc Am. 1988;83:1908–18.
63. Timm EL. The woodwinds: performance and instructional techniques. Boston: Allyn and Bacon; 1964.
64. Sataloff RT, Brandfonbrener AE, Lederman RE. Performing arts medicine. 3rd ed. Science & Medicine, Inc: Narberth; 2010.
65. Sataloff RT. Bodily injuries and their effects on the voice. In: Profesional voice: science and art of clinical care. 4th ed. San Diego: Plural Publishing; 2017. p. 1003–5.
66. Sataloff R. Professional singers: part II. J Voice. 1987;1:191–201.
67. Wolfe J, Tarnopolsky AZ, Fletcher NH, Hollenbert LCL, Smith J. Some effects of the player's vocal tract and tongue on wind instrument sound. Paper presented at: proceedings of the Stockholm music acoustic conference; August 6–9, 2003; Stockholm, Sweden.
68. Wolfe J, Smith J. Acoustical coupling between lip valves and vocal folds. Acoust Aust J. 2008;26:23–7.
69. Bianco T, Freour V, Cossette I, Bevilacqua F, Caussé R. Measures of facial muscle activation, intra-oral pressure and mouthpiece force in trumpet playing. J New Music Res. 2012;41(1):49–65.
70. Freour V, Scavone GP. Acoustical interaction between vibrating lips, downstream air column, and upstream airways in trombone performance. J Acoust Soc Am. 2013;134(5):3887–98.
71. Chen JM, Smith J, Wolfe J. Saxophonists tune vocal tract resonances in advanced performance techniques. J Acoust Soc Am. 2011;129(1):415–26.
72. Chen JM, Smith J, Wolfe J. Do trumpet players tune resonances of the vocal tract? J Acoust Soc Am. 2012;131(1):722–7.
73. Chen JM, Smith J, Wolfe J. Pitch bending and glissandi on the clarinet: roles of the vocal tract and partial tone hole closure. J Acoust Soc Am. 2009;126(3):1511–20.
74. Wolfe J, Garnier M, Smith J. Vocal tract resonances in speech, singing, and playing musical instruments. HFSP J. 2009;3(1):6–23.
75. Cammarota G, Masala G, Cianci R, et al. Reflux symptoms in wind instrument players. Aliment Pharmacol Ther. 2010;31(5):593–600.
76. Hamdan AL, Sataloff RT, Hawkshaw MJ. Obesity and voice. 1st ed. San Diego: Plural Publishing; 2020.
77. Ward CP, York KM, McCoy JG. Risk of obstructive sleep apnea lower in double reed wind musicians. J Clin Sleep Med. 2012;8(3):251–5.
78. Wardrop PJ, Ravichandran S, Hair M, Robertson SM, Sword D. Do wind and brass players snore less? A cross-sectional study of snoring and daytime fatigue in professional orchestral musicians. Clin Otolaryngol. 2011;36(2):134–8.
79. Gossett CW Jr. Electromyographic investigation of the relationship of the effects of selected parameters on concurrent study of voice and oboe. J Voice. 1989;3(1):52–64.

Part II

Acoustic Properties: Special Considerations in Patients with Dentofacial Anomalies

Orthodontic Disorders and Diagnosis

5

Anthony T. Macari

Orthodontics is the first organized dental specialty, a unique offspring of two centuries of continuous progress in the field of dentistry. It entails a deep knowledge of dental development, physical growth concepts, as well as physiologic and psychosocial development [1]. Historically orthodontists comprehensively investigated growth of the body in its general somatic and more specifically its facial aspects. The procedures performed most commonly in this specialty cover all age groups including children, adolescents, adults, and elderly. The approach to patients can be divided into two major categories:

1. Collection of diagnostic data and information through initial examination, clinical evaluation, and a series of "orthodontic" records including radiographs, dental casts (substituted more recently by less invasive oral scanning), and finally the intra-oral and extra-oral photographs.
2. Formulation of problem list and treatment planning.

Initial Orthodontic Examination

Chief Complaint

The first interaction between the orthodontist and the patient is important in developing a primary problem list. The chief complaint stated by the patient and/or his or her guardian is considered first. In many instances, an excellent standardized outcome of orthodontic treatment may not be considered successful by the patient if the initial complaint had not been addressed appropriately. Complaints about the position and alignment of the teeth usually are due to two rational motives: An abnormal function of the teeth or the jaws, and/ or impaired facial aesthetics with subsequent psychosocial problems. Younger children may face difficulties in relationships with their peers because of their smile and facial appearance [2, 3]. Aesthetic and functional problems may lead to substantial reduction in oral health-related quality of life in adolescent and adult individuals seeking orthodontic treatment [2].

The first interaction with the patient is usually a structured process. Most orthodontists use a questionnaire that helps in "extracting" the chief complaint of patients who are not able to verbalize it. The used questionnaire also has helped patients assess carefully their aesthetic preferences and articulate clearly their complaints. Orthodontists often rely on a sequence of pertinent questions, such as "Tell me what bothers you about your face or teeth" [4], in order to elucidate what is important to the patient. In few instances, the orthodontist may not agree with the patient's evaluation, and the ensuing stages of diagnosis clarify their impressions.

A.-L. Hamdan et al., *Dentofacial Anomalies*, https://doi.org/10.1007/978-3-030-69109-7_5

Dental History

Dental history constitutes an important component of the first clinical encounter. Over the years, orthodontists have developed several questionnaires aiming first to elicit as much as possible dental history of the patient and family, and second to assess potential associated concerns. It is important to evaluate the patient's attitude about dental hygiene and regular visits to a dentist. A compromised periodontal history if present also need to be noted because of the detrimental effect that orthodontic treatment may have on the teeth in patients with significant periodontal disease. Within this context, and specifically in growing children, parent's dental health may be a valid sign of the patient's predisposition to periodontal disease and/or caries. History of facial trauma also needs to be highlighted, as it is often overlooked. A common example is mandibular condylar fracture in a child with history of trauma to the chin. Such a fracture in a growing child can easily be missed leading to malocclusion in addition to facial asymmetry. In the presence of external wounds (e.g., chin, lips, or even front teeth), a fractured mandibular condyle often is overlooked, resulting in facial growth deficit.

Medical History

It is important to obtain a comprehensive medical history prior to beginning orthodontic treatment. The orthodontist should know last time the patient was checked by a physician, latest laboratory tests done and for what reasons, any hospitalizations or any long-term medications currently being taken. This information key in the design of a treatment plan given the association between overall health and oral health. These questions are important in revealing any information concerning chronic diseases that the patient or guardian failed to volunteer. Patients with uncontrolled diabetes, for instance, may experience severe loss of periodontal tissue including alveolar bone and gingiva, which in turn can induce tooth loss. The treating orthodontist also should be aware of a history of allergy, especially to latex (gloves and elastics) or nickel sensitivity (wires and brackets containing nickel). Similarly, patients should be asked about a history of blood transfusions given the associated increased risk of viral transmissions such as immunodeficiency virus (HIV) and hepatitis. Heart diseases such a mitral valve prolapse, and rheumatic fever also are of a concern. These may necessitate antibiotic prophylaxis when invasive procedures are planned (such as inserting bands under the gingiva) [5, 6]. The current guidelines from the American Dental Association (ADA), the American Heart Association (AHA), and the American Association of Cariology (ACC) support prescription of preventive premedication in infective endocarditis in only a small category of patients, because the adverse effects of treatment may outweigh the desired benefits [7, 8]. Accordingly, the American Association of Orthodontists (AAO) recommends that orthodontists communicate with the patient's physician and decide collaboratively whether antibiotics should be administered. Treatment of few chronic diseases may impinge on orthodontic treatment by decreasing or inhibiting the rate of tooth movement. Prescription of high doses of prostaglandin inhibitors or resorption-inhibiting agents in patients with arthritis and/ or osteoporosis are good examples. In rare cases, orthodontic treatment may be contraindicated.

Physical Growth – Initial Screening Assessment

Despite the steady annual increase in the number of adult subjects seeking orthodontic treatment, growing individuals remain a majority of orthodontic patients. Hence, core scientific knowledge of growth and development on therapy and their implications is essential for an orthodontist. Orthodontists are trained to evaluate physical growth of children and young adolescents, and to predict growth timing and duration particularly during pubescence. Their ability to specify patient's facial and skeletal development on a growth chart is crucial in deciding on orthodontic treatment initiation and planning. The reason why a couple of decades ago the American Association of Orthodontists modified the "Orthodontics" labeling of the specialty to "Orthodontics and Dentofacial Orthopedics" was to highlight the fact that orthodontists have the skills to alter the facial skeleton, particularly the jaws and the alveolus, with non-surgical means during the active phase of growth. Nevertheless, despite the best treatment approaches, the effect of craniofacial growth on orthodontic treatment may be unfavorable in "poor" growers.

Within these perspectives, orthodontists routinely evaluate growth through diagnostic tools which include physical measurements, growth charts, and radiographic assessment of bone age and skeletal growth (partially used by other health care professionals such as pediatricians). In addition, the initial screening must include questions related to the physical growth especially when a child development stage is around puberty. A summary of somatic growth assessment is described in Fig. 5.1.

During the first visit, the orthodontist should develop an idea of the physical growth of the patient in relation to the amount of and potential for remaining growth. For young adolescents who are approaching the pubertal peak, the orthodontist commonly questions the patient and parents about recent sudden rapid growth, changing shoe and/or clothes sizes, signs of sexual maturation (if menarche in girls occurred and when; and voice changes for males), and about the history of sexual maturation in older siblings. Inquiry about secondary sexual characteristics is considered an adjunctive screening tool which can yield equally important information about physical growth status [9]. Additional data from the growth charts in the pediatrician's record are retrieved when

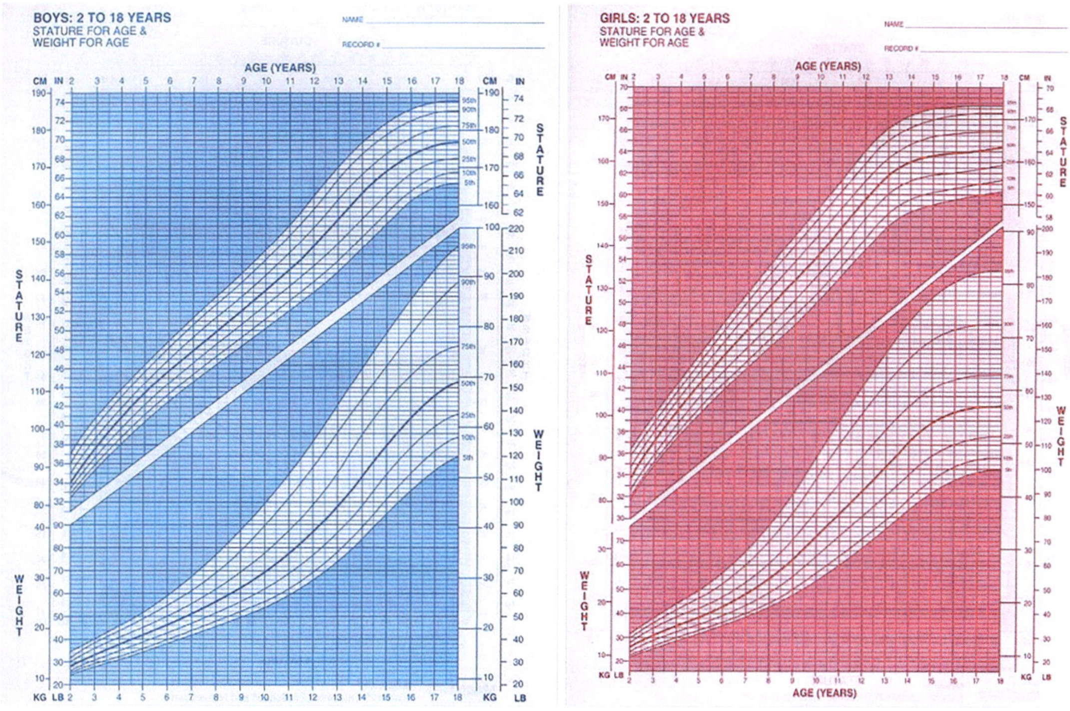

Fig. 5.1 Growth chart for boys and girls showing the different percentile curves of longitudinal growth. An individual who projects exactly at the midpoint of the normal distribution would fall along the 50% line of the graph

deemed necessary. A standard tool for bone age evaluation is the hand-wrist radiograph taken on all growing subjects. This is discussed in the section below on orthodontic records.

Clinical Evaluation

The orthodontic clinical evaluation includes examination of oral health, jaw function, and facial aesthetics. After thorough clinical assessment, the orthodontist will decide what dental and orthodontic records are needed to develop the treatment plan.

Oral Health Assessment

Oral health assessment is mandatory for all patients seeking orthodontic treatment. The first thing the practitioner does is to count the teeth to find out whether any missing or supernumerary teeth are present. This is followed by screening for any oral hygiene problems, dental caries, or dental pulp pathology that need to be addressed. Periodontal disease affecting the underlying alveolar bone and the surrounding gingiva and buccal mucosa must be ruled out. Detecting periodontal disease is usually accomplished by probing in the gingival sulci around the teeth to establish presence of periodontal pockets or identify any gingival bleeding indicating underlying inflammation. Inadequate height or thickness of attached gingiva is concerning and might be a contraindication to orthodontic treatment, which often requires expansion of the arches and may induce further loss of tissue attachments.

Jaw, Occlusal, and Other Functions

Orthodontic screening requires evaluation of many functions such as speech, sleep, mastication, and the temporomandibular joint.

Speech

As orthodontists focus mostly on mastication and temporomandibular joints, the impact of malocclusion and skeletal discrepancies on sound production and speech is often overlooked. Many investigations revealed an association between voice parameters and oral cavity dimensions, particularly arch width, length, and palatal volume [10], as reviewed elsewhere in this book. The normal process of airflow and resonance may be hindered by malocclusion, tongue posture, and lip placement, thus affecting sound production [11–14]. Malocclusions that are considered to influence sound production include the following [4]:

- Open bite characterized by a decreased overbite (gap) between the front teeth. In other words, the front teeth do not touch at all (Fig. 5.2) [15]. In this type of malocclusion, lisping can be present with distortion in producing the sibilants /s/ and /z/, and the linguodental fricatives /th/, /sh/, /ch/.
- Mandibular prognathism in which the lower jaw is more prominent with an anterior crossbite characterized by the lower front teeth being more anterior than the upper ones (Fig. 5.3a) [16]. In this malocclusion, which is

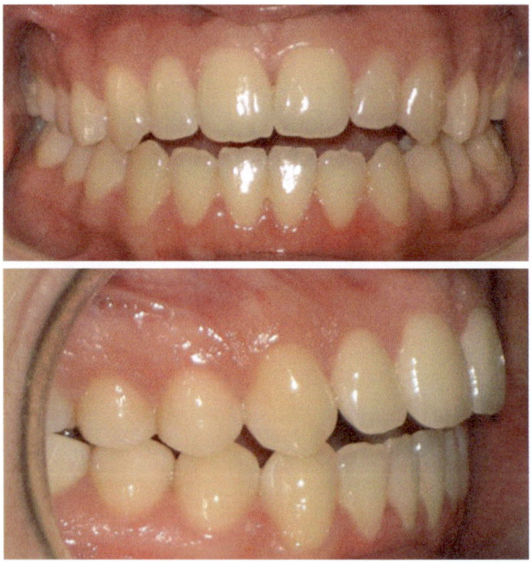

Fig. 5.2 Frontal and lateral view of an 18-year-old female with anterior open bite. The maxillary and mandibular incisors do not touch, in contrast with a normal 20–30% vertical overlap of maxillary incisors on mandibular ones

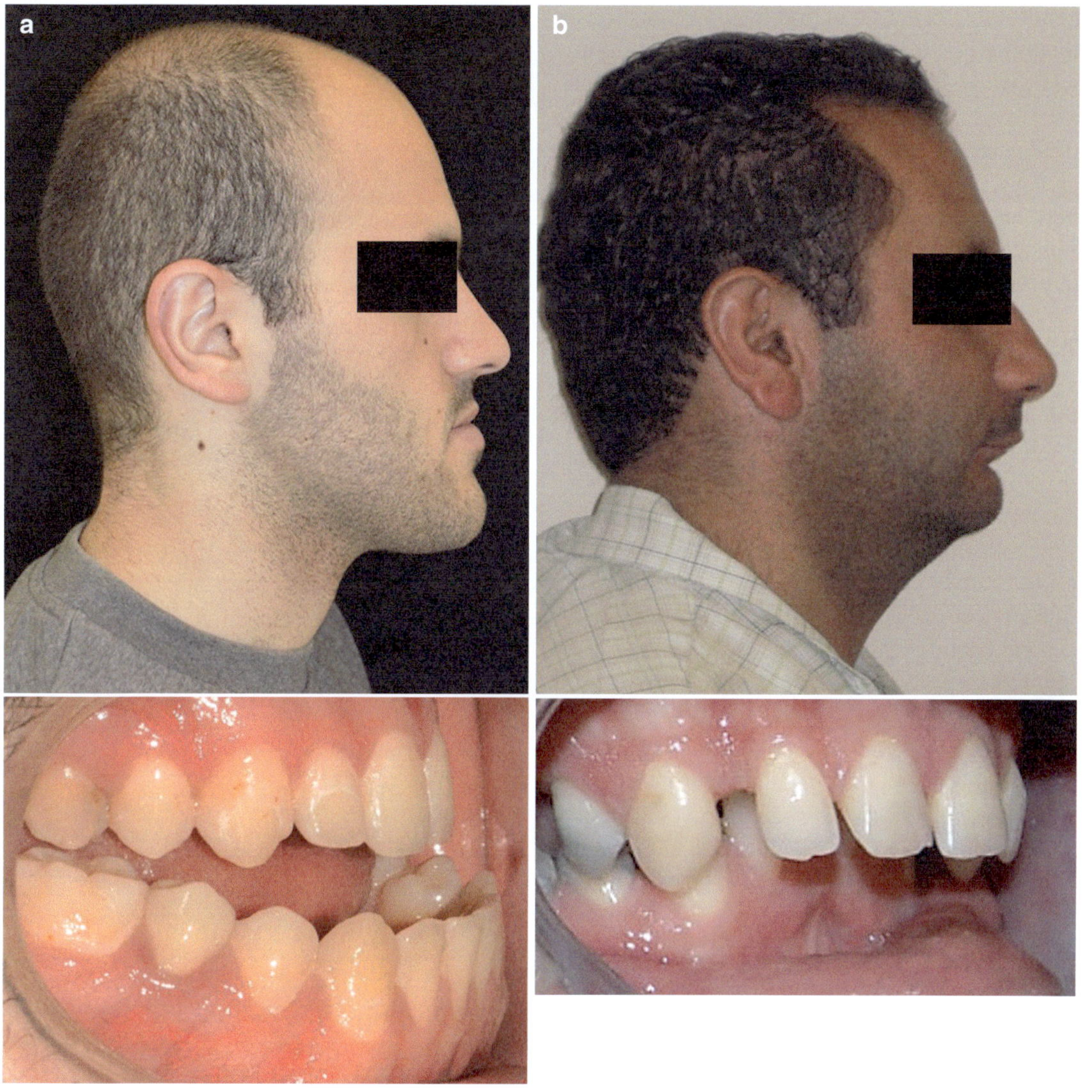

Fig. 5.3 (**a**) Mandibular prognathism in an adult male: Anterior crossbite is present. The mandibular incisors occlude in a front of the maxillary ones. The chin is positioned forward in the profile view. (**b**) Mandibular retrognathism in an adult male: increased overjet with a gap between the maxillary and mandibular incisors in the sagittal plane

labeled Class III angle malocclusion, the labiodental fricatives /f/ and /v/ are affected.

- Mandibular retrognathism characterized by backward position of the chin and lower jaw and increased overjet with maxillary anterior teeth in a forward position (Fig. 5.3b) [16].

While speech abnormalities can be associated with different types of malocclusion, normal sound production can be present even in severe dentoalveolar and skeletal discrepancies. Accordingly, not all speech difficulties can be solved by orthodontic treatment only but may need to be addressed with speech therapy.

Mastication

Patients with skeletal discrepancy may suffer from mastication disorders [17, 18]. The effect may cause a decrease in oral health-related quality of life [19] and is more pronounced in elderly who avoid chewing hard foods to minimize cheek and lip biting. As a consequence, disturbances in the digestive system often are reported in affected patients, suggesting that there is a correlation between malocclusion and gastric emptying function [20]. Notably, swallowing is rarely affected in patients with malocclusion.

Temporomandibular Joint Function

The lower face is connected to the skull base through the right and left temporomandibular joint. The clinician commonly starts by palpating these joints and the adjacent structures such as the masseter and temporalis muscles looking for symptoms of soreness or pain. The patient is asked to open his/her mouth, and the movement of the lower jaw is evaluated in its vertical, sagittal, and lateral planes. The presence of any clicking sounds and or reduction in the range of opening are signs of temporomandibular disorders (TMDs). Moreover, deviation of the jaw while opening and closing is also a sign of TMJ dysfunction that warrants attention. Given the vague relationship between orthodontic treatment and TMDs, patients are advised prior to initiation of treatment on all potential side effects associated with temporomandibular disorders, and this discussion is documented in the consent.

Breathing

Evaluating the mode of respiration is particularly important. In the medical questionnaire, questions like "do you snore at night"; "did you have adenoidectomy and/or tonsillectomy" are very common. The association between mouth breathing and malocclusion has been studied widely [21] over the last 50 years and remains a "hot" scientific topic especially with the increase in awareness of sleep disorders and sleep apnea in children and adults. Objective evaluation of airway clearance is mandatory in the cephalometric evaluation especially when symptoms are reported by the patient. We refer the readers to Chap. 6 for further information on airway space and dentofacial anomalies.

Orthodontic Records

At the end of the initial phase of consultation, the practitioner will decide whether the patient needs orthodontic treatment and what additional records he or she requires. On average, and in growing patients, extra-oral and intra-oral photographs, lateral and posteroanterior cephalometric, hand-wrist, and panoramic radiographs, and dental cast/intra-oral scans are needed. The purpose of orthodontic records is to document the initial/pretreatment dentofacial features of the patient and to extract additional information needed for diagnosis and treatment planning. In adults, additional periapical radiographs (small radiographs for individual or a group of teeth for better visualization of bone contouring) usually are requested in view of the high prevalence of periodontal diseases in adults. In children, the orthodontist may not need to ask for cephalometric and hand-wrist radiographs if the orthodontic treatment is minor and consists of simply inserting passive appliances, for instance.

Photographic Evaluation

Extra-oral/facial and intra-oral photographs are mandatory before any orthodontic treatment.

Facial Photographs

Frontal picture at rest: Taken with the patient in natural head position. The teeth should be in occlusion and the lips gently touching. If the patient has lip incompetence, two frontal photographs will be taken, one with lips together with strain of the muscles, and one with lips at rest and in open (Fig. 5.4). Using this photograph, the practitioner will evaluate the vertical proportions of the face divided into five equal distances, and the horizontal proportions divided into three equal distances (Fig. 5.5a, b). Asymmetry of the face is assessed on these photographs, and an imaginary midsagittal line is traced to relatively evaluate nose tip, lip, and chin positions. Any asymmetry detected on this view will have to be confirmed on the posteroanterior cephalometric radiograph.

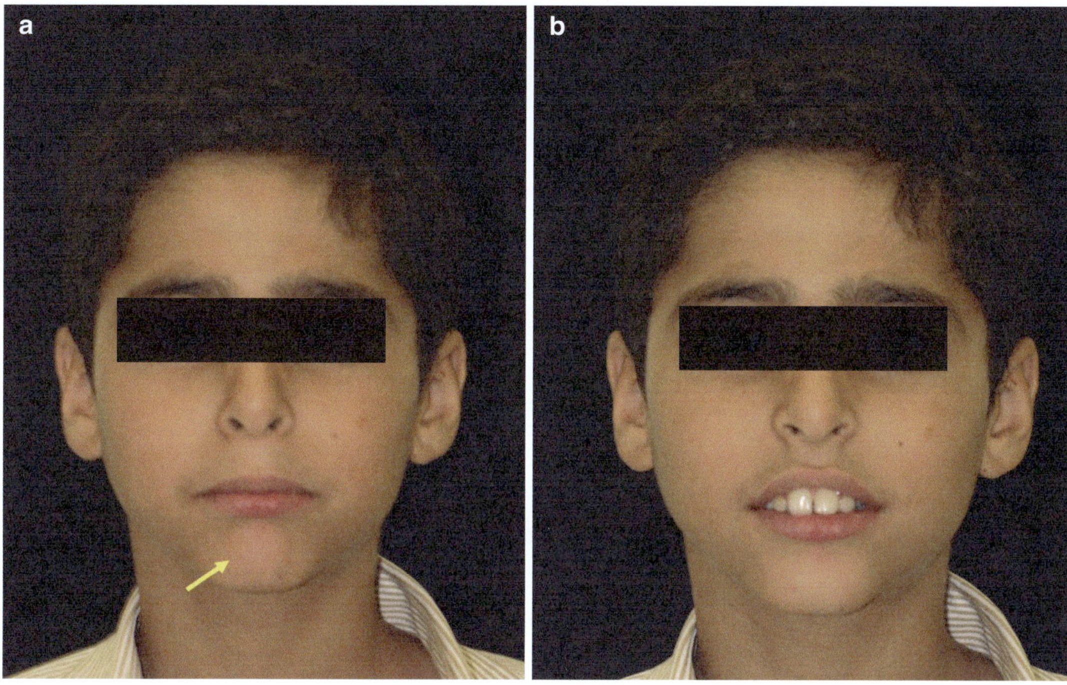

Fig. 5.4 (**a**) Frontal picture of an 11-year-old boy with mental muscle strain (arrow) because of lip incompetency. (**b**) Frontal picture of the same patient with lips at rest

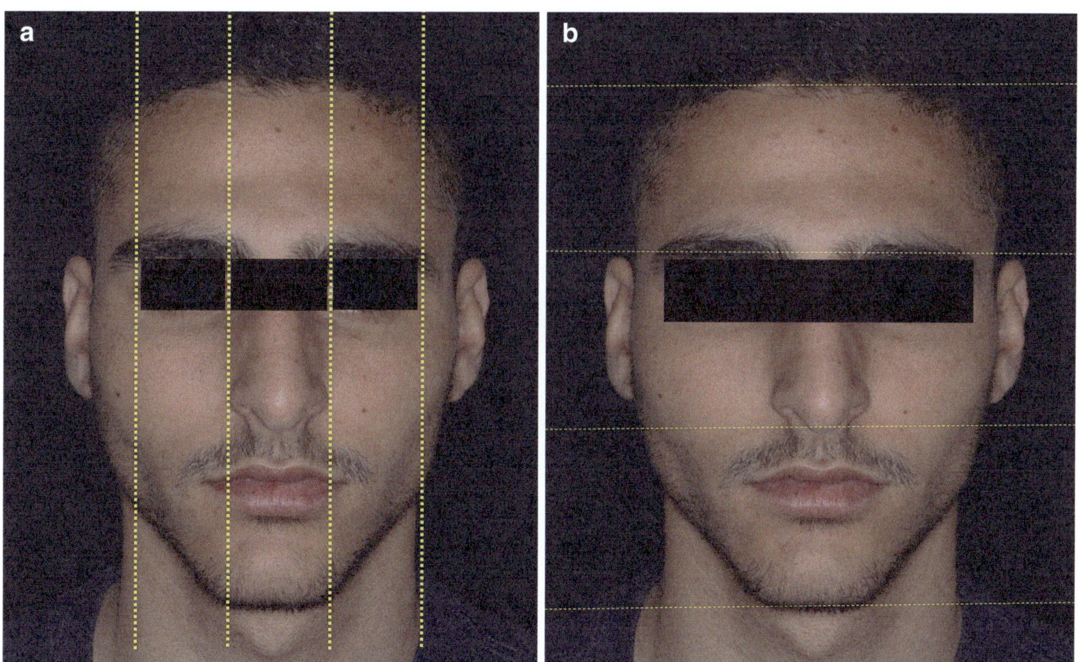

Fig. 5.5 (**a**) Vertical lines dividing the face of an 18-year-old boy into 5 equal proportions. (**b**) Horizontal lines dividing the face into equal upper, middle, and lower facial thirds

Frontal smile: The smile picture should have the lips elevated enough to show the teeth and any excessive gingival display, if present (Fig. 5.6a, b). The smile should not be a shy smile as that may differ from a spontaneous smile. An important feature of this photograph is the lip line, which shows the relationship between the upper lip and the teeth. If a lip line is low, it means that less than the full height of the tooth crown is visible. A normal lip line will show the full height of the teeth in males and an additional 2 mm of gingiva in females. If a lip line is high, more than 2 mm of the gingiva is displayed. Moreover, on this smile view, the upper midline is evaluated relative to the facial midsagittal line. Also, any asymmetry in the display of the teeth between right and left side is evaluated.

A close-up picture of the smile: This picture is taken excluding the face in order to show the teeth in a better perspective. Inclination of the clinical crowns (tip), spaces among the teeth, missing teeth, and other anatomic variable are examined in this view.

Profile picture at rest: This photograph simulates the position of the patient during acquisition of the lateral cephalometric radiograph (Fig. 5.7). The patient should be in natural head position with the teeth in occlusion and with lips touching gently. This is an important picture from which the practitioner defines the outline of the profile as convex with mandibular retrognathism,

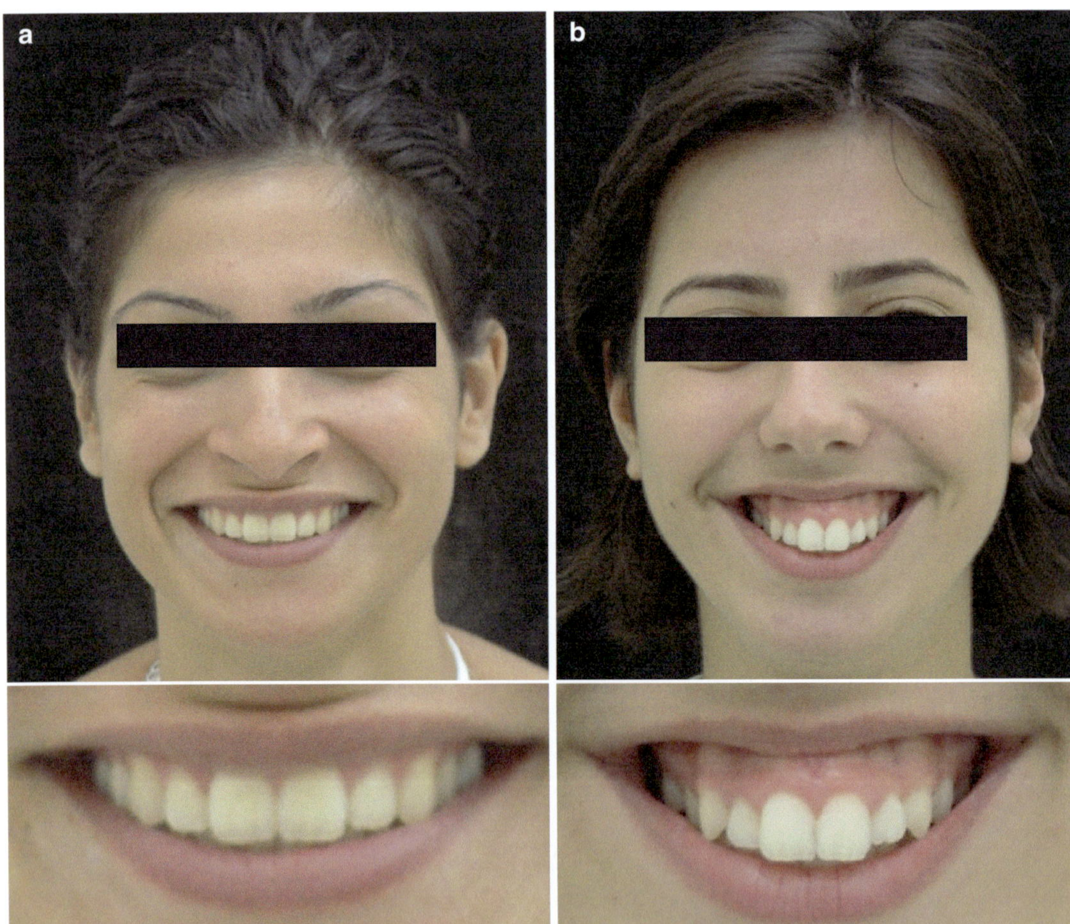

Fig. 5.6 (**a**) Frontal smile picture of a 22-year-old female with full height of the teeth indicating a normal lip line. (**b**) Frontal smile picture of an 18-year-old female with excessive gingival display by around 6–7 mm indicating a high lip line

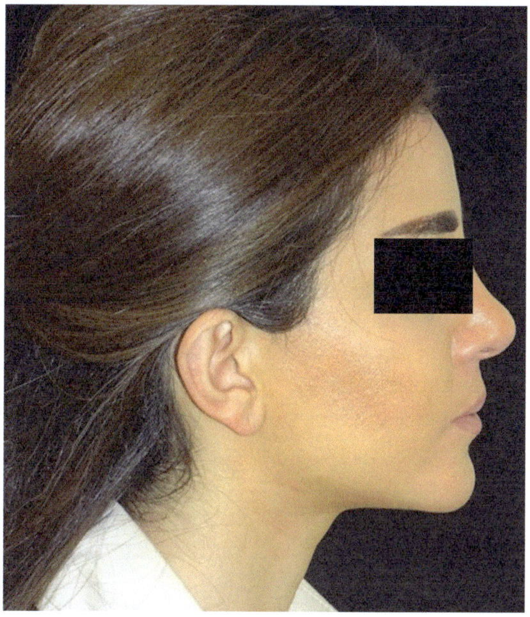

Fig. 5.7 Profile picture at rest of a 25-year-old female subject taken in natural head position, identical to the position of the patient in the cephalostat

straight, or concave with mandibular prognathism. In addition, horizontal proportions are double checked on this view. The relationships between nose, lips, and chin are determined.

Profile picture with smile: This view is similar to the frontal photograph with a smile but taken in a profile view. On this view, the inclination of the maxillary incisors relative to the upper lip and the nose is evaluated. This important information is essential for treatment planning.

A three-quarter profile smile: The patient is asked to move from a profile smile position toward the camera for a ¾ view (Fig. 5.8). This is an important view for assessment of the midface and asymmetry. A flat midface or a prognathic lower jaw is shown clearly.

A submental picture: This picture is usually taken when the orthodontist suspects facial asymmetry. The patient is asked to move his or her head up, and the photograph is taken from below the chin. (Fig. 5.9).

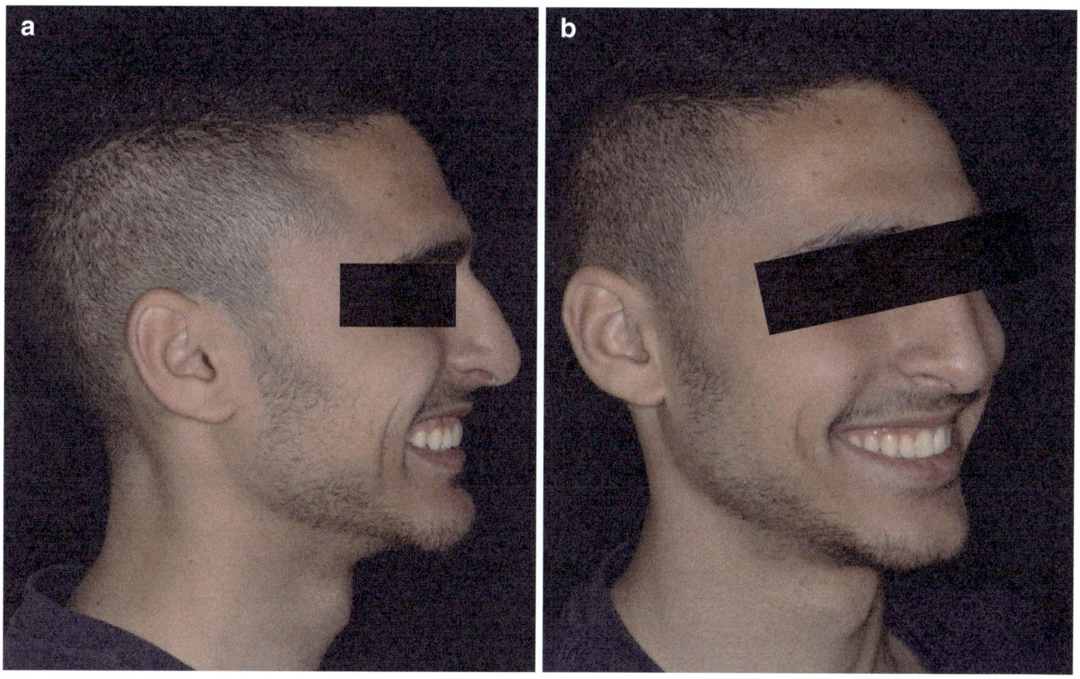

Fig. 5.8 (**a**) Profile smile picture of an 18-year-old male. (**b**) ¾ profile smile of the same subject

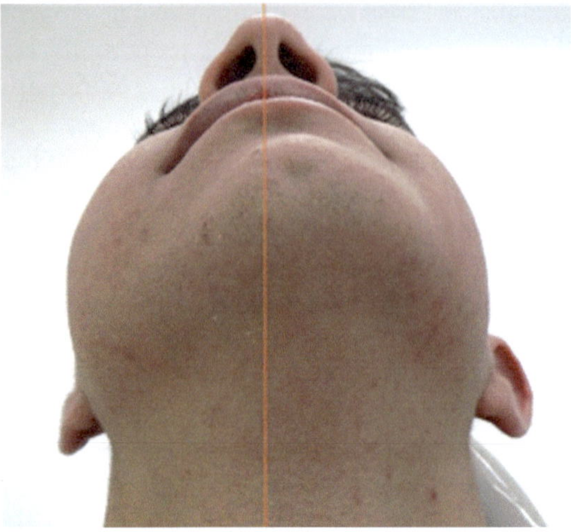

Fig. 5.9 Submental photograph of a 16-year-old boy showing facial asymmetry, namely, the deviation of the mandible/chin to the left relative to the midsagittal plane

Intra-oral Photographs

All intra-oral photographs are taken in occlusion, with frontal, right, and left views, and maxillary and mandibular arches images (Fig. 5.10).

Hand-wrist Radiograph

Maturation age of an individual may differ from chronological age. Orthodontists have been evaluating bone age on hand-wrist radiograph solely. Recently, they started to use the lateral cephalometric radiograph, as well, to evaluate the vertebral maturation stage and deduce bone age. However, hand-wrist radiographs remain the standard tool to evaluate bone age (Fig. 5.11).

Around 30 small bones are present on a hand-wrist radiograph, and none is an excellent indicator of the growth maturation. Instead, ossification of the shaft between the epiphysis and diaphysis is evaluated on all bones including the radius and ulna in order to establish the bone age. A widely used method to evaluate a hand-wrist X-ray is the comparison to standard radiographs in an atlas of the development of the hand and wrist [22]. Orthodontists label the bone age as being delayed, concomitant, or advanced relative to the chronological age of the patient.

Panoramic Radiograph

This a routine X-ray taken by orthodontists for many reasons (Fig. 5.12).

- It shows the full set of teeth whether in mixed or permanent dentition.
- It helps detect missing and supernumerary teeth.
- It visualizes the roots of the teeth in the bone and depicts any pathology around the roots or in the basal bone of the maxilla and mandible.
- It gives excellent information about the temporomandibular joints and the symmetry between the two sides.
- It helps detect dental caries and root fractures, although it is not the standard radiograph for diagnosis of those conditions.

Cephalometric Analyses

The introduction of the cephalometric radiograph in daily routine orthodontic evaluation was a major advance. Orthodontists created the cephalostat to standardize taking head radiographs. Originally, cephalometry was used for research on growth of the craniofacial complex. Later, orthodontists understood that cephalometrics could be very helpful in clinical assessment and started to rely on them to define the relationships between the jaws and cranial base, the anatomic basis of malocclusions, and dentoalveolar compensations (Fig. 5.13).

Knowing that malocclusion results from the interface between position of the jaws and the teeth, orthodontists use cephalometric measures to evaluate the major functional components of the face (cranial base, jaws, teeth) and how they are related to each other. For instance, it may be possible that two identical malocclusions (as assessed on dental casts or during the intra-oral clinical examination) have different cephalometric findings and different facial proportions. Thus, the individualization of diagnosis by a complete set of data from all orthodontic records is essential. Given that cephalometric radio-

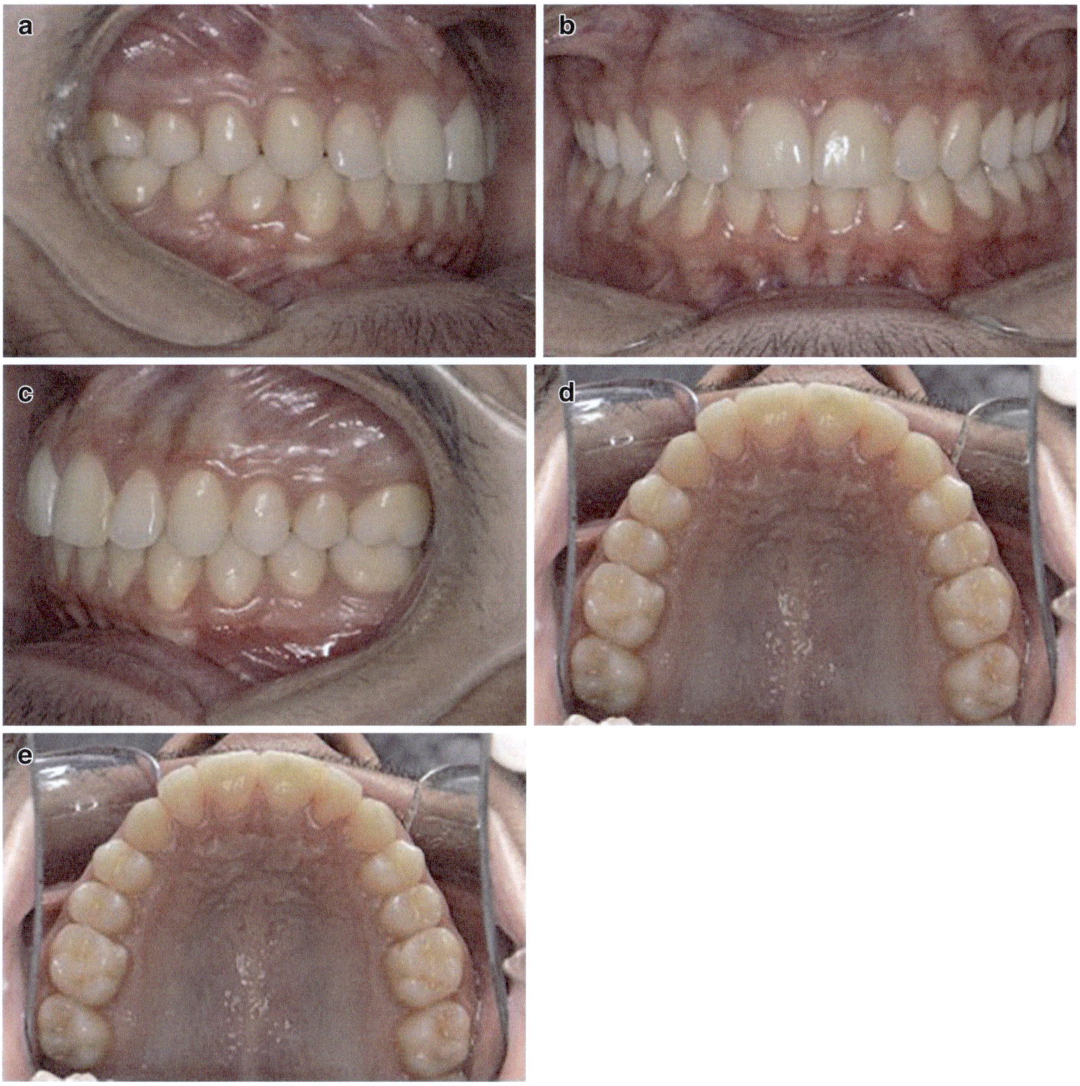

Fig. 5.10 Intra-oral photographs of an 18-year-old male subject presented in a composite picture: (**a**) right. (**b**) Frontal. (**c**) Left. (**d**) Maxillary arch. (**e**) Mandibular arch

graphs are taken pre- and post-treatment and at other times, modifications carried out by the orthodontic treatment can be evaluated by superimposition of images. In growing children, the changes that the orthodontist observes are a combination of growth and treatment effect, whether on skeleton and/or teeth. If it were not for the ability to superimpose cephalometric radiographs, those important findings would not be defined.

The historic method of manually tracing the cephalometric radiographs has been replaced recently by computerized imaging software, which has revolutionized clinical practice and facilitated cephalometric tracing, measurements, and storage [23]. Superimposition of cephalometric tracing and facial photographs was brought to clinical practice through this technological advance, allowing practitioners to simulate treatment changes prior to initiation of

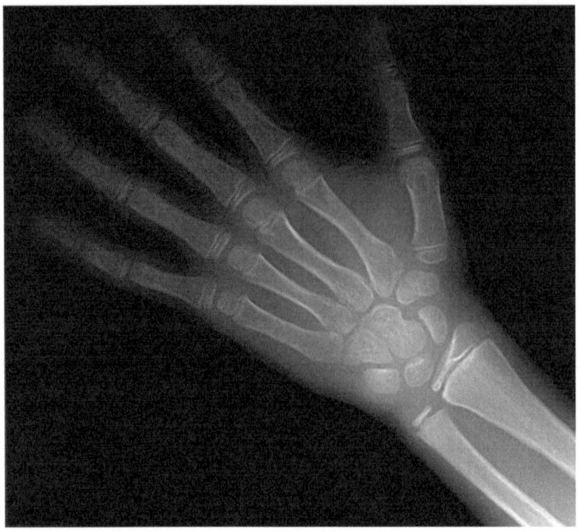

Fig. 5.11 Hand-wrist radiograph of a 10-year-old boy taken to evaluate bone age and stage of growth

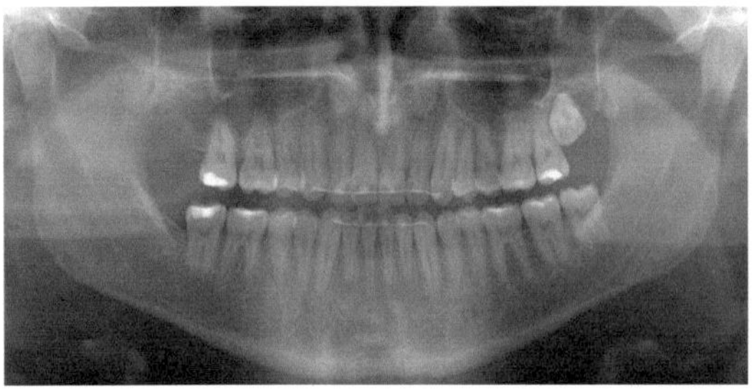

Fig. 5.12 A panoramic radiograph of a 25-year-old male subject

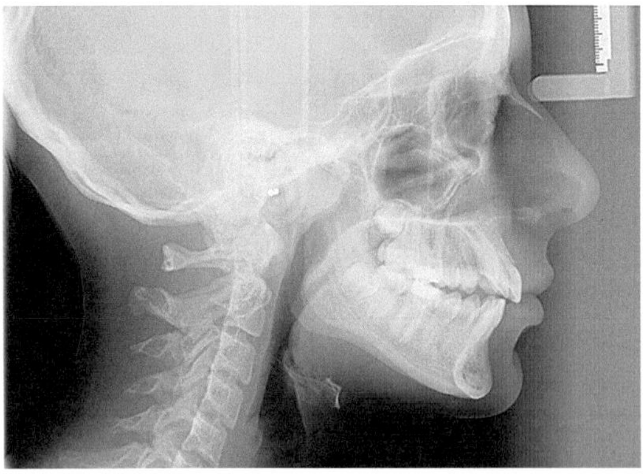

Fig. 5.13 A lateral cephalometric radiograph of a 16-year-old female patient. This radiography is taken routinely on all orthodontic patients before, during, and after treatment

orthodontic therapy and/or orthognathic surgery. In addition, patients can check the potential modifications on their jaws and teeth, and their corresponding effect on facial features, prior to treatment (Fig. 5.14).

Lateral Cephalometric Radiograph

Lateral cephalometric radiographs allow evaluation of the vertical and sagittal relationships between the following:

- The skeletal components of the face (cranial base, maxilla, and mandible).
- The teeth and the corresponding basal bones.
- The upper and lower teeth.
- The soft tissue thickness and projection in profile, and the underlying skeletal and dento-alveolar structures.

Skeletal components of the face: Skeletal evaluation on lateral cephalometric radiograph includes the relationship of the maxilla and the mandible to the cranial base, and the maxilla to the mandible separately. Both associations are considered in the vertical and sagittal planes (Fig. 5.15). In general, lateral cephalometric measurements include hundreds of analyses by different people. However, few of those analyses are used on daily basis [24–32]. In the sagittal plane, and relative to the anterior cranial base, the mandible or maxilla can be orthognathic, retrognathic, or prognathic (Fig. 5.16). Maxillary-to-mandibular angle is important to diagnose any sagittal discrepancy between the jaws and that may reflect the dental malocclusion. In the vertical plane, it is very important to assess the divergence angle of the mandible as it relates to the facial type. An open angle or hyperdivergent pattern usually is associated with a dolychofacial type and an increased lower facial type. A mesofacial type is associated with a normal divergence and an average mandibular angle rotation. A reduced divergence angle of the mandible is associated commonly with brachyfacial type and a reduced lower third of the face (Fig. 5.17).

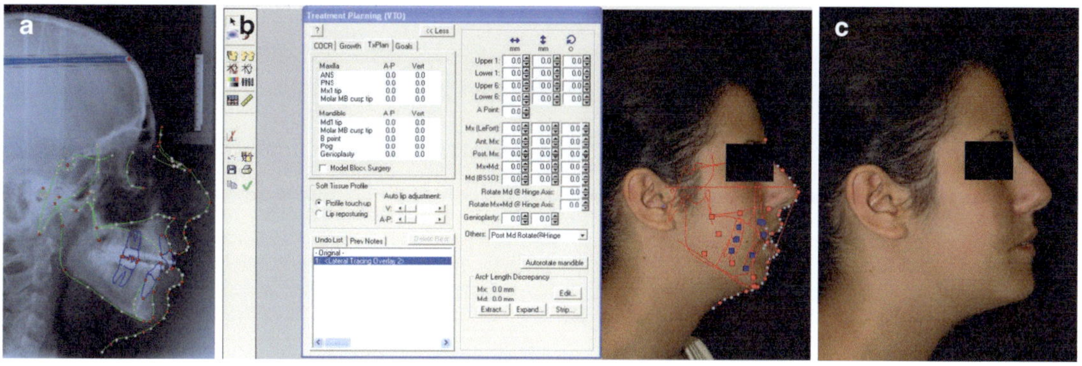

Fig. 5.14 (**a**) Digitization and tracing of pretreatment lateral cephalometric radiograph of a 17-year-old female. (**b**) Superimposition of the lateral cephalometric tracing on the profile picture of the patient. (**c**) Surgical simulation of the planned movements to predict changes in the patient's profile

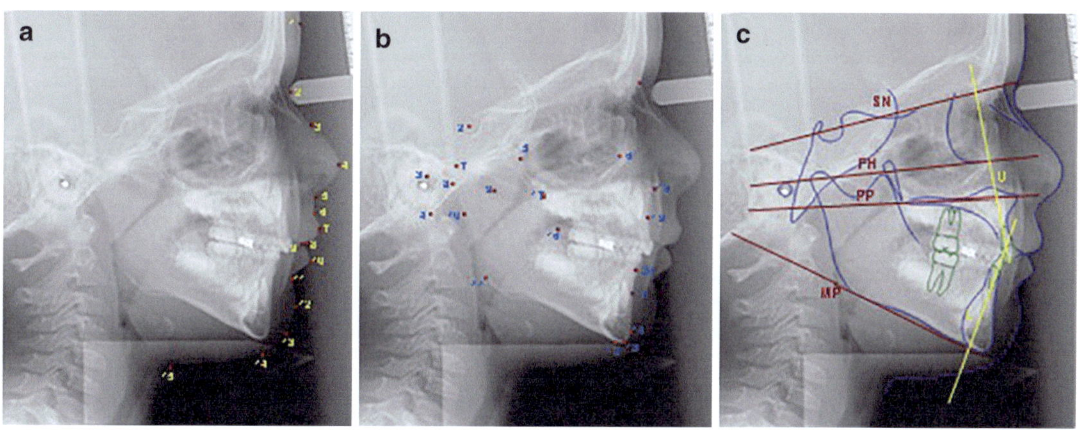

Fig. 5.15 Lateral cephalometric radiograph of a 5-year-old boy. (**a**) Soft tissue landmarks. (**b**) Hard tissue landmarks. (**c**) Summary of planes traced on the lateral cephalometric radiograph to diagnose malocclusion in the vertical and sagittal dimensions

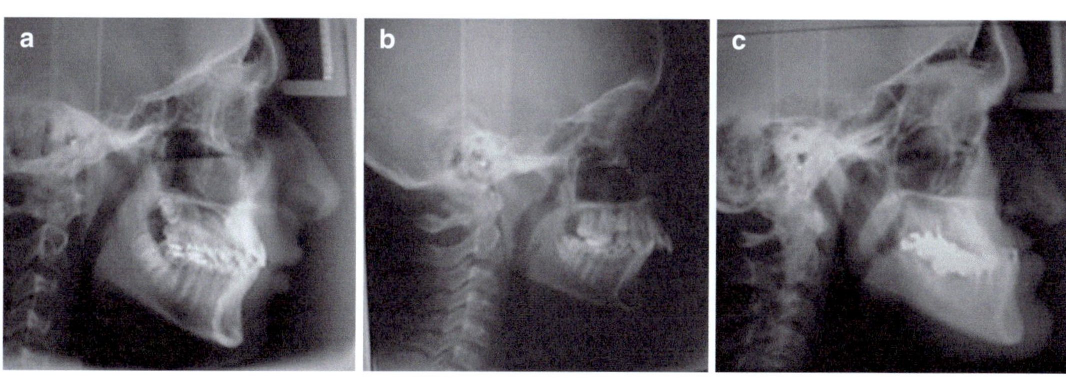

Fig. 5.16 Lateral cephalometric radiographs. (**a**) A 16-year-old boy with orthognathic position of the maxilla and mandible. (**b**) A 12-year-old boy with retrognathic mandible. (**c**) A 34-year-old male subject with prognathic mandible and retrognathic maxilla

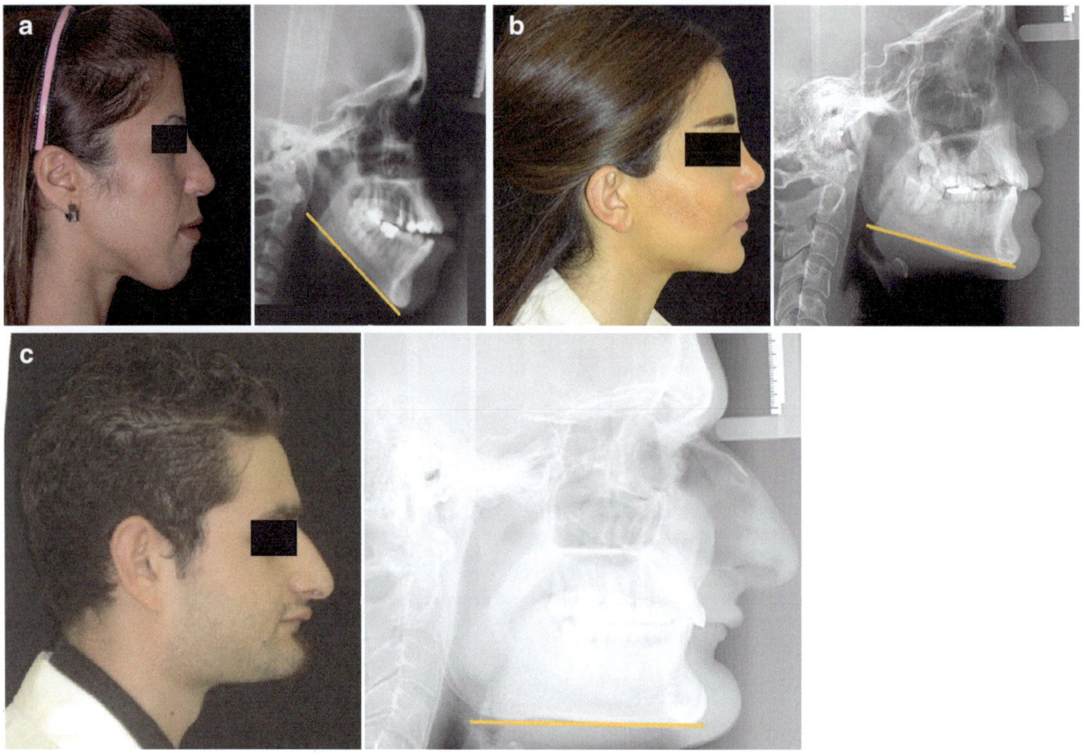

Fig. 5.17 Profile pictures and corresponding lateral cephalometric radiographs. (**a**) A 30-year-old female subject with dolychofacial type and severe clockwise rotation of the mandibular plane. (**b**) A 25-year-old woman with mesofacial type and normal inclination of the mandibular plane. (**c**) A 27-year-old male subject with brachyfacial type and flat mandibular plane

Dentoalveolar evaluation: Dentoalveolar evaluation on lateral cephalometric radiograph includes measurements of maxillary and mandibular incisors and molars. Similar to the skeletal assessment, the teeth are gauged relative to the corresponding jaw and relative to each other. This assessment indicates the position of the teeth in the sagittal and vertical planes. In summary, the maxillary and mandibular incisors can be well inclined, proclined, or retroclined in the sagittal plane relative to maxilla and the mandible. In the same plane, the maxillary and the mandibular incisors can be retruded or protruded relative to the more anterior facial planes. Many combinations can be present. For instance, the maxillary incisors can be well inclined (average incisor-to-palatal plane is 110 degrees), but at the same time they can be protruded (increased incisor to nasion/maxilla base angle). Vertical position of the incisors and molars is measured by tracing the perpendicular projection to the corresponding jaw. These measurements indicate whether the teeth are intruded, extruded, or positioned well vertically.

Soft tissue evaluation: A complete lateral cephalometric analysis includes the evaluation of soft tissues and their relationships to the underlying skeletal and dentoalveolar structures. In addition, comparisons with norms for length, thicknesses, and angulation of lips and chin usually are performed (Fig. 5.18).

Posteroanterior Cephalometric Radiograph

Despite the introduction of the posteroanterior cephalographs along with the lateral ones, and despite the fact that people present to each other by “face” [33], frontal evaluation of the face has

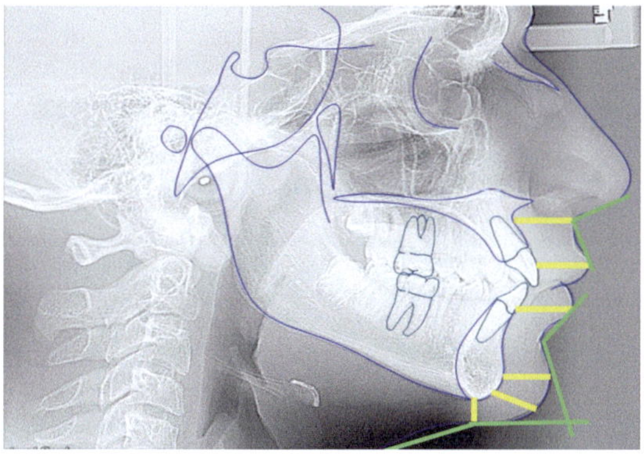

Fig. 5.18 Lateral cephalometric radiographs of 15-year-old boy with soft tissue thickness measurements of the lips and chin (yellow), and angular measurements of the nasolabial, mental sulcus, and chin throat angles (green)

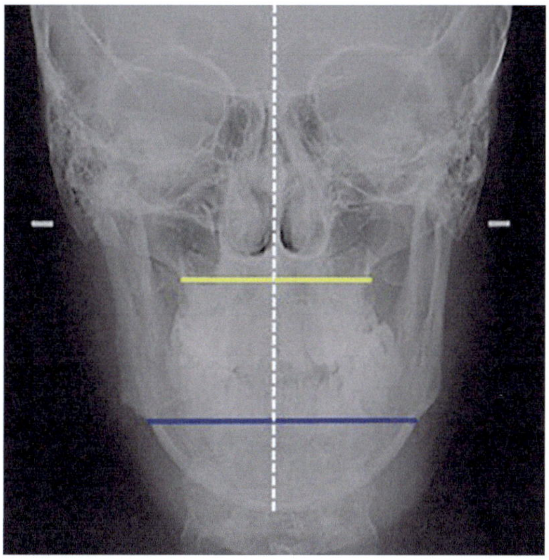

Fig. 5.19 Posteroanterior cephalometric radiographs of a 17-year-old girl. Maxillary (yellow) and mandibular (blue) widths are evaluated. In addition, the midsagittal line (white) is traced to evaluate facial symmetry

not gained popularity similar to that of the profile view [34]. The transverse dimensions evaluated on the posteroanterior cephalometric radiograph (Fig. 5.19) include the following:

- *Maxillary and mandibular width:* These measurements are important to define any discrepancy in width between the jaws. The presence of a narrow maxilla is an indication for palatal expansion.
- *Symmetry of the face*: The midsagittal plane is the reference position from which to evaluate symmetry between left and right.
- *Inclination of the maxillary and mandibular teeth to their corresponding jaws:* This evaluation describes potential compensation by the teeth in response to decrease in maxillary or increase in mandibular widths. The long axes of the maxillary and mandibular molars usually are traced and compared to average inclinations.

Intra-oral Scan Evaluation

One of the most important records for orthodontic diagnosis is cast models. Orthodontists take impressions of the teeth and arches on all patients prior to initiation of treatment. Once the gypsum molds are cut, the type of malocclusion is defined, and arch measurements are made. Arch tooth discrepancies, crowding, and interspace are measured. Other measurements including overjet and overbite also are performed (Fig. 5.20).

Recently, intra-oral scans started to replace the impressions and gypsum models (Fig. 5.21). During a period between reliance on gypsum models and development of oral scans, gypsum models were scanned digitally and later converted to the alginate impressions scanning. Orthodontists worked on digitizing the teeth so they can easily perform measurements, simulate movements within a planned orthodontic treatment, as well as design and fabricate appliances [35]. Other advantages of digital casts include improved diagnostic accuracy, better storage and retrieval, and decreased treatment time [36].

Orthodontic Diagnosis

Malocclusion Classification

In the nineteenth century, the orthodontic specialty developed into a clinical science. An increasing number of orthodontists started to be involved in treating the dentofacial deformities of growing children. Clinicians began to recognize and describe the facial features that commonly were associated with aberrant facial functions.

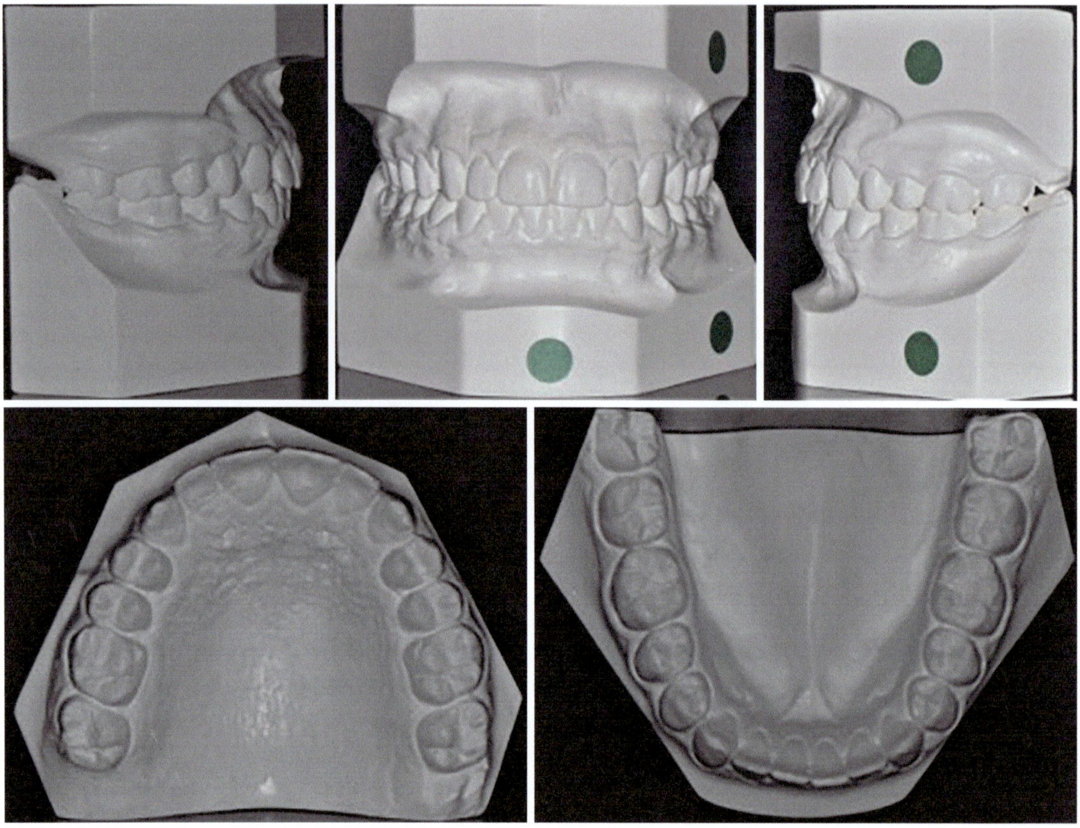

Fig. 5.20 Different views of the study models cut in gypsum of an 18-year-old male patient

Fig. 5.21 Intra-oral scan of maxillary and mandibular arches substituting the cast models shown in Fig. 5.20

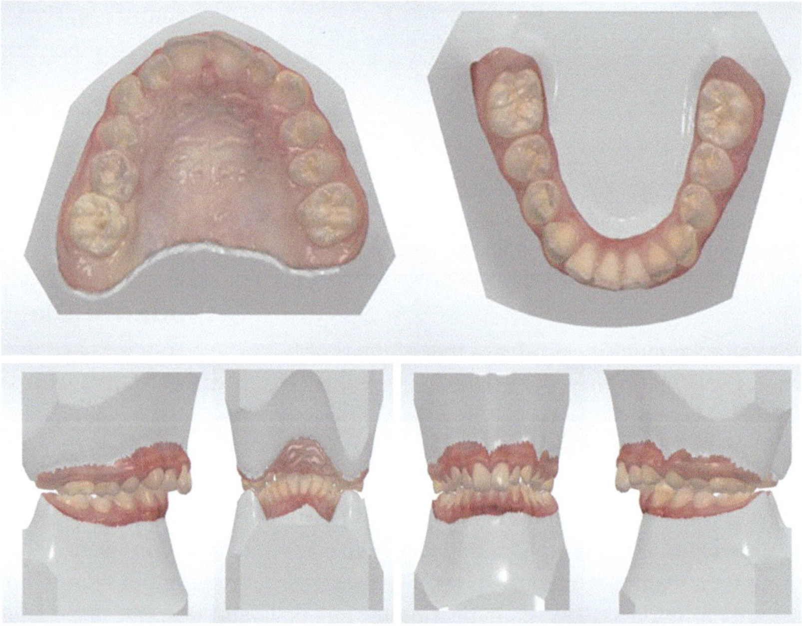

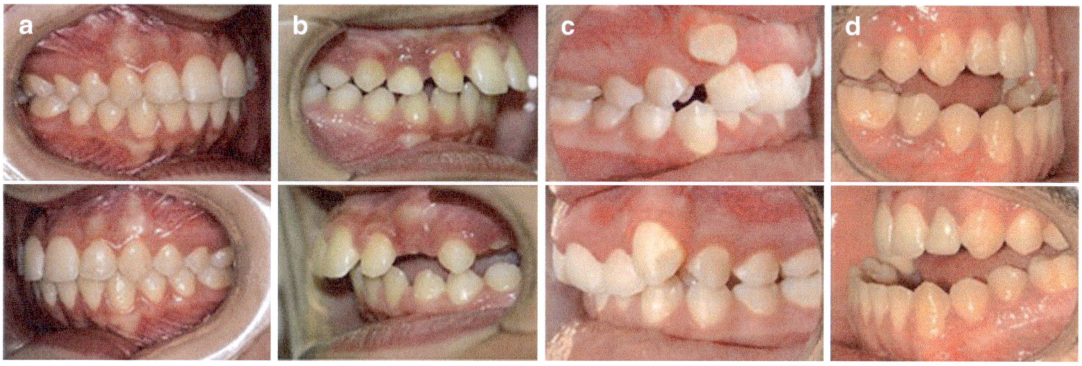

Fig. 5.22 Intra-oral photographs describing: (**a**) Class I Angle occlusion in a 16-year-old female. (**b**) Class II division 1 malocclusion in a 10-year-old boy. (**c**) Class II division 2 malocclusion in a 13-year-old girl. (**d**) Class III malocclusion in a 29-year-old male patient

At the onset of the twentieth century, Edward Angle [1], known as the father of contemporary orthodontics, classified the occlusion into three types (Fig. 5.22):

- Class I normal occlusion or neutroclusion: the mesiobuccal groove of the permanent mandibular first molar.
- Class II division 1 malocclusion or distoclusion: the mandibular teeth are distal (or posterior) to the maxillary teeth, and an overjet (anterior protrusion) is present between the anterior teeth.
- Class II division 2 malocclusion: the mandibular teeth are distal to the maxillary teeth, but the maxillary central incisors are tipped backward with no increase in overjet, accompanied usually with by deep bite.
- Class III malocclusion: the mandibular teeth are in a mesial occlusion or mesioclusion (more anterior) relative to the maxillary dentition.

The three types of malocclusion as defined by Angle, and which hold his name, were developed prior to the presence of the cephalometry. In most instances, the dental Angle malocclusions correspond to skeletal and facial appearances. However, possible discrepancy between the Angle dental malocclusion classification and the skeletal and facial appearance may occur. This highlights the importance of cephalometry along with a full clinical examination to properly diagnose the dentofacial features of any individual.

Problem List

Once the orthodontist has assembled data from the different diagnostic records, the final step is specifying the problem list. This step-by-step systematic evaluation is done on all patients to ensure that nothing is overlooked irrespective of the severity or complexity of the problems. In summary, the developmental problems related to any aspects of the patient's malocclusion constitute part of the problem list.

Various ways to compile problems exist. A widely used method is to relate problems that define facial, skeletal, and dentoalveolar separately. Another method is to link "sub-problems" from skeletal, dental, and facial in one major problem [4]. For instance, a deep overbite with decreased lower facial height and a hypodivergent mandibular plane are all different facets of one major problem which is the brachyfacial type.

Once the problem list is completed, the clinician and the patient will decide about treatment. There is only one diagnosis and corresponding problem list, but there may be several ways to approach the orthodontic treatment. Different treatment plans and tools will be discussed in a subsequent chapter.

References

1. Angle EH. Treatment of malocclusion of the teeth. 7th ed. Philadelphia: SS White; 1907. p. 46–57.
2. Shaw WC. The influence of children's dentofacial appearance on their social attractiveness as judged by peers and lay adults. Am J Orthod. 1981;79(4):399–415.
3. Sarver D, Proffit W, Ackerman J. Diagnosis and treatment planning in orthodontics. In: Graber LW, Vanarsdall RL, Vig KWL, Huang GJ, editors. Orthodontics: current principles and techniques. 6th ed. Elsevier: St. Louis Missouri; 2017. p. 208–366.
4. Proffit W, Ackerman J. Diagnosis and treatment planning. In: Proffit W, Fields H, Larson B, Sarver D, editors. Contemporary Orthodontics. St. Louis, MO: Elsevier/Mosby; 2018.
5. Nishimura RA, Otto CM, Bonow RO, et al. 2017 AHA/ACC focused update of the 2014 AHA/ACC guideline for the management of patients with valvular heart disease: a report of the American College of Cardiology/American Heart Association Task Force on Clinical Practice Guidelines. Circulation. 2017;135:e1159–95.
6. Wilson W, Taubert KA, Gewitz M, et al. Prevention of infective endocarditis: guidelines from the American Heart Association: a guideline from the American Heart Association Rheumatic Fever, Endocarditis, and Kawasaki Disease Committee, Council on Cardiovascular Disease in the Young, and the Council on Clinical Cardiology, Council on Cardiovascular Surgery and Anesthesia, and the Quality of Care and Outcomes Research Interdisciplinary Working Group. Circulation. 2007;116(15):1736–54.
7. Antibiotic Prophylaxis 2017 Update. AAE Quick Reference Guide Endocarditis Prophylaxis Recommendations.
8. ADA Council on Scientific Affairs Prepared by: Department of Scientific Information, ADA Science Institute Last Updated: August 5, 2019.
9. Perinetti G, Westphalen GH, Biasotto M, Salgarello S, Contardo L. The diagnostic performance of dental maturity for identification of the circumpubertal growth phases: a meta-analysis. Prog Orthod. 2013;14:8.
10. Hamdan AL, Khandakji M, Macari AT. Maxillary arch dimensions associated with acoustic parameters in prepubertal children. Angle Orthod. 2018;88(4):410–5.
11. Subtelny JD, Mestre JC, Subtelny JD. Comparative study of normal and defective articulation of /s/ as related to malocclusion and deglutition. J Speech Hearing Dis. 1964;29:269–85.
12. Bloomer HH. Speech defects associated with dental malocclusions and related anomalies. In: Travis LE, editor. Handbook of speech pathology and audiology. New York: Appleton-Century-Crofts; 1971. p. 715–65.
13. Jensen R. Anterior teeth relationship and speech. Acta Radiol. 1968;276(Suppl):1–69.
14. Leavy KM, Cisneros G, LeBlanc E. Malocclusion and its relationship to speech sound production: redefining the effect of malocclusal traits on sound production. Am J Orthod Dentofac Orthop. 2016;150:116–23.
15. Laine T. Associations between articulatory disorders in speech an occlusal anomalies. Eur J Orthod. 1987;9:144–50.
16. de Almeida Prado DG, Filho HN, Berretin-Felix G, Brasolotto AG. Speech articulatory characteristics of individuals with Dentofacial deformity. J Craniofac Surg. 2015;26(6):1835–9.
17. Joshi N, Hamdan AM, Fakhouri WD. Skeletal malocclusion: a developmental disorder with a life-long morbidity. J Clin Med Res. 2014;6(6):399–408.
18. Masood Y, Masood M, Zainul NN, Araby NB, Hussain SF, Newton T. Impact of malocclusion on oral health related quality of life in young people. Health Qual Life Outcomes. 2013;11:25–30.
19. Choi SH, Kim JS, Cha JY, Hwang CJ. Effect of malocclusion severity on oral health-related quality of life and food intake ability in a Korean population. Am J Orthod Dentofac Orthop. 2016;149(3):384–90.
20. Koike S, Sujino T, Ohmori H, et al. Gastric emptying rate in subjects with malocclusion examined by [(13) C] breath test. J Oral Rehabil. 2013;40(8):574–81.
21. Macari AT, Haddad RH. The case for environmental etiology of malocclusion in modern civilizations—airway morphology and facial growth. Semin Orthod. 2016;22(3):223–33.
22. Greulich WW, Pyle SI. Radiographic atlas of skeletal development of the hand and wrist. Stanford, CA: Stanford University Press; 1959.
23. Jacobson A, Jacobson R. Radiographic cephalometry: from basics to 3D imaging. 2nd ed. New Malden, Surrey, UK: Quintessence Publishing Co. Limited; 2006.
24. Downs WB. Analysis of the demo-facial profile. Angle Orthod. 1956;26:191.
25. Downs WB. The role of cephalometrics in orthodontic case analysis and diagnosis. Am J Orthod. 1952;38:162–82.
26. Steiner CC. Cephalometrics for you and me. Am J Orthod. 1953;39:729–55.
27. Steiner CC. Cephalometrics in clinical practice. Angle Orthod. 1959;29:8–29.
28. Steiner CC. The use of cephalometrics as an aid to planning and assessing orthodontic treatment. Am J Orthod. 1960;46:721–35.
29. Ricketts RM. The evolution of diagnosis to computerized cephalometrics. Am J Orthod. 1969;55(6):795–803.
30. Ricketts RM. Perspectives in the clinical application of cephalometrics. The first fifty years. Angle Orthod. 1981;51(2):115–50.
31. Reidel RA. The relation of maxillary structures to cranium in malocclusions and in normal occlusion. Angle Orthod. 1952;22:140–5.
32. Tweed CH. The Frankfort mandibular incisor. Angle (FMIA) in orthodontic diagnosis, treatment planning, and prognosis. Am J Orthod. 1954;24:121–69.

33. Ghafari JG. Posteroanterior cephalometry: craniofacial frontal analysis. In: Jacobson A, Jacobson R, editors. Radiographic Cephalometry: from basics to 3D imaging. 2nd ed. New Malden, Surrey, UK: Quintessence Publishing Co. Limited; 2006. p. 267–92.
34. Gottlieb EL, Nelson AH, Vogels DS 3rd. JCO study of orthodontic diagnosis and treatment procedures. 1. Results and trends. J Clin Orthod. 1991;25(3):145–56.
35. Kusnoto B, Evans C. Reliability of a 3D surface laser scanner for orthodontic applications. Am J Orthod Dentofac Orthop. 2002;122:342–8.
36. Burzynski JA, Firestone AR, Beck FM, Fields HW Jr, Deguchi T. Comparison of digital intraoral scanners and alginate impressions: time and patient satisfaction. Am J Orthod Dentofac Orthop. 2018;153(4):534–41.

The Upper Airway Space in Patients with Dentofacial Anomalies

6

Introduction

The upper airway space is delineated by the anatomic boundaries of the craniofacial bony and soft tissue structures. Its surface area and volume are linked to the vertical and sagittal growth of the facial bones and skull base angulation (Fig. 6.1) [1]. More than two decades ago, Trenouth et al. investigated the relation between functional oropharyngeal airway and craniofacial morphology in 70 subjects (39 females and 31 males) and proved a positive correlation between the former, mandibular length and cranial base angle. The functional oropharyngeal airway was measured on radiologic images as the minimal distance between the posterior pharyngeal wall and the most posterior part of the tongue in a sagittal plane [2]. Similarly, in 2006, Martin et al. studied the nasopharyngeal dimensions in 91 patients with ideal occlusion (mean value for facial convexity of 0.13 ± 3.06 mm and of ANB angle, (see below) of 1.08 degrees ±1.79), and they showed a strong link between the cranial base and several cephalometric measurements, among which were lower airway thickness and length of the nasal fossa. The ANB angle is defined as the angle between the line drawn from the nasion (N) to the most concave point of the maxilla (A), and the line between the nasion and the most concave point of the mandible (B). The authors emphasized the role of soft tissue patterns in outlining airway dimensions [3]. The growth of craniofacial bony structures is also paramount in delineating the changes in upper airway morphology with age. Johnston and Richardson investigated the natural growth of the

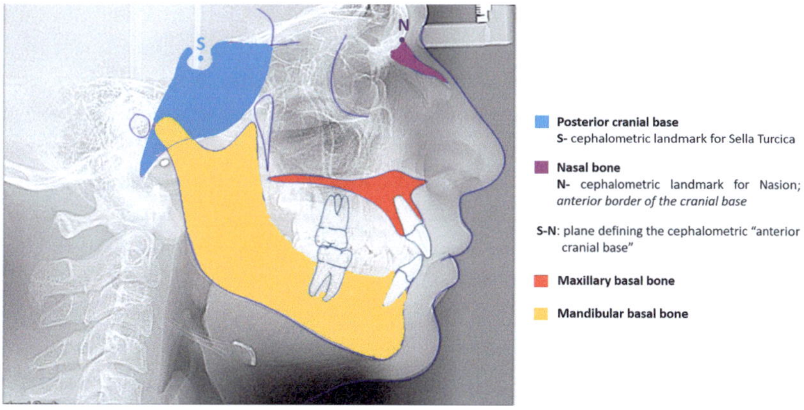

Fig. 6.1 Lateral view of the craniofacial structures showing the skeletal boundaries of the upper airway: base of skull, mandible, and maxilla

A.-L. Hamdan et al., *Dentofacial Anomalies*, https://doi.org/10.1007/978-3-030-69109-7_6

pharynx during the course of 32 years in a group of 16 young adults with a mean age of 20.2 years. Using cephalometric radiographs taken at a mean age of 20.2 years and 52.4 years, the authors showed a decrease in the sagittal depth of the oropharyngeal space and an increase in the vertical pharyngeal length (mean of 4.70 mm). The authors also noted an increase in the anteroposterior dimension of the nasopharyngeal space with age that was partially due to thinning of the posterior pharyngeal wall [4]. In 2012, Schendel et al. investigated the morphologic changes in the upper airway of 1300 subjects who were divided into three age groups, less than 20 years, greater than 50 years, and those in between. Using three-dimensional computer analysis, the authors analyzed growth-induced alterations in airway dimensions and showed an increase in upper airway volume, area, and length with age until 20 years. No changes were noted between the ages of 20 years and 50 years, whereas a decrease in upper airway dimensions was recorded after the age of 50 years. The authors attributed most of the changes in upper airway volume after the age of 50 years to the decrease in its smallest cross-sectional area [5].

The strong link between craniofacial morphology and upper airway space is also suggested by the high prevalence of breathing disorders in patients with dentofacial anomalies [6–12]. Shintani et al. in 2006 investigated facial skeletal morphology in relation to obstructive sleep apnea (OSA) and proved that mandibular protrusion was less pronounced in subjects with OSA in comparison to subjects with no OSA. Moreover, the position of the hyoid bone was lower [7]. In 2003, Endo et al. reported similar findings in their investigation on the morphologic features of 103 patients with OSA. The authors concurred that micrognathia is a risk factor for obstructive sleep disorders [8]. Lee et al. in 2010 showed a significant positive correlation between the upper airway and facial surface measurements in 69 subjects with OSA. Facial width, height, and nasal width correlated with tongue volume and thickness of the soft tissues. The authors alluded to the possible role of facial soft tissue measurements in phenotyping patients with OSA [9]. Similarly, Bruwier et al. in 2016 reported narrower maxilla-palatine core volume in 127 patients with OSA, in agreement with Poirrier et al. who also showed that maxillary width and nasal fossae angle characterize subjects with OSA [10, 11]. Last but not least, Galeotti et al. in 2019 investigated the association between cephalometric variables and OSA in children, and they reported a strong correlation between the severity of OSA and anatomic variations in maxilla-mandibular skeletal structures [12].

All the above substantiate the significant association between upper airway space dimensions and craniofacial morphology. The purpose of this chapter is to review the variations in upper airway dimensions in patients with dentofacial anomalies. Proper understanding of these variants in subjects with skeletal and non-skeletal dentofacial anomalies is important for otolaryngologists, speech-language pathologists, and voice teachers during the course of their diagnostic evaluation and treatment of patients with phonatory disorders. This information is also of importance to singers and wind instrumentalists who rely on vocal tract morphology to regulate the quality of their voice and/or musical note.

Upper Airway Morphology in Patients with Dentofacial Anomalies

There are many reports in the literature that concur about the relationship between dentofacial anomalies and the shape of the upper airway space. The impact of facial skeletal patterns on the upper airway at different levels, namely, nasopharynx, oropharynx, and hypopharynx, is important to recognize in patients with and without laryngeal or pharyngeal pathology. As early as five decades ago, Mergen and Jacobs proved that subjects with class II malocclusion had a positive correlation between nasopharyngeal dimensions and depth of the face. Depth of the face was defined as the space from the most anterior point on the occipital condyle to the anterior nasal spine. The study was conducted on 40 female subjects using cephalograms [13]. In

1992, Ceylan and Oktay examined pharyngeal size in 90 subjects with various ANB angles; less than 1 degree, between 1 and 5, and greater than 5. The authors proved that the oropharyngeal area gets larger with a decrease in the ANB angle [14]. Similarly, in 2005 de Freitas et al. showed that the upper pharyngeal airway width was narrower in class I and class II occlusion subjects with vertical growth pattern in comparison to those with class I and II and normal growth pattern. Neither the type of occlusion nor the growth pattern affected the width of the lower pharyngeal airway. The study was conducted on a total of 80 subjects stratified based on the type of occlusion (class I vs. class II) and growth pattern (vertical vs. normal) [15]. That same year, Abu Allhaija and Al-Khateeb investigated the uvulo-glosso-pharyngeal dimensions in 90 subjects with three different types of malocclusion using cephalometric radiographs. The authors proved a significant correlation between the lower pharyngeal airway space and the anteroposterior skeletal pattern. Moreover, vertical airway length was shorter in male patients with class II malocclusion vs. patients with class III and class I occlusion. The results also showed significant disparities in the dimensions of the tongue and palate among the three groups, which inevitably contributed to the variations in airway measures across the different skeletal patterns [16]. In 2008, Muto et al. compared the anteroposterior dimension of the pharyngeal airway space (PAS) in three subgroups of subjects, those with normal mandible (SNB angle between 76 and 82 degrees), retrognathism (SNB angle less than 76 degrees), and prognathism (SNB angle greater than 82 degrees). Note that SNB angle is the angle between a line drawn from the sella turcica to the nasion, and a line drawn from the nasion to the most concave point of the mandible. Using lateral cephalograms, the authors proved an association between mandibular skeletal patterns and PAS. Subjects with retrognathism had the smallest PAS, whereas those with prognathism had the largest [17]. In 2008, Alves et al. investigated the upper airway morphology of healthy subjects with skeletal class II and III deformities using three-dimensional cephalometric analysis. Aside from the significant differences in several cephalometric measurements between genders, there was no statistically significant difference between class II and III deformities except for the nasopharyngeal transverse dimension. The authors also noted that male subjects with class III malocclusion had larger retroglossal area and longer spine distance [18]. In 2009, Kecik investigated the correlation between the sagittal projection of the mandible and upper airway morphology and proved significant differences in the vertical length of the upper airway and the nasopharyngeal area across subgroups with different mandibular projection. The pharyngeal airway space (nasopharyngeal and hypopharyngeal) was found to be smaller in patients with class II malocclusion in comparison to those with class III malocclusion with mandibular protrusion [19]. In 2009, Iwasaki et al. investigated the shape of the oropharyngeal airway in patients with class III malocclusion and class I using cone beam computed tomography (CBCT). Although there was no significant difference in the nasopharyngeal airway dimensions between the two groups of subjects, those with class III had a larger oropharyngeal airway with a cross-sectional area of 168.56 mm^2 vs. 119.18 mm^2 in class I. The results also indicated significant differences in the shape of the oropharyngeal airway between the two groups. Class III subjects had a higher tendency for a flat shape, whereas a square shape was more common in class I subjects [20]. In 2009, Grauer et al. evaluated the shape as well as the volume of the pharyngeal airway in relation to the morphology of the face in 62 subjects using CBCT and three-dimensional virtual model [21]. The facial types were stratified in the anteroposterior dimension according to Angle's classification [22] and in the vertical dimension as short, long, or average. The results indicated a relationship between the inferior airway volume and both facial size and anteroposterior jaw projection. The inferior pharyngeal airway volume in the anteroposterior grouping was significantly smaller in class II subjects in comparison to class I and III subjects (9.399 mm^3 vs.13.163 mm^3 vs. 12.187 mm^3, respectively). Moreover, the pharyngeal airway was more inclined forward in class II patients in comparison to class III patients whose airway was oriented vertically [21]. In 2010, Jena et al. investigated the correlation between sagittal mandibular development and awake pharyngeal airway passage in 91 patients stratified into three groups based on the position of the mandible. Using lateral cephalograms, the authors showed that the oropharyngeal depth was greater in patients with prognathic mandible in comparison to those with normal or retrognathic mandible. However, there was statistically no significant difference in the hypopharyngeal and nasopharyngeal depth between the three groups of patients [23]. In 2011, El H and Palomo investigated the airway volume, namely, nasal passage and oropharynx, in 140 patients with different malocclusions based on the ANB, SNB, and SNA angles. SNA is the angle drawn between a line from nasion and sella turcia, and a line drawn from nasion and most concave point of the maxilla. The authors proved that the oropharyngeal volume was narrower in class II subjects in comparison to class I and class III. The smaller volume was attributed to the mandibular position and the more acute SNB angle [24]. In 2011, Oh et al. studied the volume and inclination of the pharyngeal airway in relation to the different facial patterns in the anteroposterior dimension and showed that subjects with class I and III subjects had larger pharyngeal airway in comparison to subjects with class II malocclusion [25]. Moreover, in this latter group, the pharyngeal airway had a more backward inclination as evidenced by a larger angle between the Frankfort horizontal plane (FH plane) and mid-plane of the oropharyngeal airway [26]. In conclusion, the authors commented on the interplay between the pharyngeal and laryngeal airway morphology [25]. In 2012, Ucar and Uysal investigated the differences in upper airway dimensions in patients with class I malocclusion and various degrees of vertical growth patterns. Using craniofacial and orofacial measurements, the authors showed that high-angle subjects had smaller upper posterior airway space but larger palatal tongue space in comparison to low-angle subjects, and the higher-angle subjects had larger tongue gap in comparison to those with low or normal angle [27]. The vertical growth pattern was stratified based on the SN-MP angle whether less than 26 degrees for the low angle and greater than 38 degrees for the high angle. SN-MP angle is the angle between a line drawn from the sella (S) to the nasion (N) and a line drawn along the mandibular plane (MP). In 2013, Bollhalder et al. investigated the correlation between the dimensions of the upper airway and the severity of class II in 131 males and 115 females. The severity of the malocclusion was determined by the ANB angle with a cut-point of 7 degrees, and by the extent of over-jet (distance between the upper and lower incisors in a horizontal plane) with a cut-point of 10 mm. The results indicated that subjects with retrognathia were more inclined toward having smaller upper airway [28]. In 2014, Indriksone and Jackobsone conducted a systemic review on upper airway morphology and reported controversial results. Only 5 out of 11 studies concurred that the oropharyngeal space is smaller in class II malocclusion and larger in class III malocclusion [29]. In 2015, Castro-Silva et al. investigated the pharyngeal airway space using CBCT in three groups of patients with class I, II, and III malocclusion. The results showed that patients with class III malocclusion had larger pharyngeal airway space area and volume than those with class I and class II malocclusion, and those with class I malocclusion had a larger pharyngeal airway volume than those with class II. The mean values and standard deviations for these volumes in class III, I, and II were 19.879 ± 5.066 mm^3, vs. 14.858 ± 5.719 mm^3, and 10.923 ± 3.161 mm^3, respectively [30]. In 2015, Soni et al. evaluated the nasopharynx, oropharynx, and soft palate of 30 patients with class II malocclusion secondary to retrognathic mandible and 30 patients with class II malocclusion secondary to a prognathic maxilla. The authors found no statistically significant difference in the measures of the nasopharyngeal space between the two groups of patients. However, the oropharyngeal region, measured by the distance between the soft palate and its counterpoint on the posterior pharyngeal wall, was significantly larger in patients with prognathic maxilla in comparison to those with retrognathic mandible [31]. In 2017, Uslu-Akcam evaluated angular, linear, and computed cephalometric airway measurements in subjects with skeletal class II, stratified as two patterns of division 1 and 2, along three growth periods, pre-peak, peak, and post-peak. The authors demonstrated a significant difference in oropharyngeal and nasopharyngeal airway space among the groups. Subjects with skeletal II, division 2, had the smallest measures [32].

In summary, the link between dentofacial anomalies and the shape of the upper airway space is irrefutable. The impact of skeletal and non-skeletal anomalies on upper airway dimensions varies with the type of occlusion and vertical growth pattern (Figs. 6.2, 6.3, and 6.4).

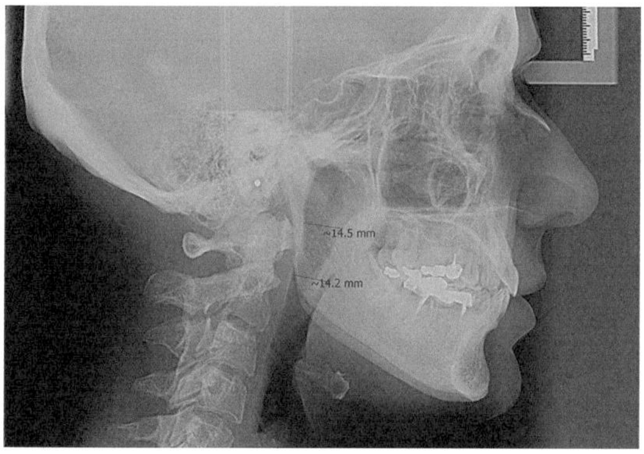

Fig. 6.2 Lateral radiographic view showing the retropalatal and retroglossal width in a 50-year-old female with class I occlusion

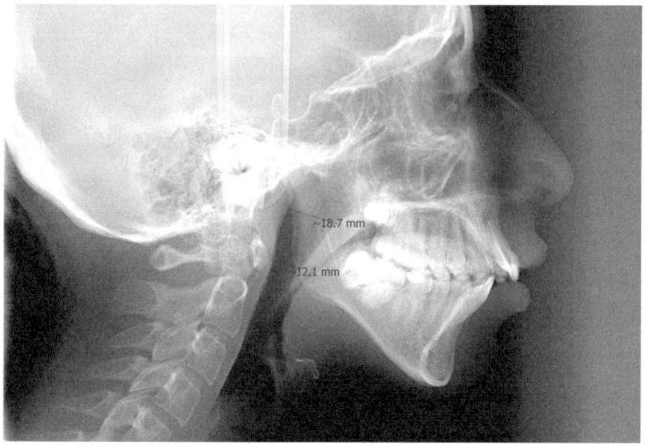

Fig. 6.3 Lateral radiographic view showing the retropalatal and retroglossal width in a 21-year-old female with class II malocclusion

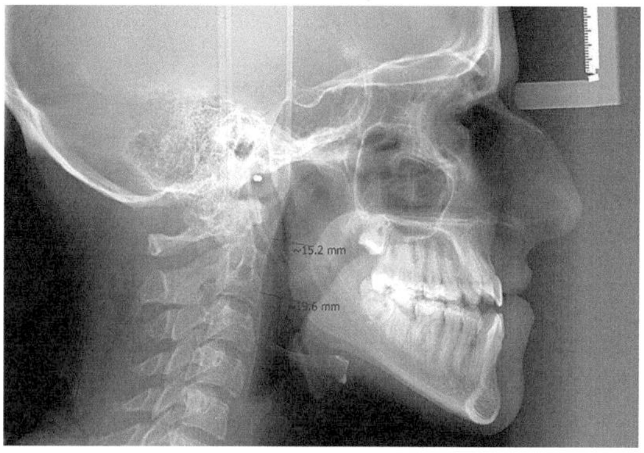

Fig. 6.4 Lateral radiographic view showing the retropalatal and retroglossal width in a 20-year-old female with class III malocclusion

The disparity in the mode of assessment used in the above studies, conventional lateral head films, computerized tomography, or three-dimensional evaluation, can explain partially the differences in results [8, 33–37]. The anatomic variations in the upper airway space should be considered in the work-up and management strategy of instrumentalists and singers with performance complaints.

Why the Association Between Dentofacial Anomalies and Upper Airway Space Morphology?

The variations in the dimensions of the upper airway space with different types of malocclusion are attributed partially to the anatomic variation of the upper and lower jaw, and partially to associated variations in the position of the uvula, palate, and hyoid bone. Anatomic changes in these structures lead to the disparities in upper airway space dimensions commonly observed in subjects with various types of malocclusion. In 2009, Kecik reported significant differences in the length, area, and angular direction of the uvula among subgroups of patients with different mandibular sagittal projection, namely, class I, class II, and class III [19]. In 2010, Jena et al. found that the soft palate was shorter and thicker in patients with mandibular prognathism, in comparison to those with retrognathism or normal mandibular projection. Interestingly, maxillary position was normal in all subjects. In their investigation on pharyngeal airway space in relation to sagittal mandibular development, the authors also showed greater depth of the oropharynx in subjects with prognathism in comparison to normal subjects [23]. Similarly, in the study by Abu Allhaija et al. in 2005, the authors showed that the soft palate was thicker in class II and class III female subjects vs. class I subjects [16]. The position of the hyoid bone also plays an important role in shaping the upper airway space in patients with dentofacial anomalies, primarily through association with the position of the tongue and mandible. Most of the studies on the correlation between upper airway shape and malocclusions type II and III corroborate the association of mandibular length and position with that of the hyoid bone, both in the cephalo-caudal or anteroposterior dimensions, and between the position of the hyoid bone and tongue. The well-known difference in upper airway inclination reported across subjects with different types of malocclusion substantiates this association further [21, 25]. In the above study by Abu Allhaija et al., the anteroposterior position of the hyoid bone was described as closer to C3, and its vertical position as closer to the mandible and to a line drawn between the retrognathion and C3 in subjects with class II, in comparison to subjects with class I and III. Moreover, the thickness of the tongue was greater in class III female subjects in comparison to class II subjects [16]. Yamaoka et al. studied the relation between hyoid bone position and tongue in 51 patients with class III malocclusion and reported a significant correlation between the two. The authors suggested the compensatory behavior of the genioglossus muscle secondary to change in the position of the hyoid bone in cases of malocclusion [38]. Similarly, in 2009, Kecik in her study on the association between upper airway dimensions and mandibular position showed that the sagittal position of the mandible affects that of the hyoid bone and tongue. The interplay is understandable given the muscular attachment of the tongue to the lingual cortex of the body of the mandible [19]. In the study by Iwasaki et al. in 2009, the authors attributed the larger cross-sectional intraoral area in subjects with class III malocclusion in comparison to those with normal occlusion (2101.52 mm^2 vs. 702.03 mm^2), respectively, to the lower position of the tongue [20]. In 2014, Jose et al. studied the relation between the pharyngeal space and hyoid bone position in subjects with normal occlusion and subjects with malocclusion. The results indicated lack of significant difference in the horizontal position of the hyoid bone between the different groups. However, the authors revealed a significant positive correlation between the distance drawn from the hyoid bone to the retrognathion in a horizontal plane, and the lower airway in subjects with class I skeletal pattern [39]. In 2019, Iwasaki et al. investigated hyoid bone position and tongue volume in 60 children with different types of malocclusion using CBCT. The authors showed a lower position of the hyoid bone in class II patients, and showed a positive correlation between hyoid position and A-nasion-B angle [40].

In summary, anatomic variations in the shape of the uvula, palate, and position of the hyoid bone and its muscular attachments play an important role in shaping the upper airway space in patients with dentofacial anomalies. In addition to its role in maintaining cranial balance and upright position of the head [41], the hyoid bone affects the position of the tongue and mandible [42]. Understanding this interplay is crucial in the work-up and management of functional voice disorders and wind instrument performance problems in patients with dentofacial anomalies. A high-positioned hyoid bone may be misinterpreted in patients with hyperfunctional voice or wind instrument disorders and malocclusion. The associated soft tissue changes are also important to consider in the interpretation of the acoustic changes in subjects with malocclusion. A thorough discussion on the fundamental frequency, formant frequencies, and dentofacial is presented in Chaps. 8 and 9.

Upper Airway Space Morphology in Wind Instrumentalists with Dentofacial Anomalies

Wind instrumentalists also should be considered as professional voice users. There is extensive literature on the laryngeal behavior during wind instrument playing with emphasis on the role of the glottis and upper airway space in modulating airflow entry into the mouthpiece of the instrument. The glottic aperture is critical for the initiation and sustainability of a musical tone, and is recognized as an indicator of experience among wind instrumentalists [43, 44]. In 1989, Mukai reported that beginners tend to have a large glottic opening while playing, whereas experts tend to have a small glottis aperture. Hence, the extent of vocal fold opening is a sign of expertise in controlling the amount of airflow during expiration, which is harder than during inspiration [43]. Adduction of the vocal folds during playing also was noted by Eckley in 2006, in her study of ten wind instrument players. The authors concurred with the findings of Mukai and noted furthermore the presence of supraglottic constriction referred to as "lateral laryngeal tension." Using flexible fiberoptic endoscopy, the authors associated the supraglottic laryngeal behavior with the degree of difficulty in performing [44].

The observations of laryngeal behavior in wind instruments by both Eckley and Mukai reveal that the larynx is very much involved in wind instrument production in describing laryngeal behaviors that are more closely associated with tension [43–45]. Therefore, we must ask whether these observed behaviors are desirable or required when playing wind instruments. For example, it is unlikely now that the above conclusion of Mukai (that the extent of the vocal fold opening shows a sign of expertise) is indicative of a desirable vocal behavior, and instead may be an indication of tension, which has been more recently reinforced through wind players indicating that they experience dry throat, pain, tiredness, discomfort and itchiness, and so forth after playing their instruments [44, 46, 47]. It is also not known if any of these wind players studied voice as well. Traditionally, wind instrument instruction has not addressed how the laryngeal area should be thought of by wind players, since it has not been a part of any instrumental pedagogical method. With students who are beginners, it is likely they are using student model instruments that may leak, that may have dents or cracks, that require them to use mouthpieces or reeds that are too resistant (especially in young brass players) or too weak (especially for younger reed players who use reeds that are too thin or are no longer functioning adequately). These problems result in embouchure and throat behaviors that produce more tension to create the desired sound. Within the past 10 years or so, consideration has been given to the laryngeal area in playing wind instruments, in promoting the notion of an "open throat" when blowing. However, this imagery as thought of by wind instrumentalists is based on the idea that the throat has an orange in it, or a tennis ball, or some such object; so, they think that the vocal folds are completely abducted, while laryngoscopic observation evaluation indicates that the folds are engaged and active. However, it is not known if this is reactive behavior or controlled.

The observations above substantiate the importance of the laryngeal behavior in wind instrumentalists and the need to understand any variations in this behavior that might be associated with dentofacial anomalies. Noting the adverse effects of facial skeletal and non-skeletal anomalies on the upper airway space is essential for the assessment and treatment planning of wind instrumentalists with difficulties in embouchure and/or performance. Although wind instrument playing has been described as helpful to orthodontist in rare selected cases, it is also considered as a predisposing factor to the development and/or worsening of a pre-existing orthodontic anomalies [45]. The pressure exerted during playing is concentrated on the teeth, oral soft tissues, or lips, with different intensities across the various mouthpieces and reeds used, and pressure can have significant effect on orofacial and dental structures. The long-term behavior of the orofacial neuromuscular complex and the extensive activity associated with it during the development of embouchure direct these pressure forces and contribute to the growth inclination of the upper and lower jaw anterior dentition and to the growth pattern of the dental arch, in a favorable or unfavorable way [45]. In a study by Brattstrom et al. on the longitudinal effect of wind instrument playing on dentofacial morphology, the authors reported wider dental arches in musicians compared to controls. Moreover, there was favorable anterior mandibular growth with a reduction in anterior facial height in wind instrumentalists. Interestingly, female musicians using single reed mouthpieces had more anteriorly displaced incisors compared with those who used cup-shaped mouthpieces [48]. Brattstrom et al. in 1989 "reported that the high intra-oral pressure in wind instrument players may explain the wider dental arch in wind instrumentalists. Moreover, the cup-shaped mouthpiece of the trumpet seems to retocline the maxillary incisors, whereas the single-reed mouthpiece of the clarinet seems to procline the maxillary incisors" [48]. This finding is important in relationship to how beginning students learn how to play these instruments. A major problem with young trumpet players is that when they start trying to play higher notes (C5/@500HZ and above) instead of using breath support and adjusting the embouchure, they usually press the mouthpiece through the lip into the upper teeth (maxillary) to force out the higher note. This seems to be an instinctive behavior, and it is noticeable because the young player will tilt the head forward to do so. Unless the teacher (usually the school band director at this level) is a trained trumpeter or other brass musician, it is unlikely that she or he will catch and remediate the behavior effectively. Therefore, the student will continue to engage in this behavior to play higher notes. For young clarinetists, there is a similar issue when they start trying to play in their upper register, but often use a reed that is too soft and will not provide the resistance needed to have those notes speak. Therefore, the students bite on the mouthpiece (which is often evidenced by tooth indentations that have been carved, through the biting, into the mouthpiece), which would likely lead to the problem of proclining maxillary incisors. As with the young trumpet players, often the child's first teacher is the school band director who may not be really familiar with playing the clarinet, and especially with adjusting reeds for the students or in recognizing when a reed is no longer suitable. While brass mouthpieces do not wear out for young players, reeds usually disintegrate and break down, and even young students should be changing out their reeds adjusted regularly. At the professional level, it is common for an oboe reed to last about 2 weeks and a bassoon reed a month or two, depending upon use, but these musicians will cycle reeds as needed. Younger players, on the other hand, do not know about this and will continue to play on reeds that are well past their prime, thus possibly leading to some of the problems Brattstrom observed.

In the study by Grammatopoulos, instruments with large mouthpieces (selected brass instruments) had an effect on occlusion, namely, lateral crossbite, whereas other wind instruments had no adverse effect. The study was conducted on 170 professional musicians and dental casts were used for assessment [49]. The same authors 3 years later also showed that large brass mouthpieces are associated with lateral crossbite [50]. The subjects investigated in both studies were adults and professional musicians. Lateral crossbite is also common in some younger tuba players who play in a kind of side-saddle position, so that they may actually at times play with more pressure on one side of the mouth than the other, because they cannot see the music with the instrument directly in front of them and have to turn their bodies to play. The same behaviors are common in those students who play larger saxophones (as the instrument hangs at the side of the body) and also young contrabassoon players, who are also forced to turn the instrument as well as the head (depending upon the model of the instrument) to the left or right, sometimes resulting in a more sideways embouchure, because the music cannot be seen due to the instrument being in the way.

In a longitudinal study by Herman on children playing musical instruments over the course of 2 years, the authors demonstrated a significant anterior tooth movement in comparison to controls [51]. Similarly, Kula et al. investigated the association between malocclusion and trumpet performance in a group of 70 trumpet students who were asked to perform specific skill tests while three-dimensional CBCT was used for evaluation [52]. The study proved that anterior crowding and maxillary protrusion correlated negatively with performance. Moreover, maxillary inter-canine width correlated positively with flutter tongue articulation and flexibility exercises, and maxillary intermolar width correlated significantly with flutter tongue articulation [53]. Shimada investigated the dentoskeletal shape of 55 wind instrumentalists and showed that class B instrumentalists (single-reed mouthpieces) had a significant increase in overjet on the horizontal plane, with an inclination of the mandibular incisors lingually, and maxillary incisors labially. The author attributed these inclinations to the pressure exerted on the mandibular anterior teeth. Moreover, there was labial inclination of maxillary and mandibular anteriors in class C (double-reed mouthpieces) and D (hole or aperture mouthpieces). Even more interesting, the dental arch and the alveolar basal arch were narrower but longer [53]. The increase in lower incisor inclination and subsequent increase in overjet also has been demonstrated by Gualtieri in his study on 82 wind instrumentalists. An increase in overjet was significantly more prominent in class B musicians in comparison to other wind instrumentalists [54]. Despite all the above reports, many authors have argued against the correlation between wind instrument playing and dentofacial anomalies. In the study by Fuhrimann et al. in 1987, which included 24 wind instrument musicians, 12 trumpet players and 12 on the clarinetists, the authors showed that wind instrument playing had no effect on occlusion despite the disproportionately high pressure exerted by the soft tissues on the upper teeth. Lip strength and activity were measured using a dysnometer and electromyography during rest and while performing [55]. Similarly, Rindisbacher et al. conducted a study on 62 wind instrument players, 31 brass instruments and 31 reed instruments, and demonstrated that the difference in overbite between musicians and a control group was non-significant. However, the width of the upper dental arch at the canines' level was less in musicians in comparison to controls [56].

In summary, wind instrument playing is associated with potential alteration in the orofacial skeletal and dental structures, particularly the anterior teeth and maxillary arch dimensions. These alterations may impact the vocal tract shape and length. Given the well-known role of the vocal tract in instrument performance, dental and or skeletal alterations associated with dentofacial anomalies need to be considered in wind instrumentalists. This may have even more impact when instrumentalists are also singers. The change in vocal tract length or shape secondary to wind instruments playing may impact voice adversely. Understanding the potential effect of wind instrument playing on voice performance is invaluable in voice pedagogy, and understanding the effect of voice and laryngeal function on wind instrument playing is similarly important and complex.

References

1. Agur AM, Dalley AF, editors. Grant's atlas of anatomy. 12th ed. Philadelphia: Lippincott Williams & Wilkins; 2009.
2. Trenouth MJ, Timms DJ. Relationship of the functional oropharynx to craniofacial morphology. Angle Orthod. 1999;69(5):419–23.
3. Martin O, Muelas L, Viñas MJ. Nasopharyngeal cephalometric study of ideal occlusions. Am J Orthod Dentofac Orthop. 2006;130(4):436.e1–9.
4. Johnston CD, Richardson A. Cephalometric changes in adult pharyngeal morphology. Eur J Orthod. 1999;21(4):357–62.
5. Schendel SA, Jacobson R, Khalessi S. Airway growth and development: a computerized 3-dimensional analysis. J Oral Maxillofac Surg. 2012;70(9):2174–83.
6. Smith RM, Gonzalez C. The relationship between nasal obstruction and craniofacial growth. Pediatr Clin N Am. 1989;36(6):1423–34.
7. Shintani T, Asakura K, Kataura A. Adenotonsillar hypertrophy and skeletal morphology of children with obstructive sleep apnea syndrome. Acta Otolaryngol Suppl. 1996;523:222–4.
8. Endo S, Mataki S, Kurosaki N. Cephalometric evaluation of craniofacial and upper airway structures in Japanese patients with obstructive sleep apnea. J Med Dent Sci. 2003;50(1):109–20.

9. Lee RW, Sutherland K, Chan AS, et al. Relationship between surface facial dimensions and upper airway structures in obstructive sleep apnea. Sleep. 2010;33(9):1249–54.
10. Bruwier A, Poirrier R, Albert A, et al. Three-dimensional analysis of craniofacial bones and soft tissues in obstructive sleep apnea using cone beam computed tomography. Int Orthod. 2016;14(4):449–61.
11. Poirrier AL, Pire S, Raskin S, Limme M, Poirrier R. Contribution of postero-anterior cephalometry in obstructive sleep apnea. Laryngoscope. 2012;122(10):2350–4.
12. Galeotti A, Festa P, Viarani V, et al. Correlation between cephalometric variables and obstructive sleep apnoea severity in children. Eur J Paediatr Dent. 2019;20(1):43–7.
13. Mergen DC, Jacobs RM. The size of nasopharynx associated with normal occlusion and Class II malocclusion. Angle Orthod. 1970;40(4):342–6.
14. Ceylan I, Oktay H. A study on the pharyngeal size in different skeletal patterns. Am J Orthod Dentofac Orthop. 1995;108(1):69–75.
15. de Freitas MR, Alcazar NM, Janson G, de Freitas KM, Henriques JF. Upper and lower pharyngeal airways in subjects with Class I and Class II malocclusions and different growth patterns. Am J Orthod Dentofac Orthop. 2006;130(6):742–5.
16. Abu Allhaija ES, Al-Khateeb SN. Uvulo-glosso-pharyngeal dimensions in different anteroposterior skeletal patterns. Angle Orthod. 2005;75(6):1012–8.
17. Muto T, Yamazaki A, Takeda S. A cephalometric evaluation of the pharyngeal airway space in patients with mandibular retrognathia and prognathia, and normal subjects. Int J Oral Maxillofac Surg. 2008;37(3):228–31.
18. Alves PV, Zhao L, O'Gara M, Patel PK, Bolognese AM. Three-dimensional cephalometric study of upper airway space in skeletal class II and III healthy patients. J Craniofac Surg. 2008;19(6):1497–507.
19. Kecik D. The effect of mandibular position on upper airway dimensions. Turk J Orthod. 2009;22:93–101.
20. Iwasaki T, Hayasaki H, Takemoto Y, Kanomi R, Yamasaki Y. Oropharyngeal airway in children with Class III malocclusion evaluated by cone-beam computed tomography. Am J Orthod Dentofac Orthop. 2009;136(3):318.e1–9.
21. Grauer D, Cevidanes LS, Styner MA, Ackerman JL, Proffit WR. Pharyngeal airway volume and shape from cone-beam computed tomography: relationship to facial morphology. Am J Orthod Dentofac Orthop. 2009;136(6):805–14.
22. Angle EH. Treatment of malocclusion of the teeth. 7th ed. Philadelphia: SS White; 1907. p. 46–57.
23. Jena AK, Singh SP, Utreja AK. Sagittal mandibular development effects on the dimensions of the awake pharyngeal airway passage. Angle Orthod. 2010;80(6):1061–7.
24. El H, Palomo JM. Airway volume for different dentofacial skeletal patterns. Am J Orthod Dentofac Orthop. 2011;139(6):e511–21.
25. Oh KM, Hong JS, Kim YJ, Cevidanes LS, Park YH. Three-dimensional analysis of pharyngeal airway form in children with anteroposterior facial patterns. Angle Orthod. 2011;81(6):1075–82.
26. Oh S, Ahn J, Nam KU, Paeng JY, Hong J. Frankfort horizontal plane is an appropriate three-dimensional reference in the evaluation of clinical and skeletal cant. J Korean Assoc Oral Maxillofac Surg. 2013;39(2):71–6.
27. Ucar FI, Uysal T. Orofacial airway dimensions in subjects with Class I malocclusion and different growth patterns. Angle Orthod. 2011;81(3):460–8.
28. Bollhalder J, Hänggi MP, Schätzle M, Markic G, Roos M, Peltomäki TA. Dentofacial and upper airway characteristics of mild and severe class II division 1 subjects. Eur J Orthod. 2013;35(4):447–53.
29. Indriksone I, Jakobsone G. The upper airway dimensions in different sagittal craniofacial patterns: a systematic review. Stomatologija. 2014;16(3):109–17.
30. Castro-Silva L, Monnazzi MS, Spin-Neto R, et al. Cone-beam evaluation of pharyngeal airway space in class I, II, and III patients. Oral Surg Oral Med Oral Pathol Oral Radiol. 2015;120(6):679–83.
31. Soni J, Shyagali TR, Bhayya DP, Shah R. Evaluation of pharyngeal space in different combinations of Class II skeletal malocclusion. Acta Inform Med. 2015;23(5):285–9.
32. Uslu-Akcam O. Pharyngeal airway dimensions in skeletal class II: a cephalometric growth study. Imaging Sci Dent. 2017;47(1):1–9.
33. Fairburn SC, Waite PD, Vilos G, et al. Three-dimensional changes in upper airways of patients with obstructive sleep apnea following maxillomandibular advancement. J Oral Maxillofac Surg. 2007;65(1):6–12.
34. Aboudara CA, Hatcher D, Nielsen IL, Miller A. A three-dimensional evaluation of the upper airway in adolescents. Orthod Craniofac Res. 2003;6:173–5.
35. Aboudara C, Nielsen I, Huang JC, Maki K, Miller AJ, Hatcher D. Comparison of airway space with conventional lateral headfilms and 3-dimensional reconstruction from cone-beam computed tomography. Am J Orthod Dentofac Orthop. 2009;135(4):468–79.
36. Degerliyurt K, Ueki K, Hashiba Y, Marukawa K, Nakagawa K, Yamamoto E. A comparative CT evaluation of pharyngeal airway changes in class III patients receiving bimaxillary surgery or mandibular setback surgery. Oral Surg Oral Med Oral Pathol Oral Radiol Endod. 2008;105(4):495–502.
37. Guijarro-Martinez R, Swennen GRJ. Cone-beam computerized tomography imaging and analysis of the upper airway: a systematic review of the literature. Int J Oral Maxillofac Surg. 2011;40(11):1227–37.
38. Yamaoka M, Furusawa K, Uematsu T, Okafuji N, Kayamoto D, Kurihara S. Relationship of the

hyoid bone and posterior surface of the tongue in prognathism and micrognathia. J Oral Rehab. 2003;30(9):914–20.
39. Jose NP, Shetty S, Mogra S, Shetty VS, Rangarajan S, Mary L. Evaluation of hyoid bone position and its correlation with pharyngeal airway space in different types of skeletal malocclusion. Contemp Clin Dent. 2014;5(2):187–9.
40. Iwasaki T, Suga H, Yanagisawa-Minami A, et al. Relationships among tongue volume, hyoid position, airway volume and maxillofacial form in paediatric patients with Class-I, Class-II and Class-III malocclusions. Orthod Craniofac Res. 2019;22(1):9–15.
41. Brodie AG. Anatomy and physiology of the head and neck musculature. Am J Orthod. 1950;36(11):831–44.
42. Bibby RE, Preston CB. The hyoid triangle. Am J Orthod. 1981;80(1):92–7.
43. Mukai S. Laryngeal movements during wind instruments playing. Nihon Jibiinkoka Gakkai Kaiho. 1989;92(2):260–70.
44. Eckley CA. Glottic configuration in wind instrument players. Rev Bras Otorrinolaingol. 2006;72(1):45–7.
45. Trollinger VL, Satallof RT. Respiratory behaviors and vocal tract issues in wind instrumentalists. In: Sataloff RT, editor. Professional voice: the science and art of clinical care. 4th ed. San Diego: Plural Publishing; 2017. p. 1017–28.
46. Cappellaro J, Beber BC. Vocal tract discomfort and voice-related quality of life in wind instrumentalists. J Voice. 2018;32(3):314–8.
47. Trollinger V. Relationships among self-reported vocal and laryngeal health and performance career success in professional wind instrumentalists. The international voice symposium 48th annual symposium "Care of the Professional Voice"; 2019; Philadelphia, PA.
48. Brattström V, Odenrick L, Kvam E. Dentofacial morphology in children playing musical wind instruments: a longitudinal study. Eur J Orthod. 1989;11(2):179–85.
49. Grammatopoulos E. A study of the effects of playing a wind instrument on the occlusion [Doctoral dissertation]. University of Birmingham, UK; 2009.
50. Grammatopoulos E, White AP, Dhopatkar A. Effects of playing a wind instrument on the occlusion. Am J Orthod Dentofac Orthop. 2012;141(2):138–45.
51. Herman E. Influence of musical instruments on tooth positions. Am J Orthod. 1981;80(2):145–55.
52. Kula K, Cilingir HZ, Eckert G, Dagg J, Ghoneima A. The association of malocclusion and trumpet performance. Angle Orthod. 2016;86(1):108–14.
53. Shimada T. A morphological study on the effect of wind instruments on the Dento-Oral region. J Nihon Univ Sch Dent. 1978;20(1–4):23–36.
54. Gualtieri PA. May Johnny or Janie play the clarinet? The Eastman Study: a report on the orthodontic evaluations of college-level and professional musicians who play brass and woodwind instruments. Am J Orthod. 1979;76(3):260–76.
55. Fuhrimann S, Schüpbach A, Thüer U, Ingervall B. Natural lip function in wind instrument players. Eur J Orthod. 1987;9(1):216–23.
56. Rindisbacher T, Hirschi U, Ingervall B, Geering A. Little influence on tooth position from playing a wind instrument. Angle Orthod. 1990;60(3):223–8.

Medical Disorders and Treatments in Professional Voice Users and Wind Instrumentalists

7

Robert Thayer Sataloff, Mary J. Hawkshaw, and Johnathan Brandon Sataloff

Physicians, dentists, music teachers, and musicians routinely encounter patients/students with medical conditions in, or distant from, the head and neck that may affect performances. Familiarity with these conditions helps optimize care. Laryngologists specializing in voice devote the majority of their practices to the medical management of benign voice disorders. Although most of us are active surgeons, the good voice specialist takes pride in avoiding the need for laryngeal surgery through expert medical management. Success depends not only on a good laryngologist but also on the availability of a voice team, including a speech-language pathologist, voice scientist, singing voice specialist, and medical consultants who have acquired special knowledge about voice disorders (neurologists, pulmonologists, endocrinologists, internists, allergists, and others). This chapter provides an overview of many of the benign voice problems encountered by health care providers and current nonsurgical management concepts.

Numerous medical conditions affect the voice adversely. Many have their origins primarily outside the head and neck. This chapter is not intended to be all inclusive but rather to highlight some of the more common and important conditions found in professional voice users and wind instrumentalists seeking medical care.

In the 2286 cases of all forms of voice disorders reported by Brodnitz in 1971 [1], 80% were attributed to voice abuse or to psychogenic factors resulting in vocal dysfunction. Of these patients, 20% had organic voice disorders. Of women with organic problems, about 15% had identifiable endocrine causes. A much higher incidence of organic disorders, particularly reflux laryngitis, acute infectious laryngitis, and benign vocal fold masses, is found in the author's (RTS) practice.

Voice Abuse

When voice abuse is suspected or observed in a patient with vocal complaints, he or she should be referred to a laryngologist who specializes in voice, preferably a physician affiliated with a voice care team.

Common patterns of voice abuse and misuse will not be discussed in detail in this chapter. They are covered elsewhere in the literature [2]. Voice abuse and/or misuse should be suspected particularly in patients who complain of voice fatigue associated with voice use or playing wind instruments, whose voices are worse at the end of a working day or week, and in any patient who is chronically hoarse. Technical errors in voice use or instrument performance technique may be the primary etiology of a voice complaint or may develop secondarily as a result of a patient's efforts to compensate for voice disturbance from another cause.

Speaking in noisy environments such as cars and airplanes is particularly abusive to the voice, as are backstage greetings, post-performance

A.-L. Hamdan et al., *Dentofacial Anomalies*, https://doi.org/10.1007/978-3-030-69109-7_7

parties, choral conducting, voice teaching, cheerleading, and many other activities. With proper training, all these vocal activities can be done safely. However, most patients, surprisingly even singers, have little or no training for their speaking voice.

If voice abuse is caused by speaking, treatment should be provided by a licensed, certified speech-language pathologist in the United States or by a phoniatrist in many other countries. In many cases, training the speaking voice will benefit singers greatly not only by improving speech but also by indirectly helping singing technique. Physicians should not hesitate to recommend such training, but it should be performed by an expert speech-language pathologist who specializes in voice. Many speech-language pathologists who are well trained in swallowing rehabilitation, articulation therapy, and other techniques are not trained in voice therapy for the speaking voice, and virtually none are trained through their speech and language programs to work with singing unless they are also singing teachers or singing voice specialists.

Specialized singing training also may be helpful to many voice patients who are not singers, and it is invaluable for patients who are singers. Initial singing training teaches relaxation techniques, develops muscle strength, and is symbiotic with standard voice therapy. Abuse of the voice during singing is an even more complex problem, as discussed elsewhere in this book.

Approaches to wind instrument technical problems that may be associated with dysphonia are discussed in Chap. 4.

Infection and Inflammation

Upper Respiratory Tract Infection Without Laryngitis

Although mucosal irritation usually is diffuse, patients sometimes have marked nasal obstruction with little or no sore throat and a "normal" voice. If the laryngeal examination showed no abnormality, a singer or professional speaker with a "head cold" should be permitted to use his or her voice and be advised not to try to duplicate his or her usual sound but rather accept the insurmountable alterations in self-perception caused by the change in the supraglottic vocal tract and auditory system. The decision as to whether performing under the circumstances is advisable professionally rests with the voice professional and his or her musical associates. The patient should be cautioned against throat clearing, as this is traumatic and may produce laryngitis. If a cough is present, nonnarcotic medications should be used to suppress it. In addition, the patient should be taught how to "silent cough," which is less traumatic. "Cold sores" or dry, split lips or tongue also may interfere with singing, although they are far more troublesome for wind instrumentalists, as are dental braces which can traumatize mucosal surfaces and affect performance in instrument (or voice) performance.

Laryngitis with Serious Vocal Fold Injury

Hemorrhage in the vocal folds and mucosal disruption associated with acute laryngitis are contraindications to speaking and singing. When these are observed, treatment includes strict voice rest in addition to correction of any underlying disease. If the patient also plays a wind instrument, laryngoscopy while playing will determine whether there is vocal fold contact during wind performance (there is in many players, but not all). If so, instrument playing should be stopped during the period of voice rest. Vocal fold hemorrhage in voice professionals is most common in premenstrual women who are using aspirin products or non-steroidal anti-inflammatory drugs (NSAIDs) for dysmenorrhea. Severe hemorrhage or mucosal scarring may result in permanent alternations in vocal fold vibratory function. In rare instances, surgical intervention may be necessary. The potential gravity of these conditions must be stressed, for singers are generally reluctant to cancel an appearance. As von

Leden observed, it is a pleasure to work with "people who are determined that the show must go on when everyone else is determined to goof off" [3]. However, patient compliance is essential when serious damage has occurred. At present, acute treatment of vocal fold hemorrhage is controversial. Most laryngologists allow the hematoma to resolve spontaneously. Because this sometimes results in an organized hematoma and scar formation requiring surgery, some physicians advocate incision along the superior edge of the vocal fold and drainage of the hematoma in selected cases. Further study is needed to determine optimal therapy guidelines (Figs. 7.1 and 7.2).

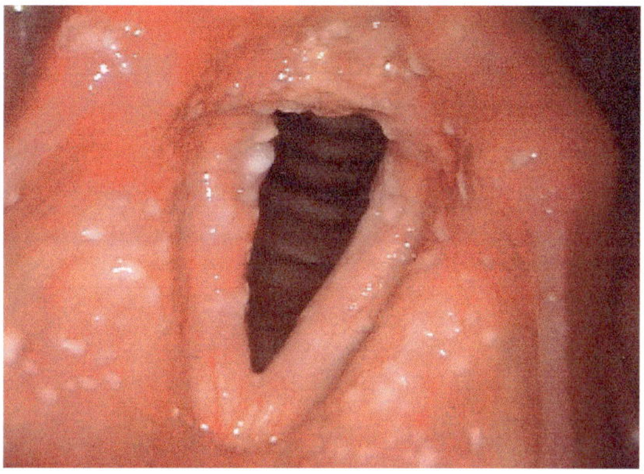

Fig. 7.2 Strobovideolaryngoscopy in this 65-year-old female shows the white, lacy, diffuse plaques embedded in inflamed mucosal surfaces. This appearance is typical of fungal laryngitis, caused most commonly by *Candida albicans*. (Figure 45.1 from Sataloff RT et al. 4). (Republished from Sataloff et al. [118]; with permission)

Laryngitis Without Serious Damage

Mild to moderate edema and erythema of the vocal folds may result from infection or from noninfectious causes. In the absence of mucosal disruption or hemorrhage, they are not absolute contraindications to voice use (including wind instrument performance in selected cases). Noninfectious laryngitis commonly is associated with excessive voice use in pre-performance rehearsals. It also may be caused by other forms of voice abuse and by mucosal irritation produced by allergy, smoke inhalation, and other causes. Mucous stranding between the anterior and middle thirds of the vocal folds is seen commonly in inflammatory laryngitis. Laryngitis sicca (dry voice) is associated with dehydration, dry atmosphere, mouth breathing, and antihistamine therapy (although antihistamines actually cause more mucous thickening than dehydration). Deficiency of mucosal lubrication causes irritation and coughing and results in mild inflammation. If no pressing professional need for performance exists, inflammatory conditions of the larynx are treated best with relative voice rest in addition to other modalities. However, in some instances, speaking and singing may be permitted. The patient should be instructed to avoid all forms of irritation and to rest the voice at all times except during warm-up and performance. Corticosteroids and other medications discussed later may be helpful. If mucosal secretions are copious, low-dose antihistamine therapy may be beneficial, but it must be prescribed with caution and generally should be avoided. Copious, thin secretions are better than scant, thick secretions or excessive dryness. The patient with laryngitis must be kept well hydrated to maintain the

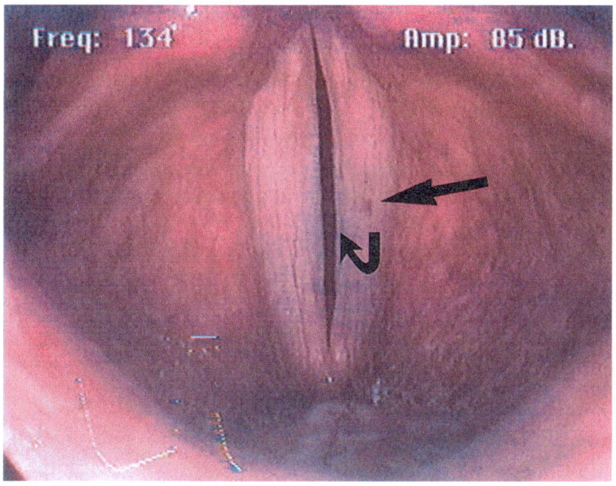

Fig. 7.1 Video print obtained from a strobovideolaryngoscopic examination shows diffuse erythema from acute laryngitis. Additionally, there is a left sulcus vocalis. Also visible is an ecstatic vessel on the superior surface of the left vocal fold (straight arrow). (Figure 40.1 from Sataloff RT et al. 4). (Republished from Sataloff et al. [118]; with permission)

desired character of mucosal lubrication. The patient should be instructed to "pee pale," consuming enough water to keep urine diluted. Psychological support is crucial. For example, it is often helpful for the physician to intercede on a singer's behalf and to convey "doctor's orders" directly to agents or theater management. Such mitigation of exogenous stress can be highly therapeutic.

Infectious laryngitis may be caused by bacteria or viruses. Subglottic involvement frequently indicates a more severe infection, which may be difficult to control in a short period of time. Indiscriminate use of antibiotics must be avoided; however, when the physician is in doubt as to the cause and when a major voice commitment is imminent, vigorous antibiotic treatment is warranted. In this circumstance, the damage caused by allowing progression of a curable condition is greater than the damage that might result from a course of therapy for an unproven microorganism while culture results are pending. When a major concert or speech is not imminent, indications for therapy are the same as for the nonsinger or nonprofessional speaker.

Voice rest (absolute or relative) is an important therapeutic consideration in any case of laryngitis. When no professional commitments are pending, a short course of absolute voice rest may be considered, as it is the safest and most conservative therapeutic intervention. This means absolute silence and communication with a writing pad or electronic device. The patient must be instructed not to whisper, as this may be an even more traumatic vocal activity than speaking softly. However, exceptions can be made for patients who do not make vocal fold contact when they whisper, as determined during flexible laryngoscopy. Whistling through the lips also involves vocal fold contact in many people and should not be permitted unless laryngoscopy has confirmed that the instrumentalist does not make vocal fold contact while playing. The playing of many musical wind instruments also should not be permitted. Absolute voice rest is necessary only for serious vocal fold injury such as hemorrhage or mucosal disruption (Fig. 7.3). Even then, it is virtually never indicated for more than 7–10 days. Three days are often sufficient. Some excellent laryngologists do not believe voice rest should be used at all. However, absolute voice rest for a few days may be helpful in patients with laryngitis, especially those gregarious, verbal singers who find it difficult to moderate their voice use to comply with relative voice rest instructions. In many instances, considerations of finances and reputation mitigate against a recommendation of voice rest. In advising performers to minimize vocal use, Punt counseled, "Don't say a single word for which you are not being paid" [4].

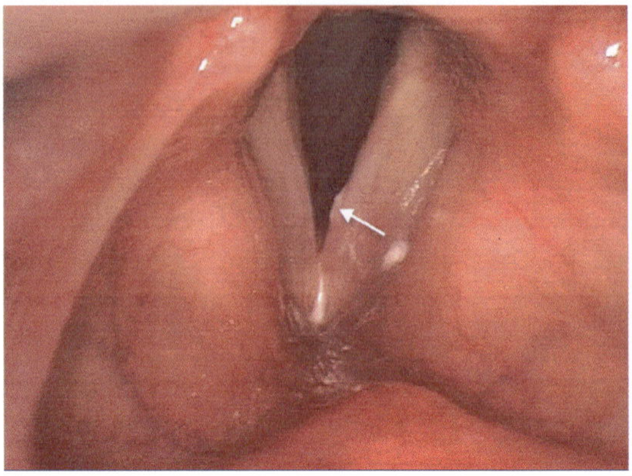

Fig. 7.3 Mucosal tear (arrow) of the vibratory margin of the left vocal fold in a 27-year-old tenor with sudden voice change. This lesion resolved completely with voice rest. (Republished from Sataloff et al. [118]; with permission)

This admonition frequently guides the ailing singer or speaker away from pre-performance conversations and backstage greetings and allows a successful series of performances. Patients also should be instructed to speak softly and as infrequently as possible, often at a slightly higher pitch than usual; to avoid excessive telephone use; and to speak with abdominal support as they would in singing. This is relative voice rest, and it is helpful in most cases. An urgent session with a speech-language pathologist is extremely helpful for discussing vocal hygiene and providing guidelines to prevent voice abuse. Nevertheless, the patient must be aware that some risk is associated with performing with laryngitis even when performance is possible. Inflammation of the vocal folds is associated with increased capillary fragility and increased risk of vocal fold injury or hemorrhage. Many factors must be considered in determining whether a given speech or concert is important enough to justify the potential consequences.

Steam inhalations deliver moisture and heat to the vocal folds and tracheobronchial tree and may be useful. Some people use nasal irrigations, although these have little proven value for voice disorders. Gargling has no proven efficacy, but it is probably harmful only if it involves loud, abusive vocalization as part of the gargling process. Some physicians and patients believe it to be helpful in "moistening the throat," and it may have some relaxing or placebo effect. Ultrasonic treatments, local massage, psychotherapy, and biofeedback directed at relieving anxiety and decreasing muscle tension may be helpful adjuncts to a broader therapeutic program. However, psychotherapy and biofeedback, in particular, must be expertly supervised if used at all.

Voice lessons given by an expert teacher are invaluable. When technical dysfunction is suggested, the singer or actor should be referred to his or her teacher or to a singing voice specialist in a medical setting. Even when an obvious organic abnormality is present, referral to a voice teacher is appropriate, especially for younger actors and singers. Numerous "tricks of the trade" permit a voice professional to overcome some of the impairments of mild illness safely. If a singer plans to proceed with a performance during an illness, he or she should not cancel voice lessons as part of the relative voice rest regimen; rather, a short lesson to ensure optimal technique is extremely useful.

Sinusitis

Chronic inflammation of the mucosa lining the sinus cavities commonly produces thick secretions known as postnasal drip. Postnasal drip can be particularly problematic because it causes excessive phlegm, which interferes with phonation, and because it leads to frequent throat clearing, which may inflame the vocal folds. Sometimes chronic sinusitis is caused by allergies and can be treated with medications. However, many medications used for this condition cause side effects that are unacceptable in professional voice users, particularly mucosal drying. When medication management is not satisfactory, functional endoscopic sinus surgery may be appropriate [5]. Acute purulent sinusitis is a different matter. It requires aggressive treatment with antibiotics, sometimes surgical drainage, treatment of underlying conditions (such as dental abscess), and occasionally surgery [5].

Lower Respiratory Tract Infection

Lower respiratory tract infection may be almost as disruptive to a voice as upper respiratory tract infection. Bronchitis, pneumonitis, pneumonia, and especially reactive airway disease impair the power source of the voice and lead to vocal strain and sometimes injury. Lower respiratory tract infections should be treated aggressively, pulmonary function tests should be considered, and bronchodilators (preferably oral rather than inhaled) should be used as necessary. Coughing is also a very traumatic vocal activity, and careful attention should be paid to cough suppression. If extensive voice use is anticipated, nonnarcotic antitussive agents are preferable because narcotics may dull the sensorium and lead to potentially damaging voice or instrument performance technique.

COVID-19

COVID-19, or SARS-CoV-2 infection, also known as the novel corona virus, may be asymptomatic, may cause mild URI symptoms, or may cause devastating symptoms including death. Cough, fever and chills, shortness of breath, sore throat, fatigue, nausea and vomiting, diarrhea, and other symptoms are common. Loss of taste and smell were recognized early as symptoms of COVID-19. However, COVID-19 also may cause many other neurological effects including vocal fold paresis and paralysis. When the disease affects the lower respiratory tract severely, it can impair respiratory function permanently. This undermines the support needed to provide power for phonation (speaking, as well as singing) and wind instrument performance. Such problems lead commonly to compensatory hyperfunction. If the respiratory compromise is severe enough, it may disable a performer permanently; and since excellent respiratory function is required for singing, projected speech and wind performance (as well as for high level athletic activity), relatively "mild" pulmonary compromise can be severe enough to impair or end a performance career.

Tonsillitis

Tonsillitis also impairs the voice through alterations of the resonator system and through technical changes secondary to pain, and it can interfere with wind instrument playing. Although there is a tendency to avoid tonsillectomy, especially in professional voice users, the operation should not be withheld when clear indications for tonsillectomy are present. These include, for example, documented severe bacterial tonsillitis 6 times per year. However, patients must be warned that tonsillectomy may alter the sound of the voice, even though there is no change at the vocal fold (oscillator) level. The implications of tonsillectomy for wind instrument players remain uncertain.

Lyme Disease

Lyme disease, as it is known today, has been reported for over a hundred years, but the bacteria responsible for the disease was not identified until 1982. It was discovered in Lyme, Connecticut, when a group of children contracted arthritis inexplicably, and research was initiated to identify the cause [6]. Due to its ability to appear similar to many other diseases and its wide range of nonspecific symptoms, Lyme disease often goes undiagnosed. If not recognized and treated, this condition can have profound consequences including damage to the inner ear, the eighth cranial nerve, and the facial nerve as reviewed by Sataloff and Sataloff (from which a portion of this section has been modified, with permission) [7]. It also can affect laryngeal nerves. Lyme disease is one of many common illnesses that can cause special problems for singers and other voice professionals, and for wind instrumentalists. Lyme disease is an increasingly prevalent infection in many parts of the United States and elsewhere. It can affect the larynx directly by causing unilateral or bilateral vocal fold paresis/ paralysis or interfere with other parts of the vocal tract by causing joint pains that impair posture and support, temporomandibular joint pain that leads to technical changes, and in other ways [8]. It is important for health care providers and music professionals to be familiar with this common problem in order to improve the chances of prompt diagnosis and treatment.

Epidemiology

In the United States, Lyme disease is known to be endemic particularly in northeastern, mid-Atlantic, and north-central states, with expansion into some parts of the southwest [9]. Approximately 60% of initial infections occur during the summer when it is warm and people are outside [10]. Lyme disease has no sex or age predilection.

Etiology

Lyme disease is an illness caused by a spirochete infection. Like syphilis, another spirochete infection, the clinical presentations may vary. Sir William Osler once termed syphilis "the great imitator," and likewise, Lyme disease has a broad clinical spectrum.

Lyme disease had many different names given to it until Steere, in 1977, recognized it as a multistage systemic disease [11]. In 1982, Burgdorfer et al. isolated the infectious organism from the belly of a tick, while studying a group of children with unexplained arthritis in Lyme, Connecticut [12]. He named this spirochete *Borrelia burgdorferi*. *Borrelia burgdorferi* is the primary cause of Lyme disease. However, *Borrelia garinii* and

Borrelia afzelii also have been implicated and reported as common causes of Lyme neuroborreliosis in Europe [13]. Many different vectors have been listed as contributors to this disease. However, the tick seems to be the main culprit transmitting the spirochete. In the Northeast, the tick *Ixodes dammini* is the most common, and in the West, *Ixodes pacificus* has been implicated [9]. The ticks carry the disease in their stomachs and transmit it while feeding on the blood of their victims which can take up to 2 days. In many cases, the ticks are noticed and removed or washed away before the disease can be spread, but sometimes a tick is small enough to avoid notice. Even when definitive symptoms occur, the tick often is not found, and the classic target rash may have been absent or gone unnoticed. Therefore, the opportunity for early diagnosis often is missed, and many people carry Lyme disease into later stages of the disorder, during which nerve and vascular problems can occur, before the condition is diagnosed [7].

The tick life cycle has three stages: larva, nymph, and adult [11]. In each stage, the tick acquires a blood meal and may obtain the spirochete from an infected host such as the white-tailed deer or white-footed mouse.

The exact nature of injury to humans is not known, but evidence exists for three possible mechanisms. These theories include direct invasion, immunological attack, and vasculitis [14].

Otolaryngologic Findings

The clinical spectrum of Lyme disease is broken down into three stages. In stage 1, a rash named erythema chronicum migrans follows the tick bite in 6–80% of cases [15]. The rash has an outer red circular or oval border with a clear central area. These lesions are called "target rash." The outer red zone is felt to represent the best area for biopsy when trying to isolate the organism for culture. This rash may follow or precede cold or flu-like symptoms. The rash usually occurs within a few days of the tick bite but may show up as long as a month later [16].

Other symptoms during this stage include fatigue, fever, chills, sore throat, headache, cough, chest pain, abdominal pain, muscle aches, loss of appetite, dizziness, lymphadenopathy, backache, conjunctivitis, enlarged liver and spleen, arthritis, and low-grade fever.

The patient usually calls on an otolaryngologist during stage 2 of Lyme disease. Although facial paralysis is the most common complaint in these patients, other symptoms may occur [10, 17]. They include hoarseness from involvement of the recurrent laryngeal nerve or inability to sustain a high note or project the voice due to injury to the superior laryngeal nerve among other symptoms. In 1988, Schroeter reported a case of a 45-year-old singer who developed left vocal fold paralysis and had positive antibodies to *Borrelia burgdorferi* [18]. The patient was treated with antibiotics for 6 weeks, during which time there was resolution of the vocal fold paralysis and dramatic reduction of the Lyme titers.

Stage 2 also may include a skin lesion called lymphadenosis benigna cutis. This lesion has another name, *Borrelia* lymphocytoma, and is characterized by lymphocytic infiltration of the dermis or subcutaneous tissue [19]. The lesion has a blue-red color with gross swelling.

Patients may have involvement of the temporomandibular joint and complain of ear pain or pain when chewing. Other joints may be involved such as the neck, knees, hips, shoulders, ankles, and elbows. Finger, wrist, elbow, shoulder, and neck involvement can be troubling particularly for wind and other instrumentalists.

Patients also may have involvement of the cardiovascular system and may develop arrhythmias and/or lightheadedness. Failure to recognize these lesions may lead to increased morbidity and possible death.

Another skin lesion is seen in stage 3 of Lyme disease. It is termed "acrodermatitis chronic atrophicans" [19]. This lesion usually is seen in elderly patients and is often misdiagnosed as scleroderma or vascular insufficiency.

Diagnosis and Treatment

The ELISA test is the most sensitive and is used widely for Lyme disease [14]. Western blot technique is used to confirm the diagnosis. Other assays such as immunofluorescence antibody and cultures have been utilized with varying success. Results of all of these studies vary from lab to lab, and blood samples should be sent to labs that do large volumes of testing and have experience. The IgM antibody is seen early and is less specific. However, it is useful when reinfection or reactivation is suspected. The IgG antibody may take 6 weeks to appear and is good for assessing stages 2 and 3. False-positive tests occur in patients with mononucleosis, syphilis, or rheumatic fever [9, 14]. False negatives may be seen in patients on antibiotics or patients who are immunocompromised by diseases such as cancer or AIDS.

Antibiotics are the recommended treatment. For adults, doxycycline or tetracycline is effective. When intolerance to these medications is encountered, amoxicillin is used. Amoxicillin is preferred in children. Chloramphenicol may be used when there is allergy to cephalosporin or penicillin. When resistance to these medications is found, intravenous medication such as ceftriaxone is used. Lyme disease is complex; with proper recognition it is treatable and has an excellent prognosis.

Autoimmune Deficiency Syndrome (AIDS)

AIDS is a potentially lethal disease that has become common. Its incidence in the artistic community is probably somewhat higher than in the general public. Physicians should consider this diagnosis along with other causes of chronic debilitation and recurrent infections in the proper clinical setting in professional voice users and instrumentalists. Dry mouth and hoarseness are common complaints in patients with HIV infection. Candida infection of the oral cavity or tracheobronchial tree should make the clinician particularly suspicious. When fungal infections are encountered, particularly fungal laryngitis, it is important not only to treat the infection, but also to rule out serious predisposing causes such as HIV infection and other conditions that suppress the immune system. Recurrent respiratory tract infection and infection with unusual organisms also raise one's suspicions, but it should be remembered that infections with Haemophilus influenza, Streptococcus pneumonia, and common viruses are the most frequent pathogens in HIV-infected patients, just as they are in patients without HIV. Acute infectious laryngitis and epiglottis may occur in AIDS patients, but they are less common than mild chronic laryngitis, dry mouth, and frequent or persistent symptoms of a "cold."

Systemic Conditions

Aging

This subject is so important that is has been covered extensively in other literature [20]. Many characteristics associated with vocal aging are actually deficits in conditioning, rather than irreversible aging changes. For example, in singers, such problems as a "wobble," pitch inaccuracies (singing flat), and inability to sing softly are rarely caused by irreversible aging changes, and these problems usually can be managed easily through voice therapy and training.

Hearing Loss

Hearing loss is often overlooked as a source of vocal problems. Auditory feedback is fundamental to speaking and singing. Interference with this control mechanism may result in altered vocal production, particularly if the person is unaware of the hearing loss. Distortion, particularly pitch distortion (diplacusis), also may pose serious problems for the singer. This appears to cause not only aesthetic difficulties in matching pitch but also vocal strain, which accompanies pitch shifts [21]. Hearing impairment can cause vocal strain, particularly if a person has sensorineural hearing loss (involving the nerve or inner ear) and is unaware of it. This condition may lead people to speak or sing more loudly than they realize.

Respiratory Dysfunction

The importance of "the breath" has been well recognized in the field of voice pedagogy. Respiratory disorders are discussed at length in other literature [22].

Even a mild degree of obstructive pulmonary disease can result in substantial voice or wind performance problems. Unrecognized exercise-induced asthma is especially problematic in singers and actors, because bronchospasm may be precipitated by the exercise and airway drying that occurs during voice performance. In such cases, the bronchospastic obstruction on exhalation impairs support. This commonly results in compensatory hyperfunction.

Treatment requires skilled management and collaboration with a pulmonologist and a voice team [23]. Whenever possible, patients should be managed primarily with oral medications; the use of inhalers should be minimized. Steroid inhalers should be avoided altogether whenever possible for professional voice users. It is particularly important to recognize that asthma can be induced by the exercise of phonation or wind playing itself [24], and in many cases a high index of suspicion and methacholine challenge test are needed to avoid missing this important diagnosis.

Allergy

Even mild allergies are more incapacitating to professional voice users and wind instrumentalists than to others. This subject can be reviewed elsewhere [25]. Briefly, patients with mild intermittent allergies can usually be managed with antihistamines, although they should never be tried for the first time immediately prior to a voice performance. Because antihistamines commonly produce unacceptable side effects, trial and error may be needed in order to find a medication with an acceptable balance between effect and side effect for any individual patient, especially a voice professional. Patients with allergy-related voice disturbances may find hyposensitization a more effective approach than antihistamine use if they are candidates for such treatment. For voice patients with unexpected allergic symptoms immediately prior to an important voice commitment, corticosteroids should be used rather than antihistamines, in order to minimize the risks of side effects (such as drying and thickening of secretions) that might make voice performance difficult or impossible. Allergies commonly cause voice problems by altering the mucosa and secretions and causing nasal obstruction.

Laryngopharyngeal Reflux

Laryngopharyngeal reflux (LPR) is extremely common among voice patients, especially singers [26]. This is a condition in which the sphincter between the stomach and esophagus is inefficient, and acidic stomach secretions reflux (reach the laryngeal tissues), causing inflammation. The most typical symptoms are hoarseness in the morning, prolonged vocal warm-up time, postnasal drip, halitosis and a bitter taste in the morning, a feeling of a "lump in the throat," frequent throat clearing, chronic irritative cough, and frequent tracheitis or tracheobronchitis. Any or all of these symptoms may be present. Heartburn is not common in these patients, so the diagnosis is often missed. Prolonged reflux also is associated with the development of Barrett esophagus, esophageal carcinoma, and laryngeal carcinoma [26].

Physical examination usually reveals erythema (redness) of the arytenoid mucosa. A barium swallow radiographic study with water siphonage may provide additional information but is not needed routinely. However, if a patient complies strictly with treatment recommendations and does not show marked improvement within a month, or if there is a reason to suspect more serious pathology, a more comprehensive evaluation should be carried out. Twenty-four-hour pH impedance monitoring of the esophagus or pharyngeal pH monitoring is often effective in establishing a diagnosis. The results are correlated with a diary of the patient's activities and symptoms. Endoscopic examination of the esophagus should be considered for many patients. Bulimia should also be considered in the differential diagnosis when symptoms are refractory to treatment and other physical and psychologic signs are suggestive.

The mainstays of treatment for reflux laryngitis are elevation of the head of the bed (not just sleeping on pillows), antacids, proton pump inhibitors and H2 blockers, low acid diet, alkaline water, alginate, and avoidance of eating for 3–4 hours before going to sleep. This is often difficult for singers and actors, as well as wind instrumentalists, because of their performance schedules, but if they are counseled about minor changes in eating habits (such as eating larger meals at breakfast and lunch), usually they can comply. Avoidance of alcohol, caffeine, and specific foods is beneficial. Medications that decrease or block acid production may be necessary. It must be recognized that control of acidity is not the same as control of reflux. In many cases, reflux is provoked during singing or wind instrument playing because of the increased abdominal pressure associated with support. In these instances, it often causes excessive phlegm and throat clearing during the first 10 or 15 minutes of a performance or lesson, as well as other common laryngopharyngeal symptoms, even when acidity has been neutralized effectively. Laparoscopic Nissen fundoplication has proven extremely effective and should be considered a reasonable alternative to lifelong medication in this relatively young patient population [26].

Endocrine Dysfunction

Endocrine (hormonal) problems warrant special attention. The human voice is extremely sensitive to endocrinologic changes. Many of these are reflected in alterations of fluid content of the lamina propria just beneath the laryngeal mucosa. This causes alterations in the bulk and shape of the vocal folds and results in voice change. Hypothyroidism is a well-recognized cause of such voice disorders, although the mechanism is not understood fully [27–30]. Hoarseness, voice fatigue, muffling of the voice, loss of range, and a sensation of a lump in the throat may be present even with mild hypothyroidism. Even when thyroid function tests results are within the low normal range, this diagnosis should be considered, especially if thyroid-stimulating hormone levels are in the high-normal range or are elevated. Thyrotoxicosis may result in similar voice disturbances [30, 31].

Voice changes associated with sex hormones are encountered commonly in clinical practice and have been investigated more thoroughly than have other hormonal changes. Although a correlation appears to exist between sex hormone levels and depth of male voices (higher testosterone and lower estradiol levels in basses than in tenors) [32], the most important hormonal considerations in males occur during the maturation process.

When castrato singers were in vogue, castration at about age 7 or 8 years resulted in failure of laryngeal growth during puberty, and voices that stayed in the soprano or alto range and boasted a unique quality of sound [33]. Failure of a male voice to change at puberty is uncommon today and is often psychogenic in etiology [1]. However, hormonal deficiencies such as those seen in cryptorchidism, delayed sexual development, Klinefelter syndrome, or Fröhlich syndrome may be responsible. In these cases, the persistently high voice may be the complaint that causes the patient to seek medical attention.

Voice problems related to sex hormones are most common in female singers [34]. Although voice changes associated with the normal menstrual cycle may be difficult to quantify with current experimental techniques, unquestionably they occur [2, 34–38]. Most of the ill effects seen in the immediate premenstrual period are known as laryngopathia premenstrualis. This common condition is caused by physiologic, anatomic, and psychologic alterations secondary to endocrine changes. The vocal dysfunction is characterized by decreased vocal efficiency, loss of the highest notes in the voice, voice fatigue, slight hoarseness, and some muffling of the voice. It is often more apparent to the singer than to the listener. It was recognized long ago that submucosal hemorrhages in the larynx are more common in the premenstrual period [36], and premenstrual vascular changes have been confirmed over the ensuing decades. In many European opera houses, singers used to be excused from singing during the premenstrual and early menstrual days ("grace days"). This practice was not followed in the United States and is no longer in vogue anywhere. Premenstrual changes cause significant vocal symptoms in approximately one-third of singers. Although ovulation inhibitors were shown long ago to mitigate some of these symptoms [37], in some women (about 5%) first-generation birth control pills used to deleteriously alter voice range and character even after only a few months of therapy [39–43]. However, modern oral contraceptives usually do not produce such problems and may even improve voice [42]. Under crucial performance circumstances, oral contraceptives may be used to alter the time of menstruation, but this practice is justified only in unusual situations. Symptoms similar to laryngopathia premenstrualis also occur in some women at the time of ovulation.

Pregnancy results frequently in voice alterations known as laryngopathia gravidarum. The changes may be similar to premenstrual symptoms or may be perceived as desirable changes. In some cases, alterations produced by pregnancy are permanent [44, 45]. Although hormonally induced changes in the larynx and respiratory mucosa secondary to menstruation and pregnancy are discussed widely in the literature, references to the important alterations in abdominal support are scarce. Abdominal distention during pregnancy also interferes with abdominal muscle function. Any singer or wind instrumentalist whose abdominal support is compromised substantially should be discouraged from strenuous practice or performance until the abdominal impairment has resolved.

Estrogens are helpful in postmenopausal singers and should be administered under the supervision of a gynecologist or endocrinologist as potential systemic side effects have been described. Under no circumstances should androgens be given to female singers even in small amounts if any reasonable therapeutic alternative exists. Clinically, these drugs are used most commonly to treat endometriosis or postmenopausal loss of libido. Androgens cause unsteadiness of the voice, rapid changes of timbre, and lowering of the fundamental frequency (masculinization) [46–50]. These changes have been known for decades but still occur not only from illicit drug use for body building, but also iatrogenically. These changes are usually permanent.

Recently, we have seen increasing abuse of anabolic steroids among bodybuilders and other athletes. In addition to their many other hazards, these medications may alter the voice. They are (or are closely related to) male hormones; consequently, they are capable of producing masculinization of the voice. Lowering of the fundamental frequency and coarsening of the voice produced in this fashion are similar to a boy's voice change at puberty and generally are irreversible.

Other hormonal disturbances may also produce voice dysfunction. In addition to the thyroid gland and the gonads, the parathyroid, adrenal, pineal, and pituitary glands are included in this system. Other endocrine disturbances may alter voice, as well. For example, pancreatic dysfunction may cause xerophonia (dry voice), as in diabetes mellitus. Thymic abnormalities can lead to feminization of the voice [51], and thymomas may cause laryngeal myasthenia gravis that produces voice instability and fatigue.

Neurologic Disorders

Numerous neurologic conditions may adversely affect the voice. They are discussed in other literature [2]. Some of them, such as myasthenia gravis, are amenable to medical therapy with drugs such as pyridostigmine (Mestinon). Such therapy frequently restores the voice to normal. An exhaustive neurolaryngologic discussion is beyond the scope of this chapter. Nevertheless, when evaluating voice dysfunction, health care providers must consider numerous neurologic problems, including Parkinson disease, essential tremor, various other disorders that produce tremor, drug-induced tremor, multiple sclerosis, dystonias, and many other conditions. Spasmodic dysphonia (SD), a laryngeal dystonia, presents particularly challenging problems. This subject is covered in detail elsewhere [2]. Focal dystonias that effect the mouth and lips can be troublesome for singers and other voice professionals, but they can be devastating for wind instrumentalists. The same is true for velopharyngeal insufficiency, a condition that is common among instrumentalists who play clarinet, oboe, saxophone, bassoon, French horn, trumpet, coronet, and other wind instruments. People who play these instruments often develop velopharyngeal insufficiency (VPI) which also is more likely to disable a wind player than a singer. In addition, wind instrumentalists (some of whom are also singers) develop a variety of other problems such as pneumoparotitis. Stuttering also provides unique challenges. Although still poorly understood, this condition is noted for its tendency to affect speech while sparing singing.

Vocal Fold Hypomobility

Vocal fold hypomobility may be caused by paralysis (no movement), paresis (partial movement), arytenoid dislocation, cricoarytenoid joint dysfunction, tumor, laryngeal fracture, and other causes. Differentiating among these conditions is often more complicated than it appears to be at first glance. A comprehensive discussion is beyond the scope of this chapter, and the reader is referred to other literature [2]. In addition to a comprehensive history and physical examination, evaluation commonly includes strobovideolaryngoscopy, objective voice assessment, laryngeal electromyography, and high-resolution computed tomography (CT) or magnetic resonance imaging (MRI) of the larynx and related neurological structures. Most vocal fold motion disorders are amenable to treatment. Voice therapy should be used first in virtually all cases. Even in many patients with recurrent laryngeal nerve paralysis, voice therapy alone is often sufficient. When therapy fails to produce adequate voice improvement in the patient's opinion, surgical intervention is appropriate and usually is effective.

General Health

As with any other athletic activity, optimal voice use requires reasonably good general health and physical conditioning. Abdominal and respiratory strength and endurance are particularly important. If a person becomes short of breath from climbing two flights of stairs, he or she certainly does not have the physical stamina necessary for proper respiratory support for a speech, let alone a strenuous musical production. This deficiency usually results in abusive vocal habits used in vain attempts to compensate for the deficiencies.

Systemic illnesses, such as anemia, Lyme disease, mononucleosis, AIDS, chronic fatigue syndrome, or other diseases associated with malaise and weakness, may impair the ability of vocal musculature to recover rapidly from heavy use and may also be associated with alterations of mucosal secretions. Other systemic illnesses may be responsible for voice complaints, particularly if they impair the abdominal muscles necessary for breath support. For example, diarrhea and constipation that prohibit sustained abdominal contraction may be reasons for the physician to prohibit a strenuous singing or acting engagement. Health care providers should be familiar with laryngeal manifestations of systemic disease [52].

Any extremity injury, such as a sprained ankle, may alter posture and therefore interfere with customary abdominothoracic support. Voice patients are often unaware of this problem and develop abusive, hyperfunctional compensatory maneuvers in the neck and tongue musculature as a result. These technical flaws may produce voice complaints such as voice fatigue and neck pain that bring the performer to the physician's office for assessment and care. They even can produce structural lesions such as hemorrhage and nodules.

Obesity

Singers, actors, and many other professional voice users are verbal, oral people. Most enjoy singing, talking, and a good bowl of pasta after the show. Many excellent wind instrumentalists have similarly gregarious personalities. However, before indulging our passions for culinary excess, it is important to understand the impact of obesity not only on singing performance, but also on general health and longevity [53].

For medical reasons, when obesity becomes extreme, serious measures may be necessary to accomplish weight loss. The most severely overweight patients have an entity called "morbid obesity." This condition is diagnosed when a person is more than 100 pounds or 100% over ideal body weight. Morbid obesity is extremely common in our society. It is estimated that 34 million adult Americans (1 of every 5 people over the age of 19) have significant obesity. As little as 20% excess over desirable body weight may be enough to constitute a health hazard. Doctors have long been aware of the difficulty in controlling weight problems with medical treatment alone. Of all patients who lose weight, 90% regain it at some point in their lives, and many even exceed their original weight. This led doctors to consider surgery as an option in treating this problem in selected cases.

In February 1985, a panel of experts from the National Institutes of Health looked at health problems associated with obesity [54]. Opinions have not changed substantially since that time. They concluded that obesity has adverse effects on health and longevity.

1. Obesity creates enormous psychological stress, which is a problem not well understood by the general population. Large people are unpopular, discriminated against in the workplace, and considered lazy.
2. Obesity is associated with high blood pressure. Obese people have high blood pressure three times more often than nonobese people.
3. Obesity is associated with higher levels of cholesterol.
4. Obesity is associated with diabetes. As with high blood pressure, this is seen three times more commonly in obese individuals.
5. Obesity is a factor in the development of heart disease.
6. Obesity increases the risk of developing certain cancers, specifically those of the uterus, breast, cervix, and gall bladder in women, and the colon, rectum, and prostate in men.
7. Obese individuals have a shorter life span.
8. Obesity is related to respiratory problems and arthritis.

With weight loss, all of these problems can be improved substantially, and prolongation of life is possible.

The best treatment for obesity is avoidance of the problem. Early in training, singers and other voice professionals, as well as all other performers, should learn the importance of good physical and aerobic conditioning. This is important to the voice professional's general health, vocal health, and art. Even a moderate degree of obesity may affect the respiratory system adversely, undermining support. Weight reduction is recommended for people who are 20% or more above ideal weight. In the singer, weight should be lost slowly through modification of eating and lifestyle habits. Loss of 2 or 3 pounds per week is plenty. More rapid loss of weight causes fluid shifts and hormonal alterations that may result in changes in vocal quality and endurance. Although these changes appear to be temporary, the effects of weight loss on vocal function have not been studied adequately; therefore, we do not have answers to all the pertinent questions. It is certainly possible for a singer to lose weight too quickly, but we are not yet sure how much weight loss is too much. Studies should be encouraged to learn more about this problem. However, it appears that maintenance of ideal body weight is probably as healthy for the voice as it is for the rest of the body. For people 20–100% above ideal body weight, weight loss can be accomplished with a medically supervised diet and exercise. However, people who are morbidly obese frequently are unable to lose weight by dietary or medical means alone. Morbidly obese patients may be candidates for surgery to help control their weight problems.

Although several kinds of obesity operations exist, the older procedures have troublesome side effects. At present, the best methods are a form of gastric restrictive surgery, known as the gastric bypass and gastric banding. Postoperatively, weight loss occurs over 12 to 18 months and stops as ideal body weight is approached. In most cases, singing may be resumed at about 6 weeks following abdominal surgery. Although the effects on the voice are not yet documented fully, there does not appear to be any significant problem associated with slow weight loss in patients with morbid obesity. Although further study is necessary to confirm these impressions, in singers or actors with this degree of weight problem, considerations of longevity, heart condition, blood pressure, and other critical health matters may outweigh immediate voice concerns.

For most singers, an extra 10, 20, or 30 pounds is not perceived as much of a problem. However, as 20 becomes 30, and 30 becomes 40, substantial adverse effects occur in the body in general and the vocal tract specifically. In training, singers and actors should be encouraged to treat their entire bodies with the same reverence with which they regard their vocal folds. Self-respect as a professional athlete is a sound basis for a long vocal career—and a long life.

Anxiety

Voice professionals, especially singers and actors, are frequently sensitive and communicative people. When the principal cause of vocal dysfunction is anxiety, the physician often can accomplish much by assuring the patient that no organic problem is present and by stating that the diagnosis of anxiety reaction. The patient should be counseled that anxiety is normal and that recognition of it as the principle problem frequently allows the performer to overcome it. Tranquilizers and sedatives are rarely necessary and often are undesirable because they may interfere with fine motor control. For example, beta-adrenergic blocking agents such as propranolol hydrochloride have become popular among performers for the treatment of pre-performance anxiety. Beta-blockers are not recommended for regular use; they have significant effects on the cardiovascular system and many potential complications, including hypotension, thrombocytopenic purpura, mental depression, agranulocytosis, laryngospasm with respiratory distress, and bronchospasm. In addition, their efficacy is controversial. Although they may have a favorable effect in relieving performance anxiety, beta-blockers may produce a noticeable adverse effect on singing performance [55]. The effect on instrumental performance seems to be less prominent, but more research is needed.

Although these drugs have a place under occasional, extraordinary circumstances, their routine use for this purpose not only is potentially hazardous but also violates an important therapeutic principle. Performers have chosen a career that exposes them to the public. If such persons are so incapacitated by anxiety that they are unable to perform the routine functions of their chosen profession without chemical help, this should be considered symptomatic of an important underlying psychologic problem. For a performer to depend on drugs to perform is neither routine nor healthy, whether the drug is a benzodiazepine, a barbiturate, a beta-blocker, or alcohol. If such dependence exists, psychologic evaluation by an experienced arts-medicine psychologist or psychiatrist should be considered [56, 57]. Obscuring the symptoms by fostering the dependence is insufficient. However, if the patient is on tour and will only be under a particular otolaryngologist's care for a week or so, the physician should not try to make major changes in his or her customary regimen. Rather, the physician should communicate with the performer's primary otolaryngologist or family physician to coordinate appropriate long-term care.

As professional voice users constitute a subset of society as a whole, all the psychiatric disorders encountered among the general public are seen from time to time in voice professionals and wind instrumentalists. In some cases, professional voice users require modification of the usual psychologic treatment, particularly with regard to psychotropic medications. Detailed discussion of this and related subjects can be found elsewhere [56, 57].

When voice professionals, especially singers and actors, have a significant vocal impairment that results in voice loss (or the prospect of voice loss), they often go through a psychologic process similar to grieving [56]. In some cases, fear of discovering that the voice is lost forever may unconsciously prevent patients from trying to use their voices optimally following injury or treatment. This can dramatically impede or prevent recovery of function following a perfect surgical result, for example. It is essential that otolaryngologists, performers, and their teachers be familiar with this fairly common scenario, and it is ideal to include an arts-medicine psychologist and/ or psychiatrist as part of the voice team.

Psychogenic voice disorders, incapacitating psychologic reactions to organic voice disorders, and other psychologic problems are encountered commonly in young voice patients. They are discussed in other literature [56].

Substance Abuse

The list of substances ingested, smoked, or "snorted" by many people is disturbingly long. Whenever possible, patients who care about vocal quality and longevity should be educated about the deleterious effects of such habits upon their voice and upon the longevity of their careers by their physicians and teachers. A few specific substances have already been discussed.

Other Diseases That May Affect the Voice

The larynx is subject to numerous acute and chronic infections. Some of them may be mistaken for malignancy and may be biopsied unnecessarily, exposing the patient (and sometimes the physician) to unnecessary risk. Tuberculosis, for example, is still seen in modern practice. Although laryngeal lesions used to be associated with extensive pulmonary infection, they are now usually associated with much less virulent disease, often only a mild cough. Laryngeal tuberculosis lesions usually are localized [58, 59]. Sarcoidosis, another granulomatous disease, causes laryngeal symptoms in roughly 3–5% of cases [60]. Noncaseating granulomas are found in the larynx, and the false vocal folds are frequently involved, producing airway obstruction rather than dysphonia. Less common diseases, including leprosy [61, 62], syphilis [63], scleroderma [64], typhoid [65], typhus, anthrax, and other conditions, can produce laryngeal lesions that might lead the laryngologist to obtain a possibly unnecessary biopsy. Confusing lesions also may be caused by a variety of mycotic infections including histoplasmosis [66–68], coccidioidomycosis [69], cryptococcosis [70], blastomycosis [68–72], actinomycosis [73, 74], candidiasis [75], aspergillosis [76–78], mucormycosis [79], rhinosporidiosis [80], and sporotrichosis [81]. Parasitic diseases may also produce laryngeal masses. The most prominent example is leishmaniasis [82]. More detailed information about most of the conditions discussed above is available in a text by Michaels [83] and elsewhere in this book [2].

Collagen vascular diseases and other unusual problems may produce laryngeal masses. Rheumatoid arthritis may produce not only fixation of the cricoarytenoid and cricothyroid joints, but also consequent neuropathic muscle atrophy [84] and rheumatoid nodules of the larynx [85]. Rheumatoid arthritis with or without nodules may produce respiratory obstruction. Gout may cause laryngeal arthritis. In addition, gouty tophi may appear as white submucosal masses of the true vocal fold. They consist of sodium urate crystals in fibrous tissue and have been documented well [86–88]. Amyloidosis of the larynx is rare but well recognized [89–91]. Urbach-Wiethe disease (lipoid proteinosis) [92] often involves the mucous membrane of the larynx, usually the vocal folds, aryepiglottic fold, and epiglottis. Other conditions, such as granulomatosis with polyangiitis (Wegener granulomatosis) and relapsing polychondritis, also may involve the larynx. They are less likely to produce discrete nodules, but the diffuse edema associated with chondritis and necrotizing granulomas may produce substantial laryngeal and voice abnormalities. Amyloidosis of the larynx is rare and usually involves the false vocal folds, but it can extend onto the true vocal folds. Unusual laryngeal masses also may be caused by trauma. Trauma is discussed in detail elsewhere [2], but the physician must be careful to inquire about laryngeal trauma, the consequences of which may not be recognized until months or years after the injury.

A few rare skin lesions also may involve the larynx producing symptomatic lesions, and sometimes airway obstruction. These include pemphigus vulgaris, seen in adults between 40 and 60 years of age. Pemphigus lesions may involve the mucosa, including the epiglottis [93]. Epidermolysis bullosa describes a group of congenital vesicular disorders usually seen at birth or shortly thereafter. This condition may cause laryngeal stenosis, or large, bleb-like vocal fold masses with detachment of the epithelium. Some viral conditions may cause laryngeal structural pathology, most notably papillomata. However, herpes, variola, and other organisms also have been implicated in laryngeal infection.

There are numerous other conditions, many of which are not covered comprehensively in this chapter, that may affect voices adversely. Most of them are not common problems among professional voice users. However, the laryngologist should remember that laryngeal manifestations of many systemic diseases may cause voice changes that bring the patient to medical attention for the first time [52, 53]. We must remain alert for their presence and think of them particularly when more common, obvious etiologies are not identified, or when patients do not respond to treatment as expected. The voice may be affected by the following problems not discussed above (among others): acromegaly, Arnold-Chiari malformations, blood dyscrasias, neurologic disease (vocal fold paralysis), collagen vascular disease (including rheumatoid arthritis, systemic lupus erythematosus, scleroderma, Sjögren's syndrome, and others), deafness, gout, Hodgkin's disease, leprosy, lymphoma, Madelung's disease, malignancies, myopathies, a myriad of infectious diseases (bacterial, viral, granulomatous, and fungal), mononucleosis, numerous syndromes (Basedow's, adrenogenital syndrome, Down's syndrome, hereditary angioedema, Kleinfelter's syndrome, Melkersson-Rosenthal syndrome, pachyonychia congenita, short stature syndromes, Shy-Drager syndrome, and many others), syphilis, sarcoidosis, tuberculosis, Crohn's disease, Wilson's disease, and other chronic diseases.

Structural Abnormalities of the Larynx

Nodules

Nodules are callous-like masses of the vocal folds that are caused by vocally abusive behaviors and are a dreaded malady of singers and actors. Occasionally, laryngoscopy reveals asymptomatic vocal nodules that do not appear to interfere with voice production; in such cases, the nodules need not be treated. Some famous and successful singers have had untreated vocal nodules throughout their careers. However, in most cases, nodules result in hoarseness, breathiness, loss of range, and voice fatigue. They may be caused by abusive speaking rather than improper singing technique. Voice therapy always should be tried as the initial therapeutic modality and will cure the vast majority of patients even if the nodules look firm and have been present for many months or years. Even apparently large, fibrotic nodules often shrink, disappear, or become asymptomatic with 6–12 weeks of expert voice therapy with good patient compliance. Even in those who eventually need surgical excision of the nodules, preoperative voice therapy is essential to prevent recurrence. Care must be taken in diagnosing nodules.

It is almost impossible to make the diagnosis accurately and consistently without strobovideolaryngoscopy and good optical magnification. Vocal fold cysts are commonly misdiagnosed as nodules, and treatment strategies are different for the two lesions. Vocal nodules are confined to the superficial layer of the lamina propria and are composed primarily of edematous tissue or collagenous fibers. Basement membrane reduplication is common. They are usually bilateral and fairly symmetric.

Caution must be exercised in diagnosing small nodules in patients who have been singing or speaking actively. In many singers, for example, bilateral, symmetric soft swellings at the junction of the anterior and middle thirds of the vocal folds develop after heavy voice use. No evidence suggests that patients with such "physiologic swelling" are predisposed to develop vocal nodules. At present, the condition is generally considered to be within normal limits. The physiologic swelling usually disappears with 24–48 hours of rest from heavy voice use. The physician must be careful not to frighten the patient by misdiagnosing physiologic swellings as vocal nodules. Nodules carry a great stigma among voice professionals, and the psychologic impact of the diagnosis should not be underestimated. When nodules are present, these patients should be informed with the same gentle caution used in telling a patient that he or she has a life-threatening mass.

Submucosal Cysts

Submucosal cysts of the vocal folds are probably also traumatic lesions that are the result of a blocked mucous gland duct in many cases. However, they also may be congenital or occur from other causes. They often cause contact swelling on the contralateral side and can be misdiagnosed as nodules. They usually can be differentiated from nodules by strobovideolaryngoscopy when the mass is observed to be fluid filled. They also may be suspected when the nodule (contact swelling) on one vocal fold resolves with voice therapy, while the mass on the other vocal fold does not resolve. Cysts may be discovered on one side (occasionally both sides) when surgery is performed for apparent nodules that have not resolved with voice therapy. The surgery should be performed superficially and with minimal trauma, as discussed in a separate chapter. Ordinarily, cysts are lined with thin squamous epithelium. Retention cysts contain mucus. Epidermoid cysts contain caseous material. Generally, cysts are located in the superficial layer of the lamina propria. In some cases, they may be attached to the vocal ligament.

Polyps

Vocal fold polyps, another type of vocal fold mass, usually occur on only one vocal fold. They often have a feeding blood vessel coursing along the superior surface of the vocal fold and joining (or originating from) the base of the polyp. The pathogenesis of polyps cannot be proven in many cases, but the lesion is thought to be traumatic and sometimes starts as a hemorrhage. Polyps may be sessile or pedunculated. Typically, they are located in the superficial layer of the lamina propria and do not involve the vocal ligament. In those arising from an area of hemorrhage, the vocal ligament may be involved with posthemorrhagic fibrosis that is contiguous with the polyp. Histologic evaluation most commonly reveals collagenous fibers, hyaline degeneration, edema, thrombosis, and often bleeding within the polypoid tissue. Cellular infiltration also may be present. In some cases, even sizable polyps resolve with relative voice rest and a few weeks of low-dose steroid therapy (e.g., methylprednisone 4 mg twice a day). However, most require surgical removal. If polyps are not treated, they may produce contact injury on the contralateral vocal fold. Voice therapy should be used to ensure good relative voice rest and prevent abusive voice behavior before and after surgery. When surgery is performed, care must be taken not to damage the leading edge of the vocal fold, especially if a laser is used. In all laryngeal surgery, delicate microscopic dissection is the standard of care. Vocal fold "stripping' is an out-of-date surgical approach formerly used for benign lesions, and it often resulted in scar and/or poor unserviceable voice function. It is no longer an acceptable surgical technique in most situations.

Granulomas

Granulomas usually occur in the cartilaginous portion of the vocal fold near the vocal process or on the medial surface of the arytenoid. They are composed of collagenous fibers, fibroblasts, proliferated capillaries, and leukocytes. They are usually covered with epithelium. Granulomas are associated with gastroesophageal reflux laryngitis and trauma (including trauma from voice abuse and from intubation). The term is a misnomer, since these lesions are inflammatory, not true granulomas as would be seen in tuberculosis or sarcoidosis. Therapy should include reflux control, voice therapy, and surgery if the granuloma continues to enlarge or does not resolve after adequate time and treatment. Granular cell tumors also can occur in the larynx [94].

Reinke's Edema

Severe Reinke's edema is characterized by an "elephant ear," floppy vocal fold appearance. It is often observed during examination in many nonprofessional and professional voice users and is accompanied by a low, coarse, gruff voice. Reinke's edema is a condition in which the superficial layer of lamina propria (Reinke's space) becomes edematous. The lesion does not usually include hypertrophy, inflammation, or degeneration, although other terms for the condition include polypoid degeneration, chronic polypoid corditis, and chronic edematous hypertrophy. Reinke's edema is often associated with smoking, voice abuse, reflux, and hypothyroidism. Underlying conditions should be treated. However, the condition may require surgery if voice improvement is desired. The surgery should be performed only if there is a justified high suspicion of serious pathology such as cancer, if there is airway obstruction, or if the patient is unhappy with his or her vocal quality. For some voice professionals, abnormal Reinke's edema is an important component of the vocal signature. Although the condition is usually bilateral, surgery should generally be performed on one side at a time. Many patients have mild Reinke's edema on one or both vocal folds that does not require treatment.

Sulcus Vocalis

Sulcus vocalis is a groove along the edge of the membranous vocal fold. The majority are congenital, bilateral, and symmetric, although post-traumatic acquired lesions occur. When symptomatic (they often are not), sulcus vocalis can be treated surgically if sufficient voice improvement is not obtained through voice therapy.

Scar

Vocal fold scar is a sequela of trauma and results in fibrosis and obliteration of the layered structure of the vocal fold. It may impede vibration and consequently cause dysphonia. Recent surgical advances have made this condition much more treatable than it used to be [95, 96], but it is still rarely possible to restore voices to normal in the presence of scar.

Hemorrhage

Vocal fold hemorrhage is a potential disaster in singers. Hemorrhages resolve spontaneously in most cases, with restoration of normal voice. However, in some instances, the hematoma organizes and fibroses, resulting in scar [97]. This alters the vibratory pattern of the vocal fold and can result in permanent hoarseness. In selected cases, it may be best to avoid this problem through surgical incision and drainage of the hematoma. In all cases, vocal fold hemorrhage usually is managed with absolute voice rest until the hemorrhage has largely resolved (usually about 1 week) and relative voice rest until normal vascular and mucosal integrity have been restored. This often takes 6 weeks and sometimes longer. Recurrent vocal fold hemorrhages usually are caused by weakness in a specific blood vessel, which may require surgical cauterization of the blood vessel using a laser or microscopic resection of the vessel [98].

Papilloma

Laryngeal papillomas are epithelial lesions caused by human papilloma virus. Histology reveals neoplastic epithelial cell proliferation in a papillary pattern and viral particles. At the present time, symptomatic papillomas are treated surgically, although alternatives have been recommended to the usual laser vaporization approach [99, 100]. Cidofovir injected into the lesion has shown considerable promise [99, 101].

Cancer

A detailed discussion of cancer of the larynx is beyond the scope of this chapter [119]. The prognosis for small vocal fold cancers is good, whether they are treated by radiation or surgery. Although it may seem intuitively obvious that radiation therapy provides a better chance of voice conservation than even limited vocal fold surgery, late radiation changes in the vocal fold may produce substantial hoarseness, xerophonia (dry voice), and voice dysfunction. Consequently, from the standpoint of voice preservation, optimal treatments remain uncertain. Prospective studies using objective voice measures and strobovideolaryngoscopy should answer the relevant questions in the future. Strobovideolaryngoscopy is also valuable for follow-up of patients who have had laryngeal cancers. It permits detection of vibratory changes associated with infiltration by the cancer long before they can be seen with continuous light. Stroboscopy has been used in Europe and Japan for this purpose for many years. In the United States, the popularity of strobovideolaryngoscopy for follow-up of patients with cancer has increased greatly since the mid-to-late 1980s.

The psychologic consequences of vocal fold cancer can be devastating, especially in a professional voice user. They may be overwhelming for nonvoice professionals, as well. These reactions are understandable and expected. In many patients, however, psychologic reactions may be as severe following medically "less significant" vocal fold problems such as hemorrhages, nodules, and other conditions that do not command the public respect and sympathy afforded to a cancer. In many ways, the management of related psychologic problems can be even more difficult in patients with these "lesser" vocal disturbances.

Laryngoceles and Pharyngoceles

The ventricle of Morgagni is located between the true and false vocal folds. The appendix of the ventricle of Morgagni is a blind pouch called the saccule in the anterior superior portion. Laryngoceles are abnormal dilations or herniations of the laryngeal saccule [101–105]. They communicate with the laryngeal lumen and generally are filled with air. They become apparent clinically when they are distended after air is forced into them or when they are filled with fluid. They are connected to the ventricle by a narrow stalk and form a sac lined with pseudostratified, ciliated columnar epithelium. The appendix of the ventricle is considered abnormal if it extends above the upper border of the thyroid cartilage.

Laryngoceles limited to the interior of the larynx are called internal; those that protrude outside the thyroid cartilage into the neck are called external. They also may be mixed (internal and external). Laryngoceles should be distinguished from pharyngoceles, which are not true pouches and which generally diminish in size in the absence of pharyngeal pressure (e.g., when not whistling or playing a wind instrument) [102]. Pharyngoceles are air-filled expansions of the pharynx that can be large enough to require musicians to wear shirts with extra-large collar sizes or to play with the collar unbuttoned. Laryngoceles and pharyngoceles are most common in brass instrumentalists. In laryngoceles, outpouchings of the laryngeal ventricle can extend through the openings in the thyrohyoid membrane for the superior laryngeal vessels and nerve, and balloon outward and upward toward the submandibular triangle [103]. External and mixed laryngoceles are really variants of the internal laryngocele. Because laryngoceles arise from the region of the saccule within the larynx, if the lesion is a laryngocele, there must be an intralaryngeal component manifested at least as a tract connecting the lateral component with the ventricle, with or without internal dilation. Hence, pure external laryngoceles do not exist. Lesions without an intralaryngeal component should be classified differently (e.g., as pharyngoceles).

There are several proposed mechanisms for laryngocele formation. In neonates, they are presumed to be remnants of the lateral air sacs seen in other primates. In adults, they can represent a congenital enlargement of the saccule or an acquired lesion associated with increased intraluminal pressure. The association of laryngoceles with occupations that involve long periods of forced expiration supports this notion, and they also are associated with laryngeal carcinomas [104].

Brass and woodwind players are at risk for a variety of head and neck abnormalities as a result of increased intraluminal pressure during musical performances. Transient ischemic attacks, temporomandibular joint dysfunction, and dental malocclusion have been reported. Injury to the orbicularis oris in brass players can require surgical repair [106]. Stress velopharyngeal incompetence has been documented in trumpeters, bassoonists, and others as noted above. Young trumpet players are at greatest risk for injury to oral and cervical tissues when they generate peak respiratory pressure averaging 151 torr [107].

Although laryngoceles usually are associated with brass instruments, several authors have examined laryngocele formation in woodwind players. Stephani and Tarab obtained plain X-rays on 25 wind instrument players and found laryngoceles in all of them [108]. Macfie found laryngoceles in 53 of 94 (56%) woodwind bandsman [109]. Subclinical laryngoceles are common among horn players, and they rarely require surgical intervention.

Surgery for laryngoceles in young musicians poses several problems. The literature offers no definitive guidance regarding the timing of surgery, the healing period before playing can be resumed, and the risk of recurrence with continued performance. Furthermore, the cervical approach used commonly for the treatment of external laryngoceles can disrupt the normal function of the strap muscles, which is important for tone generation for instrumentalists and for singers [110]. The risks of infection and progression of the defect must be balanced against a young performer's desire for musical growth.

Since Ward's early reports on this subject [103], our understanding of laryngoceles and pharyngoceles has changed slightly. Both laryngoceles and pharyngoceles can change size and appearance with variations in internal pressure. Although the classical definitions of laryngocele remain valid, combinations of both can occur. Air-filled masses that arise in the pharynx (commonly in the region of the piriform sinuses) and lack a laryngeal component or origin should be called pharyngoceles. Those that arise in the laryngeal ventricle should be called laryngoceles. Considering the origins of pharyngeal pouches as reviewed in Ward's 1963 paper [103] as well as the forces involved, it appears likely that most lesions with a laryngeal component originated in the larynx and extended in the neck rather than vice versa, but it is not always possible to prove the origin. It is also important to recognize that the therapeutic implications of the distinctions are not as clear-cut as they once were and that lesions that combine the features of laryngoceles and pharyngoceles occur [111]. The distinctions between laryngoceles and pharyngoceles were quite important when we still believed laryngoceles usually required surgery and pharyngoceles required surgery only rarely. However, as arts-medicine has evolved, experience has shown that, in most cases, neither lesion requires surgery. Contrary to our earlier understandings, the vast majority of laryngoceles are asymptomatic.

Other Conditions

Numerous other conditions could be included in this chapter. For a more comprehensive discussion of the subjects covered above, the reader is referred [2].

Medical Management for Voice Dysfunction

Medical management of many problems affecting the voice involves not only care prescribed by an otolaryngologist but also voice therapy, which is provided by an interdisciplinary team. The roles and training of the principal members of the team are covered in detail elsewhere [2]. This chapter provides a brief introduction to their roles in the medical milieu.

Speech-Language Pathologist

An excellent speech-language pathologist is an invaluable asset in caring for professional voice users and other voice patients. However, otolaryngologists and singing teachers should recognize that, like physicians, speech-language pathologists have varied backgrounds and experience in treatment of voice disorders. In fact, most speech-language pathology programs teach relatively little about caring for professional speakers and nothing about professional singers. Moreover, few speech-language pathologists have vast experience in this specialized area, and no fellowships in this specialty exist. Speech-language pathologists often subspecialize. A speech-language pathologist who expertly treats patients who have had strokes, stutter, have undergone laryngectomy, or have swallowing disorders will not necessarily know how to manage professional voice users optimally or even other less demanding voice patients. The otolaryngologist must learn the strengths and weaknesses of the speech-language pathologist with whom he or she works. After identifying a speech-language pathologist who is interested in treating professional voice users, the otolaryngologist should work closely with the speech-language pathologist to develop the necessary expertise. Assistance may be found through otolaryngologists who treat large numbers of singers or through educational programs such as the Voice Foundation's Symposium on Care of the Professional Voice. In general, therapy should be directed toward vocal hygiene, relaxation techniques, voice function exercised breath management, and abdominal support.

Speech (voice) therapy may be helpful even when a singer has no obvious problem in the speaking voice but significant technical problems in singing. Once a person has been singing for several years, a singing teacher may have difficulty convincing him or her to correct certain technical errors. However, singers are much less protective of their speaking voices. A speech-language pathologist may be able to teach proper support, relaxation, and voice placement in speaking. Once mastered, these techniques can be carried over fairly easily into singing through cooperation between the speech-language pathologist and singing teacher or singing voice specialist. This "back door" approach has been extremely useful. For the actor, coordinating speech-language pathology sessions with acting voice lessons, and especially with training of the speaking voice provided by the actor's voice teacher or coach, is often helpful. We have found this combination so helpful that we have added an acting voice trainer to our medical staff. Information from the speech-language pathologist, acting voice trainer, and singing teacher or singing voice specialist should be symbiotic and should not conflict. If major discrepancies exist, bad training from one of the team members should be suspected, and changes should be made.

Singing Voice Specialist

Singing voice specialists are singing teachers who have acquired extra training to prepare them for work with injured voices, in collaboration with a medical voice team. They are indispensable for singers and very valuable for nonsingers with voice disorders.

In selected cases, singing lessons may be extremely helpful to nonsingers with voice problems. The techniques used to develop abdominal and thoracic muscle strength, breath control, laryngeal and neck muscle strength, and relaxation are similar to those used in voice therapy. Singing lessons often expedite therapy and appear to improve the outcome in some patients.

Otolaryngologists who care for singers frequently are often asked to recommend a voice teacher. This may put them in an uncomfortable position, particularly if the singer is already studying with someone in the community. Most physicians do not have sufficient expertise to criticize a voice teacher, and we must be extremely cautious about recommending that a singer change teachers. However, no certifying agency standardizes or ensures the quality of a singing teacher. Although one may be slightly more confident of a teacher associated with a major conservatory or music school or one who is a member of the National Association of Teachers of Singing (NATS), neither of these credentials ensures excellence, and many expert teachers have neither affiliation. However, with experience, an otolaryngologist can develop valid impressions. The physician should record the name of the voice teacher of every patient and observe whether the same kinds of voice abuse occur with disproportionate frequency in the pupils of any given teacher. Technical problems can cause organic abnormalities such as nodules; therefore, any teacher who has a high incidence of nodules among his or her students should be viewed with cautious concern, but the physician also needs to determine whether the teacher attracts a student cohort that has a high incidence of nodules before the students have started lessons, as may be seen among some populations of rock and popular music singers who have performed extensively without voice training. The physician should be particularly wary of teachers who are reluctant to allow their students to consult a doctor. The best voice teachers usually are quick to refer their students to an otolaryngologist if they hear anything disturbing in a student's voice. Similarly, voice teachers and voice professionals should compare information on the nature and quality of medical care received and its success. No physician cures every voice problem in every patient, just as no singing teacher produces premiere stars from every student who walks into the studio. Nevertheless, voice professionals must be critical, informed consumers and accept nothing less than the best medical care and voice training.

After seeing a voice patient, the otolaryngologist should speak with and/or write a letter to the voice teacher (with the patient's permission) describing the findings and recommendations as he or she would to a physician, speech-language pathologist, or any other referring professional. An otolaryngologist seriously interested in caring for singers should take the trouble to talk with and meet local singing teachers. Taking a lesson or two with each teacher provides enormous insight, as well. Taking voice lessons regularly is even more helpful. In practice, the otolaryngologist will usually identify a few teachers in whom he or she has particular confidence, especially for patients with voice disorders, and should not hesitate to refer singers to these colleagues, especially singers who are not already in training.

Pop singers may be particularly resistant to the suggestion of voice lessons, yet they are in great need of training. The physician should assure patients that a good voice teacher can teach a pop singer how to protect and expand the voice without changing its quality or making it sound "trained" or "operatic." It is helpful to point out that singing, like other athletic activities, requires exercise, warm-up, and coaching for anyone planning to enter the "big league" and stay there. Just as no major league baseball pitcher would play without a pitching coach and warm-up time in the bullpen, no singer should try to build a career without a singing teacher and appropriate strength and agility exercises. This approach has proved palatable and effective. Physicians also should be aware of the difference between a voice teacher and a voice coach.

A voice teacher trains a singer in singing technique and is essential. A voice coach is responsible for teaching songs, interpretation, language, diction, style, operatic roles, and so on, but is not responsible for exercise and basic technical development of the voice.

Acting-Voice Trainer

The use of acting-voice trainers (drama voice coaches) as members of the medical team is relatively new [2]. This addition to the team has been extremely valuable to patients and other team members. Like singing voice specialists, professionals with education in theater arts use numerous vocal and body movement techniques that not only enhance physical function but also release tension and break down emotional barriers that may impede voice function. Tearful revelations to the acting-voice trainer are not uncommon, and, like the singing teacher, this individual may identify psychological and emotional problems that interfere with professional success and have been skillfully hidden from other professionals on the voice team and in the patient's life.

Others

A psychologist, psychiatrist, neurologist, pulmonologist, endocrinologist, gastroenterologist, and others with special interest and expertise in arts-medicine are also invaluable to the voice team. Every comprehensive center should seek out such people and collaborate with them, even if they are not full-time members of the voice team.

Surgery

A detailed discussion of laryngeal surgery is beyond the scope of this chapter and may be found elsewhere [2, 112]. However, a few points are worthy of special emphasis. Surgery for vocal nodules should be avoided whenever possible and should almost never be performed without an adequate trial of expert voice therapy, including patient compliance with therapeutic suggestions. A minimum of 6–12 weeks of observation should be allowed while the patient is using therapeutically modified voice techniques under the supervision of a speech-language pathologist and ideally a singing voice specialist. Proper voice use rather than voice rest (silence) is correct therapy. The surgeon should not perform surgery prematurely for vocal nodules under pressure from the patient for a "quick cure" and early return to performance. Permanent destruction of voice quality is a very real potential complication.

Even after expert surgery, voice quality may be diminished by submucosal scarring, resulting in an adynamic segment along the vibratory margin of the vocal fold. This situation produces a hoarse voice with vocal folds that appear normal on indirect examination under routine light, although under stroboscopic light, the adynamic segment is obvious. No reliable cure exists for this complication. Even large, apparently fibrotic nodules of long standing should be given a chance to resolve without surgery. In some cases, the nodules remain but become asymptomatic, and voice quality is normal. Stroboscopy in such patients usually reveals that the nodules are on the superior surface rather than the leading edge of the vocal folds during proper, relaxed phonation (although they may be on the contact surface and symptomatic when hyperfunctional voice technique is used and the larynx is forced down).

When surgery is indicated for vocal fold lesions, it should be limited as strictly as possible to the area of abnormality. Virtually no place exists for "vocal fold stripping" in patients with benign disease. Submucosal resection through a laryngeal microflap used to be advocated. The technique was introduced and first published by the author (RTS). Microflap technique involved an incision on the superior surface of the vocal fold, submucosal resection, and preservation of the mucosa along the leading edge of the vocal fold. The concept that led to this innovation was based on the idea that the intermediate layer of the lamina propria should be protected to prevent fibroblast proliferation. Consequently, it seemed reasonable to preserve the mucosa as a biologic dressing. This technique certainly produced better results than vocal fold stripping.

However, close scrutiny of outcomes revealed a small number of cases with poor results and stiffness beyond the limits of the original pathology. Consequently, the technique was abandoned in favor of a new technique called minimicroflap, or a method of local resection strictly limited to the region of pathology [113]. Lesions such as vocal nodules should be removed to a level even with the vibratory margin rather than deeply into the submucosa. This minimizes scarring and optimizes chances for return to good vocal function. Naturally, if concern about a serious neoplasm exists, proper treatment takes precedence over voice preservation. Surgery should be performed under microscopic control. Preoperative and postoperative objective voice measures are essential to allow outcome assessment and self-critique. Only through such study can we improve surgical technique. Outcome studies are especially important in voice surgery as all our technical pronouncements are anecdotal because there is no experimental model for vocal fold surgery. The human adult is the only species with our complex, layered lamina propria.

Lasers are an invaluable adjunct in the laryngologists' armamentarium, but they must be used knowledgeably and with care. Considerable early evidence suggested that healing time was prolonged and the incidence of adynamic segment formation was higher with the laser on the vibratory margin than with traditional instruments. Two early studies raised serious concerns about dysphonia after laser surgery [114, 115]. Such complications may result from using too low a wattage causing dissipation of heat deeply into the vocal fold; thus, high power density for short duration has been recommended. Small spot size is also helpful. More recent experience has shown that expert laser surgery on the vibratory margin can produce excellent results. Nevertheless, many laryngologists caring for voice professionals avoid laser surgery to eliminate the risk of thermal injury to the vocal ligament. If a laser is used when biopsy specimens are needed, they should be taken before vaporizing the lesion with a laser. If a lesion is to be removed from the leading edge, the laser beam should be centered in the lesion, rather than on the vibratory margin, so that the beam does not create a divot in the vocal fold. The CO_2 laser was used previously for cauterizing isolated blood vessels responsible for recurrent hemorrhage or other problems, and it still is used occasionally. At the suggestion of Jean Abitbol, MD, the author (RTS) has placed a small piece of ice on the vocal fold immediately before CO_2 laser use to help dissipate the heat and help prevent edema (personal communication, 1983). No studies on the efficacy of this maneuver exist, but the technique appears helpful.

Such vessels are often found at the base of a hemorrhagic polyp. Vascular lasers are better than CO_2 lasers for management of these lesions and other vascular abnormalities. They include the 532 nm KTP (Nd-YAG) laser and the 445 nm Blue Laser.

Voice rest after vocal fold surgery is controversial. Although some laryngologists do not recognize its necessity at all, many physicians recommend voice rest for approximately 1 week or until the mucosal surface has healed. Even after surgery, silence for more than 7–10 days is nearly never necessary and represents a real hardship for many patients.

Too often, the laryngologist is confronted with a desperate patient whose voice has been "ruined" by vocal fold surgery, recurrent or superior laryngeal nerve paralysis, trauma, or some other tragedy. Occasionally, the cause is as straightforward as a dislocated arytenoid that can be reduced [116, 117]. However, if the problem is an avulsed vocal process, an adynamic segment, decreased bulk of one vocal fold after "stripping," bowing caused by superior laryngeal nerve paralysis, or some other complication in a mobile vocal fold, great conservatism should be exercised. None of the available surgical procedures for these conditions are effective consistently. If surgery is considered, the procedure and prognosis should be explained to the patient realistically and pessimistically. The patient must understand that the chances of returning the voice to professional quality are very slim and that it might be made worse. Nevertheless, procedures for vocal fold scar have improved, and surgery is often possible (including vocal fold injection and other procedures) to at least decrease the severity of dysphonia and to lessen vocal effort.

Occasionally, voice professionals inquire about surgery for pitch alteration. Such procedures have been successful in specially selected patients (such as those undergoing gender modification surgery), but they do not consistently provide good enough voice quality and range to be performed on a professional voice user in most situations.

Discretion

The excitement and glamour associated with caring for voice patients and wind instrumentalists, particularly famous performers, naturally tempt the physician to talk about a distinguished patient. However, this tendency must be tempered. Having it known that he or she has consulted a laryngologist, particularly for treatment of a significant vocal problem, is not always in a voice professional's or instrumentalist's best interest. Famous singers, actors, politicians, and other professional voice users, as well as instrumentalists, are entitled ethically and legally to the same confidentiality we ensure for our other patients.

Voice Maintenance

Prevention of voice dysfunction should be the goal of all professionals involved in the care of professional voice users. Good vocal health habits should be encouraged in childhood. Screaming, particularly outdoors at athletic events, should be discouraged. Promising young singers who join choirs should be educated to compensate for the Lombard effect. The youngster interested in singing, acting, debating, or other vocal activities should receive enough training to prevent voice abuse and should receive enthusiastic support for performing works and activities suitable for his or her age and voice. Training should be continued during or after puberty, and the voice should be allowed to develop naturally without pressure to perform operative roles prematurely. Young instrumentalists should be managed with similar care, as discussed in Chap. 4.

Excellent regular training and practice are essential, and avoidance of irritants, particularly smoke, should be stressed early. Educating voice professionals and wind instrumentalists about hormonal and anatomic alterations that may influence the voice allows them to recognize and analyze voice dysfunction, compensating for it intelligently when it occurs. The body is dynamic, changing over a lifetime, and the voice is no exception. Continued voice education, training, and monitoring are necessary throughout a lifetime, even in the most successful and well-established voice professionals and instrumental musicians. Voice problems even in premiere singers commonly are caused by cessation of lessons, excessive schedule demands, and other correctable problems, rather than by irreversible alterations of aging. Anatomic, physiologic, and serious medical problems may affect the voices of patients of any age. Cooperation among the laryngologist, speech-language pathologist, acting teacher, voice specialist, music teacher, and singing teacher provides an optimal environment for cultivation and protection of the vocal artist and for voice presentation in wind instrumentalists.

References

1. Brodnitz F. Hormones and the human voice. Bull NY Acad Med. 1971;47:183–91.
2. Sataloff RT. Professional voice: the science and art of clinical care. 4th ed. San Diego, CA: Plural Publishing; 2017. p. 1–2099.
3. von Leden H. Presentation at: Seventh Symposium on Care of the Professional Voice. New York, NY: The Juilliard school; 1978.
4. Punt NA. Applied laryngology—singers and actors. Proc R Soc Med. 1968;61:1152–6.
5. Anderson TD, Sataloff RT. Rhinosinusitis. In: Sataloff RT. Professional voice: the science and art of clinical care. 4th ed. San Diego, CA: Plural Publishing; 2017. p. 747–50.
6. Nachman SA, Pontrelli L. Central nervous system Lyme disease. Semin Pediatr Infect Dis. 2003;14(2):123–30.
7. Sataloff JB, Sataloff RT. Otologic manifestations of Lyme disease. In: Kountakis SE, editor.

Encyclopedia of otolaryngology, head and neck surgery. New Delhi: Springer; 2013. p. 2015–20.
8. Goldfarb D, Sataloff RT. Lyme disease: a review for the otolaryngologist. ENT. 1994;73(11):824–9.
9. Kugeler KJ, Farley GM, Forrester JD, Mead P. Geographic distribution and expansion of human Lyme disease, United States. Emerg Infect Dis. 2015;21(8):1455–7.
10. Clark JR, Carlson RD, Sasaki CT, Pachner AR, Steere AC. Facial paralysis in Lyme disease. NATS J. 1995;95:1341–5.
11. Steere AC, Grodzick MS, Kornblatt AN, et al. The spirochetal etiology of Lyme disease. New Engl J Med. 1983;308:733–40.
12. Burgdorfer WA, Barbour AG, Hayes SF, Benach JL, Grunwaldt E, David JP. Lyme disease-tick-borne spirochetosis. Science. 1982;216:1317–9.
13. Strle F, Ruzic-Sablijic E, Cimperman J, Lotric-Furlan S, Maraspin V. Comparison of findings for patients with Borrelia garinii and Borrelia afzelii isolated from cerebrospinal fluid. Clin Infect Dis. 2006, 43(6):704–10.
14. Magnarelli LA. Serologic diagnostics of Lyme disease. Ann N Y Acad Sci. 1988;539:154–61.
15. Sehgal VN, Khurana A. Lyme disease/borreliosis as a systemic disease. Clin Dermatol. 2015;33:542–50.
16. Barbour AG. Diagnosis of Lyme disease: rewards and perils. Ann Intern Med. 1989;11(7):501–2.
17. Glassock ME, Pensak ML, Gulia AJ, Baker DC. Lyme disease: a cause of bilateral facial paralysis. Arch Otolaryngol. 1985;111:47–9.
18. Schroeter V. Paralysis of recurrent laryngeal nerve in Lyme disease. Lancet. 1988;2(8622):1245.
19. Steere AC, Malaawista SE, Hardin JA, Ruddy S, Askenase PW, Andiman WA. Erythema chronicum migrans and Lyme arthritis: the enlarging clinical spectrum. Ann Intern Med. 1988;86:685–98.
20. Sataloff RT, Johns MM, Kost KM. Geriatric otolaryngology. New York, NY: Thieme; 2015.
21. Sundberg J, Prame E, Iwarsson J. Replicability and accuracy of pitch patterns in professional singers. In: David PJ, Fletcher NH, editors. Vocal fold physiology: controlling Chaos and complexity. Sydney, Australia: Singular Publishing; 1996. p. 291–306.
22. Sataloff RT, Cohn JR, Hawkshaw MJ. Respiratory dysfunction. In: Sataloff RT. Professional voice: the science and art of clinical care. 4th ed. San Diego, CA: Plural Publishing; 2017. p. 751–64.
23. Spiegel JR, Sataloff RT, Cohn JR, et al. Respiratory function in singers. Medical assessment, diagnoses and treatments. J Voice. 1988;2(1):40–50.
24. Cohn JR, Sataloff RT, Spiegel JR, et al. Airway reactivity-induced asthma in singers (ARIAS). J Voice. 1991;5(4):332–7.
25. Cohn JR, Padams PA, Hawkshaw MJ, Sataloff RT. Allergy. In: Sataloff RT. Professional voice: the science and art of clinical care. 4th ed. San Diego, CA: Plural Publishing; 2017. p. 737–42.
26. Sataloff RT, Katz PO, Sataloff DM, Hawkshaw MJ. Reflux laryngitis and related disorders. 4th ed. San Diego, CA: Plural Publishing; 2013. p. 1–210.
27. Ritter FN. The effect of hypothyroidism on the larynx of the rat. Ann Otol Rhinol Laryngol. 1964;67:404–16.
28. Ritter RN. Endocrinology. In: Paparella M, Shumrick D, editors. Otolaryngology, vol. 1. Philadelphia, PA: Saunders; 1973. p. 727–34.
29. Michelsson K, Sirvio P. Cry analysis in congenital hypothyroidism. Folia Phoniat. 1976;28:40–7.
30. Gupta OP, Bhatia PL, Agarwal MK, Mehrotra ML, Mishr SK. Nasal pharyngeal and laryngeal manifestations of hypothyroidism. Ear Nose Throat J. 1977;56(9):10–21.
31. Malinsky M, Chevrrie-Muller C, Cerceau N. Etude Clinique et electrophysiologique des alterations de la voix au cours des thyrotoxioses. Ann Endocrinol. 1977;38:171–2.
32. Meuser W, Nieschlag E. Sexual hormone und Stimmlage des Mannes. Deutsch Med Wochenschr. 1977;102:261–4.
33. Brodnitz F. The age of the castrato voice. J Speech Hearing Disord. 1975;40:291–5.
34. Anderson TD, Anderson DD, Sataloff RT. Endocrine function. In: Sataloff RT. Professional voice: the science and art of clinical care. 4th ed. San Diego, CA: Plural Publishing; 2017. p. 655–70.
35. Schiff M. The influence of estrogens on connective tissue. In: Asboe-Hansen G, editor. Hormones and connective tissue. Copenhagen, Denmark: Munksgaard Press; 1967. p. 282–341.
36. Lacina V. Der Einfluss der Menstruation auf die Stimme der Sangerinnen. Folia Phoniatr. 1968;20:13–24.
37. Wendler J. Cyclically dependent variations in efficiency of the voice and its influencing by ovulation inhibitors. Zyklusabhangige Leistungsschwankungen der Stimme und ihre Beeinflussung durch Ovulationshemmer. Folia Phoniatr. 1972;24(4):259–77.
38. Abitbol J, Abitbol P. The larynx: a hormonal target. In: Rubin J, Sataloff RT, Korovin G. Diagnosis and treatment of voice disorders. 4th ed. San Diego, CA: Plural Publishing, Inc; 2014. p. 431–56.
39. Dordain M. Etude Statistique de l'influence des contraceptifs hormonaux sur la voix. Folia Phoniat. 1972;24:86–96.
40. Pahn V, Goretzlehner G. Stimmstorungen durch hormonale Kontrazeptiva. Zentralb Gynakol. 1978;100:341–6.
41. Schiff M. "The pill" in otolaryngology. Trans Am Acad Opthalmol Otolaryngol. 1968;72:76–84.
42. Rodney JP, Sataloff RT. The effects of hormonal contraception on the voice: history of its evolution in the literature. J Voice. 2016;30(6):726–30.
43. Brodnitz F. Medical care preventative therapy (panel). In: Lawrence V, editor. Transcripts of the seventh annual symposium, care of the professional voice, vol. 3. New York, NY: Voice Foundation; 1978. p. 86.

44. Flach M, Schwickardi H, Simen R. Welchen Einfluss haben Menstruation and Schwangershaft auf die augsgebildete Gesangsstimme? Folia Phoniatr. 1968;21:199–210.
45. Deuster CV. Irreversible Stimmstorung in der Schwangersheft. HNO. 1977;25:430–2.
46. Damste PH. Virilization of the voice due to anabolic steroids. Folia Phoniatr. 1964;16:10–8.
47. Damste PH. Voice changes in adult women caused by virilizing agents. J Speech Hear Disord. 1967;32:126–32.
48. Saez S, Francoise S. Recepteurs d'androgenes: mise en evidence dans la fraction cytosolique de muqueuse normale et d'epitheliomas pharyngolarynges humains. C R Acad Sci (Paris). 1975;280:935–8.
49. Vuorenkoski V, Lenko HL, Tjernlund P, Vuorenkoski L, Perheentupa J. Fundamental voice frequency during normal and abnormal growth, and after androgen treatment. Arch Dis Child. 1978;53:201–9.
50. Bourdial J. Les troubles de la voix provoques par la therapeutique hormonale androgene. Ann Otolaryngol. 1970;87:725–34.
51. Imre V. Hormonell bedingte Stimmstorungen. Folia Phoniatr. 1968;20:394–404.
52. Hamdan A, Sataloff RT, Hawkshaw MJ. Laryngeal manifestations of systemic diseases. San Diego, CA: Plural Publishing, Inc; 2019.
53. Hamdan A, Sataloff RT, Hawkshaw MJ. Obesity and voice. San Diego, CA: Plural Publishing, Inc; 2020.
54. National Institutes of Health. Health implications of obesity. Bethesda, MD: Consensus Development Conference Statement; 1986.
55. Gates GA, Saegert J, Wilson N, Johnson L, Sheperd A, Hearnd EM. Effects of beta-blockade on singing performance. Ann Otol Rhinol Laryngol. 1985;94:570–4.
56. Rosen DC, Sataloff JB, Sataloff RT. Psychology of Voice Disorders, Second Edition. San Diego, CA: Plural Publishing; 2020.
57. Sataloff RT, Brandfonbrener A, Lederman R. Performing arts medicine. 3rd ed. Narberth, PA: Science and Medicine; 2010.
58. Bull TR. Tuberculosis of the larynx. Br Med J. 1966;2:991–2.
59. Hunter AM, Millar JW, Wrightman AJ, Horne NW. The changing pattern of laryngeal tuberculosis. J Laryngol Otol. 1981;95:393–8.
60. Divine KD. Sarcoidosis and sarcoidosis of the larynx. Laryngoscope. 1965;75:533–69.
61. Munor MacCormick CE. The larynx in leprosy. Arch Otolaryngol. 1957;66:138–49.
62. Binford CH, Meyers WM. Leprosy. In: Binford CH, Conor DH, editors. Pathology of tropical and extraordinary diseases, vol. 1. Washington, DC: Armed Forces Institute of Pathology; 1976. p. 205–25.
63. MacKenzie M. A manual of diseases of the throat and nose, Vol. 1 diseases of the pharynx, larynx, and trachea. J.& A. Churchill: London, UK; 1884.
64. Astacio JN, Goday GA, Espinosa FJ. Escleroma. Experiences en El Salvador. Seconda Mongrafia de Dermatologia iberolatino-americana. Suplemento AO No. 1, Lisboa, Portugal, 1971.
65. Hajek M. Pathologie unde Therapie der Erkrankungen des Kehlkopfes, der Luftrohre und der Bronchien. Leipzig: Verlag von Curt Kabitzsch; 1932.
66. Withers BT, Pappas JJ, Erickson EE. Histoplasmosis primary in the larynx. Report of a case. Arch Otolaryngol. 1977;77:25–8.
67. Calcaterra TC. Otolaryngeal histoplasmosis. Laryngoscope. 1970;80:111–20.
68. Sataloff RT, Wilborn A, Prestipino A, Hawkshaw M, Heuer RJ, Cohn JR. Histoplasmosis of the larynx. Am J Otolaryngol. 1993;14(3):199–205.
69. Friedmann I. Diseases of the larynx. Disorders of laryngeal function. In: Paparella MM, Shumrick DA, editors. Otolaryngology. 2nd ed. Philadelphia, PA: WB Saunders; 1980. p. 2449–69.
70. Reese MC, Conclasure JB. Cryptococcosis of the larynx. Arch Otolaryngol. 1975;101:698–701.
71. Bennett M. Laryngeal blastomycosis. Laryngoscope. 1964;74:498–512.
72. Hoffarth GA, Joseph DL, Shumrick DA. Deep mycoses. Arch Otolaryngol. 1973;97:475–9.
73. Brandenburg JH, Finch WW, Kirkham WR. Actinomycosis of the larynx and pharynx. Otolaryngology. 1978;86:739–42.
74. Shaheen SO, Ellis FG. Actinomycosis of the larynx. J R Soc Med. 1983;76:226–8.
75. Tedeschi LG, Cheren RV. Laryngeal hyperkeratosis due to primary monilial infection. Arch Otolaryngol. 1968;82:82–4.
76. Rao PB. Aspergillosis of the larynx. J Laryngol Otol. 1969;83:377–9.
77. Ferlito A. Clinical records. Primary aspergillosis of the larynx. J Laryngol Otol. 1974;88:1257–63.
78. Keir SM, Flint A, Moss JA. Primary aspergillosis of the larynx simulating carcinoma. Hum Pathol. 1983;14:184–6.
79. Anand CS, Gupta MC, Kothari MG, Anand TS, Singh SK. Laryngeal mucormycosis. Indian J Otolaryngol. 1978;30:90–2.
80. Pillai OS. Rhinosporidiosis of the larynx. J Laryngol Otol. 1974;88:277–80.
81. Khabie N, Boyce TG, Roberts GD, Thompson DM. Laryngeal sporotrichosis causing stridor in young child. Int J Pediatr Otorhinolaryngol. 2003;67(7):819–823.
82. Zinneman HH, Hall WH, Wallace FG. Leishmaniasis of the larynx. Report of a case and its confusion with histoplasmosis. Am J Med. 1961;31:654–8.
83. Michaels L. Pathology of the larynx. New York, NY: Springer-Verlag; 1984.
84. Wolman L, Darke CS, Young A. The larynx in rheumatoid arthritis. J Laryngol. 1965;79:403–34.
85. Bridger MWN, Jahn AF, van Nostrand AWP. Laryngeal rheumatoid arthritis. Laryngoscope. 1980;90:296–303.
86. Virchow R. Seltene Gichtablagerungen. Virchows Arch Path Anat. 1868;44:137–8.

87. Marion RB, Alperin JE, Maloney WH. Gouty tophus of the true vocal cord. Arch Otolaryngol. 1972;96:161–2.
88. Epstein SS, Winston P, Friedmann I, Ormerod FC. The vocal cord polyp. J Laryngol Otol Lond. 1957;71:673–88.
89. Stark DB, New GB. Amyloid tumors of larynx, trachea or bronchi: report of 15 cases. Ann Otol Rhinol Laryngol. 1949;58:117–34.
90. Michaels L, Hyams VJ. Amyloid in localized deposits and plasmacytomas of the respiratory tract. J Pathol. 1979;128(1):29–38.
91. Pribtkin E, Friedman O, O'Hara B, et al. Amyloidosis of the upper aerodigestive tract. Laryngoscope. 2003;113:2095–101.
92. Urbach E, Wiethe C. Lipoidosis cutis et mucosae. Virchows Arch Path Anat. 1929;273:285–319.
93. Charow A, Pass F, Ruben R. Pemphigus of the upper respiratory tract. Arch Otolaryngol. 1971;93:209–10.
94. Sataloff RT, Hawkshaw MJ, Ressue J. Granular cell tumor of the larynx. Ear Nose Throat J. 1998;77(8):582–4.
95. Moore JE, Hawkshaw MJ, Sataloff RT. Vocal fold scar. United Kingdom: Compton Publishing, Ltd; 2016.
96. Moore JE, Sataloff RT. Vocal fold scar. In: Sataloff RT. Professional voice: the science and art of clinical care. 4th ed. San Diego, CA: Plural Publishing; 2017. p. 1605–10.
97. Sataloff RT, Hawkshaw MJ. Vocal fold hemorrhage. In: Sataloff RT. Professional voice: the science and art of clinical care. 4th ed. San Diego, CA: Plural Publishing; 2017. p. 1587–604.
98. Hochman I, Sataloff RT, Hillman R, Zeitels S. Ectasias and varices of the vocal fold: clearing the striking zone. Ann Otol Rhinol Laryngol. 1999;108(1):10–6.
99. Zeitels SM. Phonomicrosurgical techniques. In: Sataloff RT. Professional voice: the science and art of clinical care. 4th ed. San Diego, CA: Plural Publishing; 2017. p. 1479–500.
100. Zeitels SM, Sataloff RT. Phonomicrosurgical resection of glottal papillomatosis. J Voice. 1999;13(1):123–7.
101. Wellens W, Snoeck R, Desloovere C, et al. Treatment of severe laryngeal papillomatosis with intralesional injections of cidofovir [(S)-1-(3-Hydroxy-Phospho nylmethoxypropyl) Cytosine, HPMPC, Vistide]. In: McCafferty G, Coman W, Carroll R, editors. Proceedings of the XVI world congress of otorhinolaryngology head and neck surgery. Bologna, Italy: Monduzzi Editor; 1997. p. 455–549.
102. Holinger LD, Barnes DR, Smid LJ, Holinger PH. Laryngocele and saccular cysts. Ann Otol Rhinol Laryngol. 1978;87:675–85.
103. Ward PH, Frederickson J, Strandjord NM, Valvessori GE. Laryngeal and pharyngeal pouches. Surgical approach and the use of cinefluorographic and other radiologic techniques as diagnostic aids. Laryngoscope. 1963;73:564–82.
104. DeSanto LW. Laryngocele, laryngeal mucocele, large saccules, and laryngeal saccular cysts: a developmental spectrum. Laryngoscope. 1974;84:1291–6.
105. Norris CW. Pharyngoceles of the hypopharynx. Laryngoscope. 1979;89:1788–807.
106. Papsin BC, Maaske LA, McGrail JS. Orbicularis oris muscle injury in brass players. Laryngoscope. 1996;106:757–60.
107. Fiz JA, Aguilar J, Carreras A, et al. Maximum respiratory pressure in trumpet players. Chest. 1993;104:1203–4.
108. Stephani A, Tarab S. [Obscure and ventricular laryngocele.] Schweiz Rundsch Med Prax 1972;61:1520–1523.
109. Macfie DD. Asymptomatic laryngoceles in wind instrument bandsmen. Arch Otolaryngol. 1966;83:270–5.
110. Backus J. The effect of the player's vocal tract on wood wind instrument tone. J Acoust Soc Am. 1985;78:17–20.
111. Isaacson G, Sataloff RT. Bilateral laryngoceles in a young trumpet player: case report. Ear Nose Throat J. 2000;4:272–4.
112. Sataloff RT, Chowdhury F, Portnoy J, Hawkshaw MJ, Joglekar S. Surgical techniques in otolaryngology – head and neck surgery: laryngeal surgery. New Delhi, India: Jaypee Brothers Medical Publishers; 2014.
113. Sataloff RT, Spiegel JR, Heuer RJ, et al. Laryngeal mini-microflap: a new technique and reassessment of the microflap saga. J Voice. 1995;9(2):198–204.
114. Abitbol J. Limitations of the laser in microsurgery of the larynx. In: Lawrence VL, editor. Transactions of the twelfth symposium: care of the professional voice. New York, NY, The Voice Foundation; 1984. p. 297–302.
115. Strong MS, Jako GJ. Laser surgery in the larynx. Early clinical experience with continuous CO_2 laser. Ann Otol Rhinol Laryngol. 1972;81:791–8.
116. Sataloff RT, Feldman M, Darby KS, Carroll LM, Spiegel JR. Arytenoid dislocation. J Voice. 1988;1(4):368–77.
117. Sataloff RT, Bough ID, Spiegel JR. Arytenoid dislocation: diagnosis and treatment. Laryngoscope. 1994;104(10):1353–61.
118. Sataloff RT, Hawkshaw MJ, Sataloff JB, DeFatta RA, Eller RL. Atlas of laryngoscopy. 3rd ed. San Diego, CA: Plural Publishing, Inc; 2012.
119. Hamdan A, Sataloff RT, Hawkshaw MJ. Non-Laryngeal Cancer and Voice. San Diego, CA: Plural Publishing; 2020.

8 Fundamental Frequency and Dentofacial Anomalies

Fundamental frequency (F0) is one of many acoustic indices considered to be an indicator to body morphology. This consideration stems from the assumption that laryngeal and body structures usually grow in parallel. The hormonal influence accentuated mostly at puberty underscores the larynx as an end-organ hormonal target. Similarly, the pubertal upsurge in craniofacial and skeletal growth highlights the impact of sex and growth hormones on body morphology. Nevertheless, despite the parallel growth of the laryngeal framework with the craniofacial and body skeleton, the correlation between F0 and body size remains controversial. The free position of the larynx in the neck and its prepubertal descent have complicated the understanding of the hormonal effect and lead to uncertainties on the predictive role of F0 in estimating body stature and facial morphology [1, 2].

In this chapter, the authors review the current literature on the association between F0 and dentofacial morphology. The association between F0 and body size is presented as a prelude to the discussion on why F0 should or should not correlate with dentofacial anomalies. This information is useful to laryngologists, speech-language pathologists, and voice teachers in their assessment and management of dysphonic patients with malocclusion. Wind instrumentalists also need to be aware of the interplay between F0 and dentofacial morphology considering the contribution of the vocal folds and vocal tract in music tone. This information is even more relevant when wind instrumentalists are singers as well.

Fundamental Frequency and Body Morphology

The predictive role of F0 in estimating body size and shape has been an issue of debate in the literature. Since the early report by Lass and Davis in 1976, showing a 48–65% probability of guessing body weight using vocal cues, a considerable number of authors explored the relationship between F0 and body attributes such as weight, height, and circumferential measurements, with no clear consensus [3]. In 2006, Evans et al. reported a significant negative correlation between F0 and body weight in 50 heterosexual subjects ($r_p = -0.34$, $p = 0.02$), and a negative correlation between F0, and shoulder and chest circumferences ($r_p = -0.29$, $p = 0.04$; $r_p = -0.28$, $p = 0.04$, respectively). The authors reiterated on the important role of acoustic cues in competitive behavior among males [4]. In another study on 29 subjects by Barsties et al., the authors reported a higher percentage of low F0 in underweight subjects in comparison to normal weight subjects. This difference was attributed to the inverse correlation between vocal fold mass and pitch, with a decrease in vocal fold mass leading to an increase in vocal fold rate of vibration [5]. These

A.-L. Hamdan et al., *Dentofacial Anomalies*, https://doi.org/10.1007/978-3-030-69109-7_8

results were in agreement with Da Cunha et al. who also reported lower maximum phonation time and higher prevalence of vocal tract tension in obese subjects. The authors interpreted these findings in the context of breathing impairment and the known impact of low respiratory volume on vocal tract morphology [6]. However, there are several reports that challenged the correlation between F0 and body weight and height. In 1989, Künzel HJ reported no significant correlation between average F0 and weight and height. The authors argued that acoustic parameters carry little information on the somatic features of the speaker [7]. These findings were supported by Gunter and Manning, who stressed the differences between actual and estimated body weight and height. In their methodology, 40 listeners evaluated filtered and non-filtered voices of 20 speakers [8]. In 1995, Van Dommelen and Moxness investigated the role of acoustic parameters in identifying a speakers' weight and height using sustained vowels and spoken paragraphs. The authors found no correlation between F0 and the actual speakers' height or weight, and abandoned use of this acoustic parameter to estimate a speaker's body dimensions [9]. In 2005, Rendall et al. studied the relationship between F0 and body size in 68 subjects (34 males and 34 females) with a mean age of 23 years. The subjects produced isolated vowel sounds and single-syllable words, thus allowing the extraction of 23 vowels for analysis. Using multiple regression, F0 failed to correlate with body size [10]. In 2011, Hamdan et al. investigated body weight, mass composition, and F0 in a group of 40 male subjects and reported the absence of any correlation between these parameters. The concentration of fat in the body did not correlate with any of the acoustic parameters except for shimmer, and cycle-to-cycle variation in intensity [11]. These findings were in agreement with a study by De Souza et al. conducted on 74 female subjects divided as 44 morbidly obese and 30 non-obese. The authors also reported no significant difference in F0 between the two groups, although the prevalence of voice complaints was higher in the obese group in comparison with the control group [12].

In summary, the correlation between F0 and body size is controversial. Its predictive role in estimating body weight and height is limited when used as an isolated acoustic cue. Larger studies on the association between F0 and body size are needed in order to draw a definitive conclusion.

Fundamental Frequency and Dentofacial Anomalies

The controversial link between F0 and body morphology did not deter many authors from studying the association between F0 and facial morphology. The impetus is not surprising given the contribution of the dentofacial skeleton, particularly the shape and depth of the palate, to vocal tract morphology. Nevertheless, there is no consensus in the literature on the link between F0, voice classification, and the types of malocclusion. In 1949 and 1958, Gutzman reported a correlation between voice registers and the depth of the palate. The authors pointed that bass singers tend to have a flat palate, whereas soprano singers tend to have a high palate [13, 14]. However, in 1967 Ackermann showed no association between palatal measurements and voice classification. The study included 164 singers, and the measurements were extracted using palatal impressions [15]. In 2000, Marunick and Menaldi studied the predictive value of maxillary dental arch form and dimensions in voice classification in nine professional female singers using maxillary dental impressions. Two palatal depths were measured in that study, one from the first molar and the second from the first bicuspid. Similarly, two palatal widths were used, one from the cuspid and the second from the second molar. The voice range for each singer was classified as Soprano, Mezzo-soprano or Alto based on sustained vowel /ɑ/, speaking sample "Rainbow passage," and singing sample "Are you sleeping." Using discriminant analysis, the authors showed that a single palatal measurement was not a predictor of voice classification, but when depth and width measurements were combined, the predictive value was very high (proportions correct = 1.000) [16]. In 2009, Roers et al. investigated the correlation between vocal tract dimensions and voice classification by analyzing the vocal tract images of student singers. Among the various measurements taken was the depth of the palatal arch extracted as the maximum distance between the contour of the palate and a line drawn along the lower contour of the molars. The authors found no significant variation in the depth of the palate across the different voice classifications dentofacial anomalies. However, the depth of the palate varied with the total vocal tract length, with male singers having higher palates than female singers. Moreover, the vocal tract length was found to be shorter in sopranos compared to mezzos and altos. The variation of the vocal tract is dependent on the length of the pharyngeal cavity than on that of the oral cavity. The pharyngeal segment was measured from the most-anterior point of the laryngeal prominence to the lower anterior point of the second vertebra [17]. That same year, Jorge et al. investigated the effect of orthognathic surgery on F0 in one female subject with class III malocclusion who underwent bilateral sagittal osteotomy of the mandibular ramus, total maxillary osteotomy, and modified osteotomy for chin advancement. There was an increase in F0 3 months after surgery, followed by a decrease 1 year later (215.99 Hz preoperatively, vs. 228.08 Hz at 3 months, vs. 216.85 Hz after 1 year). The short-term increase in F0 was attributed to the anterior and forward displacement of the hyolaryngeal complex. With a forward and cephalic displacement of the larynx, there is shortening of the vocal tract with subsequent increase in tension within the intrinsic laryngeal muscles and vocal folds. Similarly, the drop in F0 after 1 year was attributed to the posterior and inferior drop of the hyolaryngeal complex. Though the authors did not compare F0 in patients with mandibular retrognathism vs. patients with normal mandibular projections, the F0 reported preoperatively was within normal range for women (215.99 Hz) [18]. In 2013, Mishima et al. studied the impact of mandibular setback on voice using acoustic analysis in a group of 16 patients (8 males and 8 females) with class III malocclusion without cleft palate in comparison with 50 controls (25 males and 25 females). The authors reported significantly lower F0 preoperatively for the vowels /α/, /i/, /u/, and /o/ in the female study group compared to controls. Moreover, there were significant differences in the resonance characteristics between the two groups [19]. In 2014, in a study by Macari et al. that included 45 subjects with a mean age of 15.4 + 7.07 years, the authors reported a negative moderate correlation between F0, habitual pitch, and the length of the mandible ($r = -0.528$, and $r = -0.577$, respectively). Similarly, there was a negative moderate correlation between F0, habitual pitch, and the length of the maxilla ($r = -0.473$ and -0.519, respectively). The length of the mandible was measured from the condyle to the most-anterior part of the chin, and the length of the maxilla was measured from the most-anterior point of the nasal spine to the most-posterior point of the nasal spine (Fig. 8.1). There was no correlation between the remaining acoustic parameters and the sagittal projection parameters, extracted from the SNA angle and SNB angle. The SNA angle is the angle drawn between a line that extends from the sella turcica to the nasion and a line that extends from the nasion to the deepest

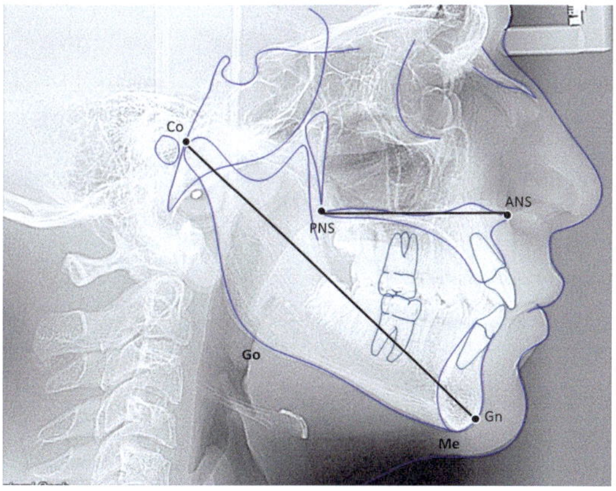

Fig. 8.1 Lateral cephalometric tracing showing the landmarks and length of mandible and maxilla. ANS: anterior nasal spine; PNS: posterior nasal spine; ANS-PNS; maxillary length. Co: condylion—anterosuperior point of the condyle; Gn: gnathion—midpoint between the most protruded and the lowest points of the symphysis. Co-Gn: mandibular length

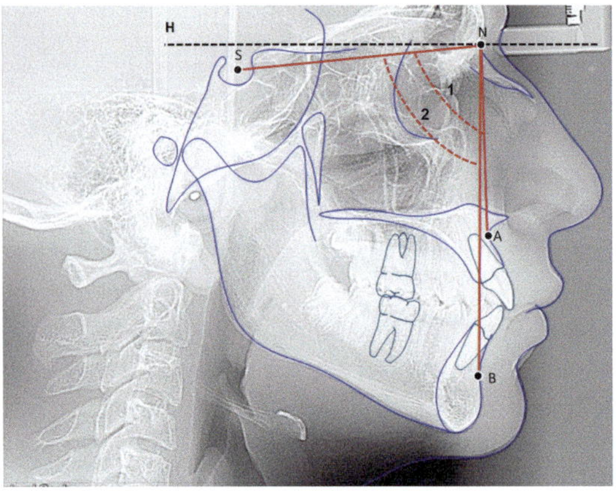

Fig. 8.2 Lateral cephalometric tracing showing the landmarks and angles. S: sella turcica; N: nasion; A: deepest point on the premaxilla between anterior nasal spine and dental alveolus; B: deepest point on anterior part of the mandible. SNA (1) and SNB (2) angles: position of the maxilla and the mandible relative to the anterior cranial base in the sagittal plane; ANB angle: indicates inter-jaws relationship and is computed by subtraction of SNA and SNB; H: true horizontal

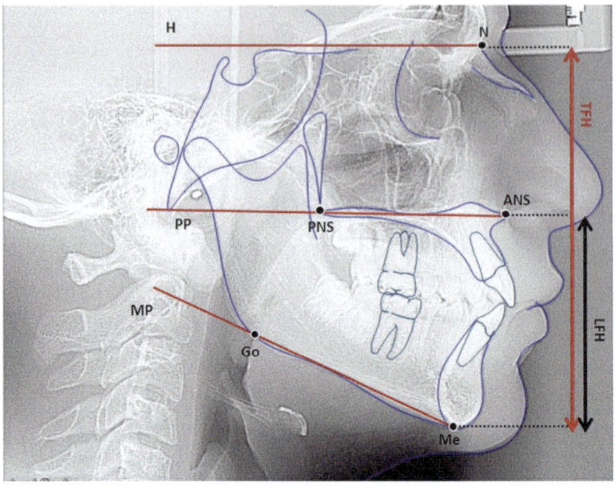

Fig. 8.3 Lateral cephalometric radiographs, Sowing N-Me, the distance between the nasion and Me, and the lower face height-to-total face height (LFH-to-TFH) ratio

point of the premaxilla. The SNB angle is the angle drawn between a line that extends from the sella turcica to the nasion and a line that extends from the nasion to the deepest point of the mandible (Fig. 8.2). It is also worth noting that the correlation between F0, mandibular length, and maxillary length remained significant even after excluding pubertal subjects, indicating that the longer the maxilla and the mandible, the low is the fundamental frequency and the habitual pitch [20]. The authors attributed this correlation to the parallel growth of the facial bones and vocal folds at puberty secondary to the change in the hormonal climate [20]. In 2017, Macari et al. investigated the association between F0, facial width, and facial length using different posteroanterior and lateral cephalometric measurements in a group of 50 subjects with a mean age of 14.19 ± 6.49 years. The authors showed a significant negative correlation between facial length and width, and F0 and habitual pitch. Subjects with wider faces had lower F0 and habitual pitch, and subjects with longer faces had lower habitual pitch. The correlation was more significant in males compared to females (Figs. 8.3 and 8.4). When the study group was stratified as prepubertal vs. postpubertal, the authors showed a negative correlation between maxillary width, mandibular width, total facial height, and habitual pitch in the prepubertal group. In the postpubertal group, there was a negative correlation between F0 and mandibular width. The negative correlation between these lateral and anteropos-

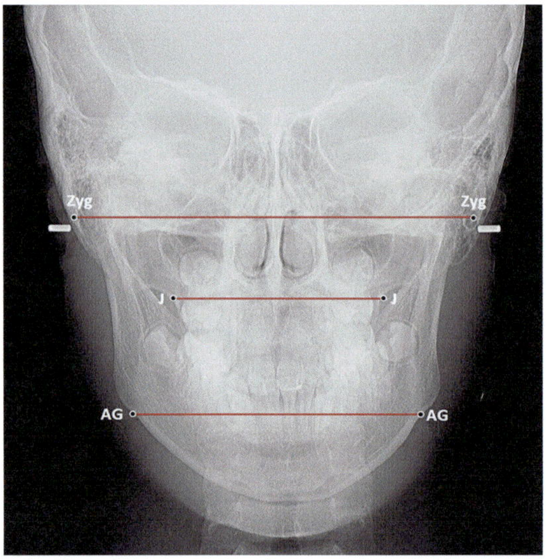

Fig. 8.4 Posteroanterior cephalometric radiograph showing landmarks and planes used in this study: Zyg: zygion—the most laterally situated point on the zygomatic arch; J: jugale—at the jugal process, the intersection of the outline of the maxillary tuberosity and the zygomatic buttress. AG: antegonion—the lateral inferior margin of the antegonial protuberances

terior facial measurements and F0 was based on the concomitant growth of facial and laryngeal structures and on the correlation between cephalo-facial anthropometry, body size, and F0 [21]. Similarly, in 2018 Hamdan et al. investigated the correlation between maxillary arch dimensions and voice characteristics and showed a moderate negative correlation between maxillary arch width and both habitual pitch and F0 ($r = -0.51$ and $r = -0.52$, respectively). Moreover, there was a moderately negative correlation between maxillary arch perimeter, habitual pitch, and F0 ($r = -0.34$ and $r = -0.39$, respectively) (Fig. 8.5). The study was conducted on 35 prepubertal subjects undergoing orthodontic treatment. The maxillary arch dimensions, namely, depth, width, and perimeter were taken from a template of the maxillary arch (Figs. 8.5 and 8.6) [22]. In 2020, Viegas et al. investigated the difference in F0 and the first three formants in subjects with skeletal class III malocclusion in comparison with subjects with normal occlusion. The results showed higher (more acute) F0 in the malocclusion group for all seven oral vowels that were assessed [23]. The authors attributed the high F0 to the high-positioned hyoid bone and shortening of the vocal tract during sound production. These findings disagree with the results of Mishami et al. who reported lower F0 in subjects with class III malocclusion undergoing orthognathic surgery [19].

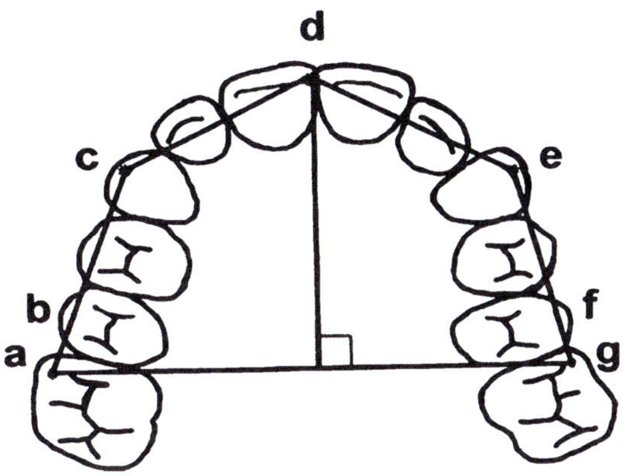

Fig. 8.5 Arch width: distances bf and ag;
Arch length: distance d to line ag
Arch perimeter: ac + cd + de + eg

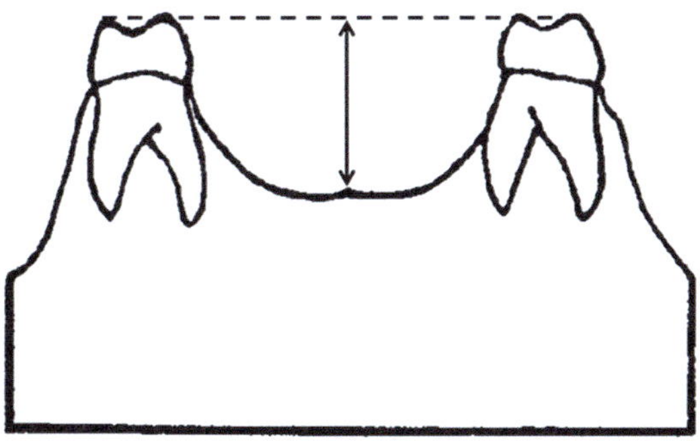

Fig. 8.6 Arch depth

Why the Correlation Between the Fundamental Frequency and Dentofacial Structures?

The Hormone Climate

The correlation between F0 and dentofacial measurements is partially based on the parallel growth of the larynx and facial bones under the influence of hormones. This chapter begins with a discussion of the effect of hormonal changes on laryngeal structures, and on facial and body skeleton (Fig. 8.7).

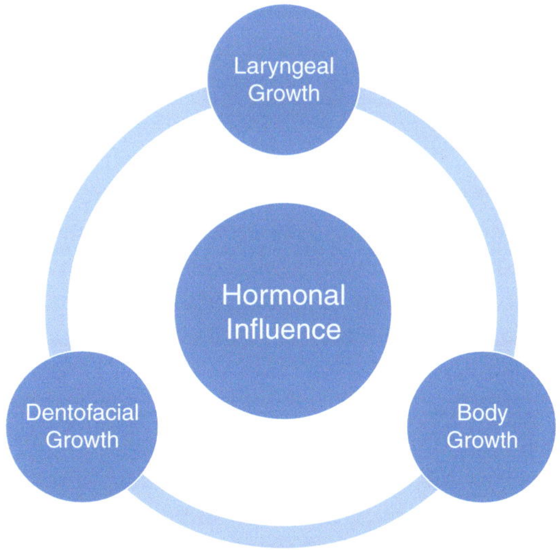

Fig. 8.7 Hormone impact on laryngeal structures

The larynx is a hormone target. Numerous authors identified different types of hormone receptors in laryngeal structures. In 2003, Altman et al. performed immunohistochemical staining using antibodies reactive to thyroid hormone receptors, alpha and beta, (TR-alpha, TR-beta) in two human cadaveric larynges. The authors demonstrated the presence of these receptors in the fibrous connective tissue of the lamina propria. Moreover, TR-alpha receptor was found in the thyroid cartilage and in the glandular structures, but not in the mucosal lining or muscles. These findings helped explain the known impact of thyroid hormones on the vocal folds and their adverse effect on phonation [24]. Similarly, alteration in growth hormone is known to impact phonation [2, 25]. In a study by Barreto et al., abnormal perceptual rating of breathiness, strain, and roughness were reported in patients with idiopathic growth hormone deficiency ($n = 23$) in comparison to controls [25]. Additionally, there were evidence of laryngeal constriction on endoscopy and abnormal acoustic findings, namely, an increase in harmonic to noise ratio and fundamental frequency, and a decrease in cycle-to-cycle variation in intensity (shimmer) [25]. Similarly, elevation in growth hormone has been associated with laryngeal dysfunction and respiratory symptoms. Stridor, dyspnea, and shortness in breath are reported often in addition to edematous changes of the glottic and supraglottic structures. In rare cases, stridor may occur as a result of unilateral and/or bilateral vocal fold fixation, which may necessitate a tracheotomy followed by a vocal fold lateralization procedure [26–28]. In 2016, Cooper et al. reported a 56-year-old man with acromegaly who presented with stridor and dyspnea secondary to bilateral immobility of the vocal folds. The patient underwent tracheotomy and unilateral laser arytenoidectomy for the relief of his airway obstructive symptoms [27].

The larynx is recognized particularly as an end-target for sex hormones. There are numerous reports with conflicting results on the presence of sex hormone receptors in different structures of the larynx. In 2000, Newman et al. investigated the presence of sex hormone receptors in the larynges of 42 fresh cadavers with a mean age of 37.7 years. Hormone receptors, mostly androgen and progesterone, were found in the glandular structures using immunohistochemical staining. These age- and gender-specific receptors were detected in both the cytoplasm and nuclei of cells within the vocal folds [29]. In 2008, Voelter et al. supported these findings in their study of 140 slides taken from 104 patients with benign and malignant laryngeal pathologies. Using monoclonal antibodies directed against androgen, progesterone, and estrogen-alpha receptors, the authors detected hormone receptors, mostly androgen and estrogen [30]. However, in 2007, Schneider et al. investigated the presence of sex hormones receptors using immunohistochemical staining in a group of 15 autopsied patients and failed to identify any, thus contradicting previous reports [31].

Despite the controversies in the above reports, voice sexual dimorphism at puberty occurs with a differential increase in vocal fold mass and length in males compared to females [32]. There are also sex hormone-induced laryngeal changes post-puberty. Abitbol proved the presence of morphologic vocal fold changes in women during their childbearing years and after menopause [33, 34]. These changes were held responsible for a constellation of vocal symptoms often reported in affected subjects and referred to as "the premenopausal vocal syndrome" and the "postmenopausal vocal syndrome," respectively.

Hormone impact on facial and somatic growth

Similar to the laryngeal framework, the facial and skeletal structures are under the influence of the hormonal environment [35, 36]. Both vertebral and mandibular growth accelerate in the first three decades of life, with peak mandibular growth at puberty. A low growth hormone level can lead to short stature, small-sized base of skull, and reduction in mandibular dimensions and facial heights [37], whereas a high hormone level results in tall stature and an increase in facial height and posterior cranial base. Affected patients tend to have broader faces and accentuated zygomatic arches. Sex hormones play an extremely important role in craniofacial and skeletal growth. In addition to being growth hormone catalysts, sex steroids have a direct effect on the linear skeletal craniofacial growth [38]. Sexual precocity has been shown to result in advanced growth of the craniofacial structures and skeletal bones, similar to the effect seen following an increase in androgen exposure, be it drug-induced or physiologic, as in cases of adrenal hyperplasia [38, 39]. In a study by Verdonck et al. on the impact of low testosterone treatment on facial growth and body, the authors reported significant increase in mandibular length, facial heights, and body height in comparison to untreated height-matched controls. Moreover, the above facial measurements were significantly lower than controls before treatment. The delayed growth of the mandible, cranial base, and facial height is based on the similar delay in stature attributed to the delayed pubertal spurt [40]. Their findings agreed with the study by Spiegel et al. in 1971 which asserted a strong association between craniofacial measures and stature [39]. The study was conducted on 7 boys with delayed puberty who were treated with testosterone propionate 25 mg twice monthly for 6 months. Additionally, thyroid hormones also may affect skeletal and facial growth. Hypothyroidism can lead to growth retardation with a delayed growth of the cranium and facial features [2].

In summary, one can conclude that the hormone climate dominates the growth of laryngeal structures, as well as body and facial skeleton. This parallel growth of the vocal folds and craniofacial structures may explain partially the association between the fundamental frequency and dentofacial anomalies.

Vocal Tract Development

Another possible explanation for the correlation between F0 and dentofacial anomalies is the difference in vocal tract length in patients with type II and III malocclusion, in comparison to subjects with normal occlusion. Xue et al. investigated vocal tract development in eight patients with class III malocclusion using acoustic reflection technology and showed greater oral length and volume in affected subjects in comparison to their cohorts. Though the authors reported higher values for F1/u/ in class III patients in comparison to controls, there was no difference in F0 between the two groups (F0 = 114.34 Hz vs. 113/36 Hz, respectively) [41]. In the study by Viegas et al. on acoustic analysis of 20 men with Angle's class III skeletal malocclusion in comparison to 40 with normal occlusion, the authors attributed the higher F0 in the former group to the shorter vocal tract, secondary to high-positioned hyoid bone [23]. Undoubtedly, the hyoid bone plays an important role in determining the width and length of the vocal tract in patients with or without malocclusion. In a study by Abu Alhajia et al., subjects with class III malocclusion had a higher hyoid bone positioned to the mandible [42]. Similarly, Iwasaki demonstrated a positive correlation between facial projection, namely, the anteroposterior positions of the maxilla and mandible as well as the craniocervical inclinations, and oropharyngeal measurements. The authors showed a lower position of the tongue in class III malocclusion children. Note that the volumetric oropharyngeal dimensions were partially extracted from the position of the epiglottis at the level of the hyoid bone [43]. Kecik also attributed the larger intraoral cross-sectional area to the lower position of the hyoid bone in class III malocclusion subjects in comparison to those with normal occlusion [44]. All the above confirm that dentofacial anomalies are associated with the position of the hyoid bone and the length of the vocal tract.

According to numerous authors, although F0 is more indicative of vocal fold and laryngeal growth rather than vocal tract development, when combined with other acoustic parameters linked to vocal tract length, it may serve as an acoustic cue to body and craniofacial morphology [7, 45]. This is in agreement with the source-filter theory, which asserts the strong correlation between vocal tract length and voice classification across singers, with emphasis on the oral and pharyngeal divisions of the vocal tract as being the most determinants in that classification [17, 46–48]. It also agrees with the study by Rendall et al., which argues against dimorphism in vocal fold length and mass as the sole reason for the vocal dimorphism in the fundamental frequency between the two genders [10].

In summary, the association between F0 and dentofacial anomalies may be interpreted in the context of the differential development of the vocal tract in patients with malocclusion class II and III in comparison with subjects with normal occlusion. Nevertheless, it is important to recognize that there is not enough evidence in the literature on vocal tract length across patients with different types of malocclusion, nor on the correlation between vocal tract length and F0 in patients with dentofacial anomalies. To draw definitive conclusions, further research on this topic is warranted.

References

1. Hamdan AL, Sataloff RT, Hawkshaw MJ. Obesity, body size and voice. In: Hamdan AL, Sataloff RT, Hawkshaw MJ. Obesity and voice. San Diego, CA: Plural Publishing; 2019. p. 115–30.
2. Hamdan AL, Sataloff RT, Hawkshaw MJ. Laryngeal manifestations of endocrine disorders. In: Hamdan AL, Sataloff RT, Hawkshaw MJ. Laryngeal manifestations of systemic diseases. San Diego, CA: Plural Publishing; 2018. p. 313–40.
3. Lass NJ, Davis M. An investigation of speaker height and weight identification. J Acoust Soc Am. 1976;60(3):700–3.
4. Evans S, Neave N, Wakelin D. Relationships between vocal characteristics and body size and shape in human males: an evolutionary explanation for a deep male voice. Biol Psychol. 2006;72(2):160–3.
5. Barsties B, Verfaillie R, Roy N, Maryn Y. Do body mass index and fat volume influence vocal quality, phonatory range, and aerodynamics in females? Codas. 2013;23(4):310–8.
6. Da Cunha MG, Passerotti GH, Weber R, Zilberstein B, Cecconello I. Voice feature characteristic in morbid obese population. Obes Surg. 2011;21(3):340–4.
7. Künzel HJ. How well does average fundamental frequency correlate with speaker height and weight? Phonetica. 1989;46(1–3):117–25.
8. Gunter CD, Manning WH. Listener estimations of speaker height and weight in unfiltered and filtered conditions. J Phon. 1982;10(3):251–7.
9. Van Dommelen WA, Moxness BH. Acoustic parameters in speaker height and weight identification: sex-specific behaviour. Lang Speech. 1995;38(Pt 3):267–87.
10. Rendall D, Kollias S, Ney C, Lloyd P. Pitch (F 0) and formant profiles of human vowels and vowel-like baboon grunts: the role of vocalizer body size and voice-acoustic allometry. J Acoust Soc Am. 2005;117(2):944–55.
11. Hamdan AL, Al-Barazi R, Tabri D, et al. Relationship between acoustic parameters and body mass analysis in young males. J Voice. 2012;26(2):144–7.
12. de Souza LB, Pereira RM, dos Santos MM, de Almeida Godoy CM. Fundamental frequency, phonation maximum time and vocal complaints in morbidly obese women. Arq Bras Cir Dig. 2014;27(1):43–6.
13. Gutzmann H. Über das Erkennen der Stimmgattung On the identification of voice classification. Folia Phoniatr Basel. 1949;2:1–5.
14. Gutzmann H. Über die Voraussetzungen eines Erfolgversprechenden Gesangsstudiums On the requirements for a successful singer education. Arch Ohren Nasen Kehlkopfheilkd. 1958;173:546–50.
15. Ackermann R. Zur frage von gaumenform und stimmqualität On the question of palate shape and voice quality. Z Laryngol Rhinol Otol. 1967;46:280–4.
16. Marunick MT, Menaldi CJ. Maxillary dental arch form related to voice classification: a pilot study. J Voice. 2000;14(1):82–91.
17. Roers F, Mürbe D, Sundberg J. Voice classification and vocal tract of singers: a study of x-ray images and morphology. J Acoust Soc Am. 2009;125(1):503–12.
18. Jorge TM, Brasolotto AG, Gonçales ES, Nary Filho H, Berretin-Felix G. Influence of orthognathic surgery on voice fundamental frequency. J Craniofac Surg. 2009;20(1):161–4.
19. Mishima K, Moritani N, Nakano H, Matsushita A, Iida S, Ueyama Y. Voice characteristics before versus after mandibular setback surgery in patients with mandibular prognathism using nonlinear dynamics and conventional acoustic analyses. J Craniomaxillofac Surg. 2013;41(8):706–9.
20. Macari AT, Karam IA, Tabri D, Sarieddine D, Hamdan AL. Correlation between the length and sagittal projection of the upper and lower jaw and the fundamental frequency. J Voice. 2014;28(3):291–6.
21. Macari AT, Karam IA, Ziade G, et al. Association between facial length and width and fundamental frequency. J Voice. 2017;31(4):410–5.
22. Hamdan AL, Khandakji M, Macari AT. Maxillary arch dimensions associated with acoustic parameters in prepubertal children. Angle Orthod. 2018;88(4):410–5.
23. Viegas F, Viegas D, Guimarães GS, Ritto F, Simões-Zenari M, Nemr K. Acoustic analysis of voice and speech in men with skeletal class III malocclusion: a pilot study. Folia Phoniatr Logop. 2020;7:1–9.
24. Altman KW, Haines GK III, Vakkalanka SK, Keni SP, Kopp PA, Radosevich JA. Identification of thyroid hormone receptors in the human larynx. Laryngoscope. 2003;113(11):1931–4.
25. Barreto VM, D'Ávila JS, Sales NJ, et al. Laryngeal and vocal evaluation in untreated growth hormone deficient adults. Otolaryngol Head Neck Surg. 2009;140(1):37–42.
26. Saussez S, Mahillon V, Chantrain G, Thill MP, Lequeux T. Acromegaly presented as a cause of laryngeal dyspnea. Auris Nasus Larynx. 2007;34(4):541–3.

27. Cooper T, Dziegielewski PT, Singh P, Seemann R. Acromegaly presenting with bilateral vocal fold immobility: case report and review of the literature. J Voice. 2016;30(6):758.e13–6.
28. Lerat J, Lacoste M, Prechoux JM, et al. An uncommon case of dyspnea with unilateral laryngeal paralysis in acromegaly. Auris Nasus Larynx. 2016;43(1):105–7.
29. Newman SR, Butler J, Hammond EH, Gray SD. Preliminary report on hormone receptors in the human vocal fold. J Voice. 2000;14(1):72–81.
30. Voelter C, Kleinsasser N, Joa P, et al. Detection of hormone receptors in the human vocal fold. Eur Arch Otorhinolaryngol. 2008;265(10):1239–44.
31. Schneider B, Cohen E, Stani J, et al. Towards the expression of sex hormone receptors in the human vocal fold. J Voice. 2007;21(4):502–7.
32. Fitch WT, Giedd J. Morphology and development of the human vocal tract: a study using magnetic resonance imaging. J Acoust Soc Am. 1999;106(3):1511–22.
33. Abitbol J, Abitbol P, Abitbol B. Sex hormones and the female voice. J Voice. 1999;13(3):424–46.
34. Abitbol J, de Brux J, Millot G, et al. Does a hormonal vocal cord cycle exist in women? Study of vocal premenstrual syndrome in voice performers by videostroboscopy-glottography and cytology on 38 women. J Voice. 1989;2:157–62.
35. Daughaday WH, Rotwein P. Insulin like growth factors −1 and −2. Peptide, messenger, ribonucleid acid and gene structures, serum and tissue concentrations. Endocrine Rev. 1989;10:68–91.
36. Albertsson-Wikland K, Rosberg S. Analyses of 24 hour growth hormone profiles in children: relation to growth. J Endocrinol Metab. 1988;67:493–500.
37. Pirinen S, Majurin A, Lenko H-L, Koski K. Craniofacial features in patients wth deficient and excessive growth hormone. J Craniofac Gen Devel Biol. 1994;14(3):144–52.
38. Cara JF, Kreiter ML, Rosenfield RL. Height prognosis of children with true precocious puberty and growth hormone deficiency: effect of combination therapy with gonadotrophin releasing hormone agonist and growth hormone. J Pediatr. 1992;120:709–14.
39. Spiegel R, Sather H, Hayles A. Cephalometric study of children with various endocrine diseases. Am J Orthod. 1971;59:362–75.
40. Verdonck A, Gaethofs M, Carels C, de Zegher F. Effect of low-dose testosterone treatment on craniofacial growth in boys with delayed puberty. Eur J Orthod. 1999;21(2):137–43.
41. Xue SA, Lam CW, Whitehill TL, Samman N. Effects of Class III malocclusion on young male adults' vocal tract development: a pilot study. J Oral Maxillofac Surg. 2011;69(3):845–52.
42. Abu Allhaija ES, Al-Khateeb SN. Uvulo-glosso-pharyngeal dimensions in different anteroposterior skeletal patterns. Angle Orthod. 2005;75(6):1012–8.
43. Iwasaki T, Hayasaki H, Takemoto Y, Kanomi R, Yamasaki Y. Oropharyngeal airway in children with Class III malocclusion evaluated by cone-beam computed tomography. Am J Orthod Dentofac Orthop. 2009;136(3):318.e1–9.
44. Kecik D. The effect of mandibular position on upper airway dimensions. Turk J Orthod. 2009;22:93–101.
45. Smith DR, Walters TC, Patterson RD. Discrimination of speaker sex and size when glottal-pulse rate and vocal-tract length are controlled. J Acoust Soc Am. 2007;122(6):3628–39.
46. Titze IR. Principles of vocal production. Englewood Cliffs, NJ: Prentice Hall; 1994.
47. Cleveland TF. Acoustic properties of voice timbre types and their influence on voice classification. J Acoust Soc Am. 1977;61(6):1622–9.
48. Dmitriev L, Kiselev A. Relationship between the formant structure of different types of singing voices and the dimensions of supraglottic cavities. Folia Phoniatr. 1979;31(4):238–41.

9 Formant Frequencies and Dentofacial Anomalies

The dentofacial skeleton is an important component of the phonatory apparatus. The sagittal and vertical growth of the upper and lower jaw establish the boundaries of the oropharyngeal division of the vocal tract. Based on the Source-Filter theory, the vocal tract acts as a resonator for the sound fed into it by oscillation of the vocal folds. Its resonance peaks are referred to as formants, and they occur at various frequencies. Their position and interspace vary with the length and shape of the vocal tract. The longer the vocal tract, the lower are these formants, and the shorter the vocal tract, the higher these formants. The formant structure is determined and limited partially by the individual's anatomy, but within those structural limits, formant adjustments are possible. Elongation and shortening of the vocal tract can be achieved by lowering or elevating the larynx, and/or by protruding or reducing the lip opening during phonation. Among the formant frequencies, the third, fourth, and fifth are the most important in defining the speaker's voice timbre [1]. Subjects with skeletal and non-skeletal dentofacial anomalies often present with distinctive vocal tract dimensions leading to distinctive acoustic properties. Understanding the vocal characteristics of these patients is imperative for patient counselling, particularly in professional voice users who are considering orthodontic and/or orthognathic surgery. It is equally important in wind instrumentalists who rely heavily on the vocal tract for creating the tone that emanates from their instrument.

This chapter reviews the current literature on formant frequencies in patients with class II and class III malocclusion. The link between dentofacial anomalies and formant frequencies is explored in the context of vocal tract development and the growth of craniofacial structures and the body. The association between formant frequencies and body size, as well as that between craniofacial structures and body stature, is reviewed.

Correlation Between Formant Frequencies and Body Size

Formant frequencies are important acoustic cues to our identities. Many authors investigated the correlation between formant frequencies and physical attributes, namely, height, weight, and body measurements, with no clear consensus. The lack of consensus has been attributed in part to the debate on laryngeal growth and development in relation to base of skull and body. In 2000, Collins reported no correlation between acoustic measures and body characteristics, although weight was estimated successfully from voice in male subjects. The acoustic analysis included harmonic peaks and harmonic spacing [2]. Similarly, Gonzalez reported a weak correlation between body height, weight, and formant frequencies. The study included 82 speakers who were asked to sustain five vowels, and 92 speakers who were asked to read a para-

A.-L. Hamdan et al., *Dentofacial Anomalies*, https://doi.org/10.1007/978-3-030-69109-7_9

graph [3]. However, other authors showed that formant frequencies can be used to predict body morphology with an acceptable error of estimation. Rendall et al. in their study of vocalizer body size and voice-acoustic allometry reported a correlation between variations in formant frequencies and height in male subjects, whereas fundamental frequency failed to correlate with any body-size variation. The study group consisted of 68 students, and the study included isolated vowels, single-syllable words, and four sentences [4]. Evans et al. showed a significant and moderate correlation between formant dispersion and body weight ($r = -0.43$) and height ($r = -0.32$) in a group of 50 heterosexual men. Subjects who were tall and/or heavier had smaller formants' dispersion [5]. These results were in agreement with those of Pisanski et al., who also showed that vocal tract resonance can predict height and weight. The authors reported statistical significance in 93% of the derived mean-weighted correlations between body size and formants [6]. Similarly, Roers et al., in their study on the voices of 340 student singers, reported differences in body weight in singers with different voice classification. There was a trend toward an increase in body weight as voice got deeper. Subjects classified as bass singers were heavier that those classified as baritone singers or tenors. Similarly, women classified as alto singers were heavier that those classified as mezzo singers. However, those classified as mezzo singers were not heavier than those classified as soprano singers. Subjects classified as bass were also taller than those classified as baritone or tenor [7] (Table 9.1).

Table 9.1 Summary of studies on the association between formant frequencies and body characteristics

Author/s & year	Number of subjects	Singers vs. non-singers	Acoustic samples	Findings
Collins (2000)	34 subjects	Non-singers	Five vowels: A, as in normal; E, as in say; I, as in see; O, as in no; U, duel (the Dutch U is not a sound used in English; duel is the closest approximation)	No correlation between acoustic measures and body characteristics
Gonzalez (2004)	82 subjects (Experiment I) 91 subjects (Experiment II)	Non-singers	A sustained phonation of each Spanish vowel (/a/, /e/, /i/, /o/, /u/) and the reading of a paragraph	A weak correlation between body height, weight, and formant frequencies
Rendall et al. (2005)	68 subjects	Non-singers	Isolated vowels, single-syllable words, and four sentences	Significant correlation between formant variation and height in male subjects
Evans et al. (2006)	50 subjects	Non-singers	English vowels: "a," "e," "i," and "o"	Significant and moderate negative correlation between formant's dispersion and measures of body size and shape
Roers et al. (2009)	340 subjects	Singers	None (tidal breathing)	Differences in body weight in relation to voice classifications. There was a trend toward an increase in body weight as voice got deeper
Pisanski et al. (2016)	700 subjects	Non-singers	For the Canadian and German samples, the five vowels were /ɑ/, /i/, /ɜ/, /o/, and /u/ (International Phonetic Alphabetic notation) For the Scottish sample, the vowels were /eI/, /i/, /aI/, /o/, and /ju/	Vocal tract resonance can predict height and weight. There was statistical significance in 93% of the derived mean-weighted correlations between body size and formants

In summary, formant frequencies may be used in the estimation of body size, but with uncertainty. Their predictive role is based on their inherent link to vocal tract morphology, and its parallel growth with body skeleton [8, 9].

The Correlation Between Formant Frequencies and Dentofacial Anomalies

There is little literature on the association between dentofacial anomalies and formant frequencies, despite the inclusion of the upper and lower jaw in the oropharyngeal division of the vocal tract. Only a few reports examined the correlation between cephalometric measurements and vocal characteristics of patients with dentofacial anomalies. Moreover, most of the studies are on non-professional voice users, though formants are more important in singers who invariably learn to modulate the length and shape of their vocal tract to tailor the sound of their voice and to be heard better. Additionally, the acoustic samples usually used for analysis are limited to vowels and/ or read paragraphs and not songs. In 1985, Bowers et al. investigated formant frequencies in three patients with class II malocclusion and two patients with class III malocclusion who underwent orthognathic surgery. The authors reported significant shifts in the second formants for the vowel /e/ but not /ɑ/ and /u/. Though there were no control subjects, the speech of all patients was judged preoperatively by their treating orthodontists as normal [10]. Lee et al. analyzed acoustically the sound /s/ derived from six words, before and after osteotomy in patients with class III malocclusion. The analysis included the first two spectral peaks, in addition to three other acoustic variables. The study group had higher means of spectral peak I and II, and wider bandwidth in comparison with the control group prior to surgery (9.09 vs. 7.36, and 9.26 vs. 7.91, respectively) [11]. In 2006, Niemi et al. investigated the impact of mandibular advancement, on quality of speech in five subjects with retrognathic mandible. The acoustic sample consisted of eight vowels, and acoustic analysis included the lower two formants F1 and F2, in addition to F0. The authors reported no significant changes in the acoustic parameters up to 1 year. The study did not include a control group with which to compare the preoperative values [12]. In 2011, Xue et al. investigated formant variations in eight patients with class III malocclusion, in comparison to eight subjects with normal occlusion. Except for F1/u/ which was higher in patients with class III malocclusion, there was no significant difference between the two groups in any of the first three formants for all four vowels [13]. In 2013, Mishima et al. investigated the effect of bilateral sagittal split ramus osteotomy on voice in a group of 16 patients with class III malocclusion. The authors reported significantly lower values preoperatively for F1/ɑ/ and F2/ɑ/ in males, and F1/u/ and F2/i/ in females in comparison to a control group of 50 healthy adults [14]. In 2015, Macari et al. examined the association between the sagittal projection and length of the upper and lower jaw and formant frequencies F1, F2, F3, and F4 of vowels /ɑ/, /i/, /o/, and /u/. The study group consisted of 46 consecutive patients presenting to the orthodontic and dentofacial orthopedist, with a typical distribution in terms of occlusion (51% class I, 40.5% class II, and 8.5% class III). Following cephalometric skeletal measurements of the upper and lower jaw in both sagittal and vertical planes, each subject underwent acoustic analysis using real-time spectrography. The results showed a moderate negative correlation between the fourth formants for all the vowels tested and the length of the maxilla. Similarly, there was a moderate negative correlation between the length of the mandible and F4/o/ and F4/u/. There was also a negative correlation between the length of the mandible and F3/i/, F3/o/, and F3/u/, and a negative correlation between the length of the maxilla and F3 for the vowels /ɑ/, /i/, and /o/. Moreover, there was a negative association between the length of the mandible and maxilla and formant dispersion, namely F2-F3, and F4-F3, for the vowel /i/ and /u/ [15]. In summary, the authors concluded that the longer the lower jaw and the longer the upper jaw, the lower the position of the third and fourth formants, and the narrow is the interspace of

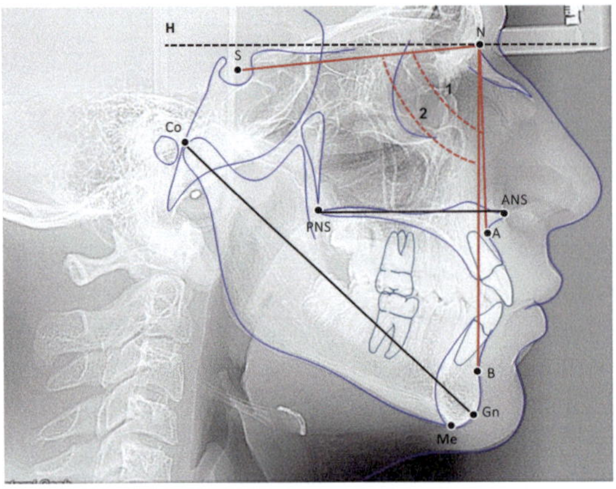

Fig. 9.1 Lateral cephalometric tracing showing the landmarks and angles measured in the study. S: sella turcica; N: nasion; A: deepest point on the premaxilla between anterior nasal spine and dental alveolus; B: deepest point on anterior part of the mandible; ANS: anterior nasal spine; PNS: posterior nasal spine; Co: condylion—anterosuperior point of the condyle; Gn: gnathion—midpoint between the most protruded and the lowest points of the symphysis. Me: menton—most inferior point on the symphysis of the mandible. SNA (1) and SNB (2) angles: position of the maxilla and the mandible relative to the anterior cranial base in the sagittal plane; ANB angle: indicates inter-jaws relationship and is computed by subtraction of SNA and SNB; ANS-PNS: maxillary length; Co-Gn: mandibular length. H: true horizontal

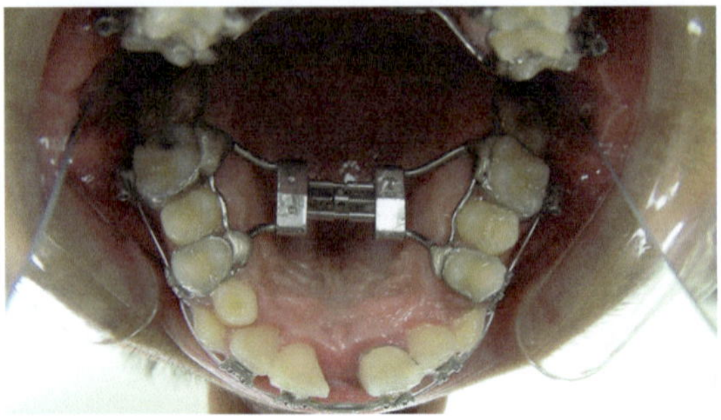

Fig. 9.2 View of the palatal expander during treatment of a patient with a constricted maxilla

these formants [15] (Fig. 9.1). In 2018, Hamdan et al. studied the association between maxillary arch dimensions and several acoustic parameters among which were the first four formants. The study group consisted of 35 prepubertal patients who had maxillary arch measurements and had their voices analyzed while sustaining four vowels /α/, /i/, /o/, and /u/. The authors reported a significant negative correlation between arch depth and F3 for vowels /α/, /i/, and /u/, and a positive correlation with F2 for the vowel /o/. Similarly, there was a negative correlation between arch length and F4 for the vowels /α/, /o/, and /u/. Notably, F3 correlated most consistently with all maxillary arch measurements [16] (Fig. 9.2). In 2020, Viegas et al. assessed formant characteristics of 7 oral vowels in 20 patients with class III skeletal malocclusion in comparison to 40 patients with class I occlusion. The results showed lower first and third formants for the vowel /u/, higher first two formants for the vowels /α/ and /ɛ/, and higher F2 /e/ and F2/i/ in the former group [17]. Table 9.2 presents a summary of the studies.

In summary, there is a negative correlation between the length of the upper and lower jaw, and F3 and F4. The longer the mandible and the longer the maxilla, the lower these formants, and the narrower the dispersion among them. Similarly, there is a negative correlation between maxillary arch length, depth, and F3.

Why the Correlation Between Dentofacial Anomalies and Formant Frequencies?

The correlation between formant frequencies and dentofacial anomalies can be attributed to the known association between formant frequencies and vocal tract morphology, and to the known association between vocal tract morphology, facial skeleton dimensions, and body size (Fig. 9.3).

Formant Frequencies and Vocal Tract Size

The position and dispersion of formant frequencies is determined by the physiologic and anatomic boundaries of the vocal tract, mostly its length and shape. At puberty, there is a difference in the descent of the larynx in men compared to women, with subsequent differential elongation of the vocal tract that is partially

Table 9.2 Summary of studies on formant frequencies in patients with dentofacial anomalies

Author/s & year	Number of subjects	Singers vs. non-singers	Acoustic samples	Findings
Bowers et al. (1985)	5 subjects (3 patients with malocclusion class II and 2 patients with malocclusion class III)	Non-singers	Sentences in the form, "Here is a ____ again." The blanks were filled with target words whose initial consonants varied between "s" and "sh." There were three vowel choices—"a" as in "sat," "u" as in "shoot," and "e" as in "sheet." The final consonant was always "t"	Significant shifts in the second formants for the vowel /e/ but not /a/ and /u/. The speech of all patients was judged as normal preoperatively
Lee et al. (2002)	9 subjects	Non-singers	The sound /s/ derived from six words. The analysis included the first two spectral peaks in addition to other three acoustic variables	Higher means of spectral peak I and II pre-surgery in the study group compared to the control group. The study group had wider bandwidth in comparison with the control group
Niemi et al. (2006)	5 subjects	Non-singers	Eight vowels in sentence context	No significant changes in formants F1 and F2 on the long term up to 1 year following surgery
Xue et al. (2011)	8 subjects with class III malocclusion in comparison to 8 subjects with normal occlusion	Non-singers	A continuous speech sample and four sustained vowels (/a/, /æ/, /i/, and /u/) were recorded	Higher value for the F1/u/ in patients with malocclusion III
Lammert et al. (2012)	5 subjects (American English speakers	Non-singers	High-front vowels while real-time magnetic resonance imaging were collected	With an increase in palatal concavity, there is an increase in F1 and a decrease in F2 and F3. Similarly, palatal anteriority had a substantial impact on the second and third formants
Mishima et al. (2013)	50 subjects	Non-singers	As voice samples, the Japanese vowels /a/, /i/, /u/, /e/, and /o/were phonated naturally three times before and at 6 months after the BSSRO	Significant lower values preoperatively for F1/a/ and F2/a/ in males and F1/u/ and F2/i/ in females in comparison to a control group
Macari et al. (2014)	46 consecutive subjects, with a normal distribution in terms of malocclusion (51% class I, 40.5% class II, and 8.5% class III)	Non-singers	Four vowels /a/, /i/, /o/, and /u/	The results showed a moderate negative correlation between the fourth formants for all the vowels tested and the length of the maxilla (R value greater than 0.3) There was a moderate negative correlation between the length of the mandible and F4/o/ and F4/u/ There was also a negative correlation between the length of the mandible and F3/i/, F3/o/, and F3/u/, and a negative correlation between the length of the maxilla and F3 for the vowels /a/, /i/, and /o/ There was a negative association between the length of the mandible and maxilla and formant dispersion, namely, F2-F3, and F4-F3, for the vowel /i/ and /u/
Hamdan et al. (2015)	35 prepubertal patients who had maxillary arch measurements	Non-singers	Four sustained vowels /a/, /i/, /o/, and /u/	A significant negative correlation between arch depth and F3 for vowels /a/, /i/, and /u/, and a positive correlation with F2 for the vowel /o/ There was a negative correlation between arch length and F4 for the vowels /a/, /o/, and /u/ F3 correlated the most with all maxillary arch measurements
Viegas et al. (2020)	20 subjects with class III skeletal malocclusion in comparison to 40 patients with class I malocclusion	Non-singers	Seven oral vowels	Lower first and third formant for the vowel /u/, higher first two formants for the vowel /a/, and /Ɛ/, and higher F2 /e/ and F2 /i/

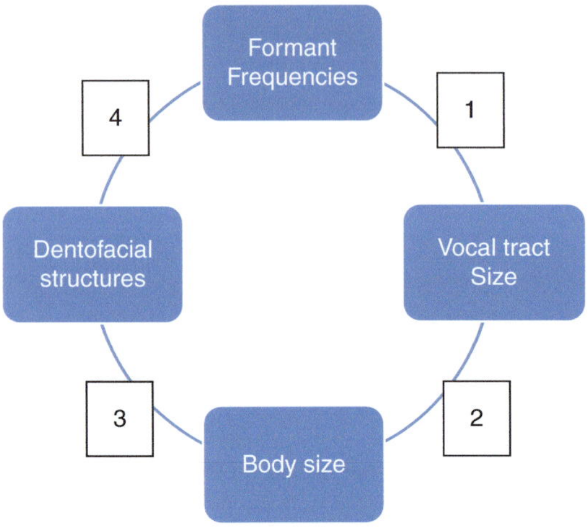

Fig. 9.3 The link between formant frequencies, vocal tract size, body size, and dentofacial structures

responsible for vocal dimorphism [18–21]. In 1966, Fant reported the difference in vocal tract length between men and women as a physiologic scaling factor that contributes to 20% higher formant frequencies in women in comparison to men [21]. Similarly, in 1999 Fitch and Giedd reported a difference of 7.5 mm between vocal tract length in prepubertal males in comparison to prepubertal females, and a difference of 12.9 mm between vocal tract lengths in pubertal males vs. females [18]. The difference in vocal tract length between genders and across speakers of the same gender, as well as the inverse relationship between vocal tract length and formants, partially explain voice classification among singers. In 1977, Cleveland reported that vocal tract length and formant frequencies distinguish the vocal characteristics of a singer. The study was done using long-term average spectral analysis of five common vowels sang by eight professional voice users, in addition to vowel synthesis [22]. In 1979, Dmitriev and Kiselev studied the association between formant frequencies and supraglottic laryngeal behavior in different styles of singing, and demonstrated that for every type of voice or classification, the singer adjusts the buccopharyngeal tract to a fixed length. For instance, for a soprano singer in a frequency range of 760 Hz to 3.500 Hz (frequency of the low singing formant to the high singing formant), the distance between the lips and vocal folds is 15.3 to 16.3 cm. However, for a bass singer using a frequency range of 450 Hz to 2.500 Hz (frequency of the low singing formant to the high singing formant), the estimated buccopharyngeal tract length is 23.3 cm to 25.0 cm. In summary, for every voice type, there is a corresponding supraglottic dimension determined by the physiologic position of the vocal tract [23]. Similarly, Sulter et al. reported an association between the spatial configuration of the vocal tract and the acoustic signal produced (F1 for the vowel /ɛ/, and F1, F2 for the vowels /ɑ/ and /i/). The study was conducted on a male singer who was asked to perform various phonatory tasks while being evaluated using magnetic resonance imaging [24]. In 2009, Roers et al. investigated the association between vocal tract dimensions and voice classifications by reviewing 132 radiologic images taken from the medical records of students classified as soprano, mezzosoprano, alto, tenor, baritone, and bass singers. The images included the larynx, pharynx, trachea, vertebrae, and base of skull. The vocal tract was measured by adding the dimensions of the oral, velar, and pharyngeal components. The authors found differences in vocal tract length among different voice classifications, with bass singers having the longest vocal tract in comparison with other singers. The pharyngeal division of the vocal tract contributed the most to these differences. It was computed as the distance from the lower most anterior edge of the second vertebra to the anterior most prominent point of the laryngeal prominence [7].

In summary, there is strong interplay between vocal tract shape/ length, and formant position and dispersion. Anatomic and/or physiologic alterations in vocal tract morphology, as in patients with dentofacial anomalies, is expected to lead to changes in the acoustic properties of the speaker or singer. Similar effect on tone production for instrumentalists seems likely but requires study.

Vocal Tract Morphology and Body Size

The association between vocal tract shape/length, and body size has been supported by many authors [25–28]. In 1993, Shelton et al. reported variations in the configuration of the vocal tract in heavy subjects, alluding to the interplay between vocal tract morphology and obesity. The variation was credited to the increased volume of pharyngeal adipose tissue secondary to excessive weight [25]. In 1998, Mortimore et al., in their study on neck and total fat deposition in obese vs. non-obese subjects with obstructive sleep apnea/hypopnea syndrome (SAHS), reported larger neck tissue volume in subjects with large body mass index vs. subjects with normal body mass index, in comparison with the control group (28% vs. 10%). The difference in neck volume was attributed to fat deposition in the retro-palatal and retro-glossal regions [26]. These findings corroborate those of Horner et al. in 1989, in their radiologic examination of vocal tract morphology of subjects with large body mass index and history of obstructive sleep apnea (OSA). In addition to the significantly higher prevalence of fat deposits in the palate of obese subjects with OSA in comparison with weight-matched controls, the authors showed alterations in the configuration of the laryngopharyngeal airspace in all subjects with large body mass index. Moreover, there was excessive fat deposition in the tongue in 50% of the cases (3 out of 6 patients) [27]. Similarly, there is strong evidence in the literature to support the presence of a correlation between body size and vocal tract length. In 1999, Fitch and Giedd demonstrated a strong correlation between vocal tract length, measured from the lips to the vocal folds, and body size. The study was conducted on 129 subjects who were investigated using magnetic resonance images [18]. Similarly, in 2002 Shen et al. showed strong correlation between body weight and the distance between the nostril and the vocal folds (N-V) in 413 infants. Vocal tract segment was measured using a fiberoptic endoscope, and body weight was used as an anthropometric measure [28].

In summary, there is substantial evidence to support a strong correlation between body size and vocal tract shape/length. The taller the individual, the longer the vocal tract, and the heavier the individual, the more crowded the vocal tract. In singers with large body mass index (BMI), this may entail a higher subglottic pressure in order to compensate for the supraglottic constriction and achieve the same loudness as a singer with normal body weight. Further research is needed to elucidate the clinical implication of the differences in vocal tract morphology in subjects with high BMI vs. those with low BMI.

The Parallel Growth of Facial Bones and Body Skeleton

Based on the above, formant frequencies, vocal tract size, and body size are interlinked. A review of the literature also supports the link between body and craniofacial growth. Most reports are derived from forensic science in which identification of the deceased individual using skeletal remnants is of crucial importance. Several studies using regression analysis have confirmed the strong correlation between craniofacial development and skeletal maturation [29–31]. The consensus is that body reconstruction can be estimated reasonably well using cranio-cephalic measurements. In 1960, Rose compared the growth of facial areas with body measurements using 125 cephalometric profiles. In that study, the author concluded that body weight and length increase concomitantly with facial growth, except for the orbito-ethmoidal area, the development of which corresponds the least with the rest of facial measures [29]. In 1961, Bambha reported commonality in the growth of the face and body skeleton. The study was conducted on 50 subjects (25 boys and 25 girls) and included eight cephalometric skull measurements [32]. In another study by Hunter in 1966, carried on 25 males and 34 females, eight of whom were undergoing orthodontic treatment, the authors reported association between the maximum facial growth and height in the majority of the study group. The anteroposterior length of the mandible had the strongest relationship with the height growth during adolescence [33]. In 1981, Bishara et al. studied the relationship between various mandibular measures and standing height in a group of 35 subjects. The authors showed significant differences between height growth and mandibular growth, and unlike previous authors, concluded that the "growth profile of height has little predictive role in determining the growth profile of any of the mandibular parameters…" [34]. In 1993, Introna et al. studied the correlation between body height and cranial measurement, specifically the anteroposterior and lateral cranial diameters in a group of 358 males. The authors derived a mathematical formula that proved useful in the evaluation of stature in forensic investigations [35]. Similarly, in 1998, Chiba and Terazawa investigated the ability to estimate stature from skull measurements in 124 Japanese cadavers. The authors reported a standard error of estimates in 7.95 cm for both sexes and concluded that cranial diameter and circumference are helpful in identifying stature but with uncertainty [36]. In 2005, Cozza et al. investigated the growth of the craniofacial structures and body in 100 prepubertal subjects. Thirty measurements were used among which were head height, circumference, breadth and length, in addition to facial height (upper and lower). The authors reported less growth of the skull and face in comparison to body, and they failed to identify any body parameter as an indicator of craniofacial growth in the prepubertal period [37]. In 2007, Krishan and Kumar estimated body statures using 16 cephalo-facial measurements in a group of 252 Koli male adolescents. The authors reported a significant correlation between these measurements and stature. The correlation with stature was stronger in relation to the cephalic measures in comparison to the facial measures [38]. That same year, Ryan and Bidmos investigated the correlation between total skeletal height and six skull measurements. The study was conducted on 99 skeletons available in a school of anatomic science. The standard errors of estimates ranged between 4.37 and 6.24, and the correlation coefficient ranged between 0.40 and 0.54 [39]. In 2008, Krishan investigated the ability to estimate stature using five anthropometric measurements of the cephalo-facial region in a group of 996 adult males. The measurements included maximum head length measured by the straight distance between the glabella and the most prominent portion of the occiput posteriorly; maximum head breadth measured as the maximum distance between the most lateral points of the parietal bones, the horizontal circumference of the head, maximal breadth of the lower jaw, i.e., bigonial diameter; and the morphological facial length. The results of his investigation showed a significant correlation between all five cephalo-facial measures and stature. The correlation was more significant for the cephalic measures vs. the facial measures [40].

In summary, there is evidence to support a strong association between craniofacial and skeletal measures. The parallel growth of the body and craniofacial structures allow us to conclude that several body measures can be used to estimate craniofacial measures and vice versa.

Dentofacial Growth and Formant Frequencies

Given the known interplay between formant frequencies and vocal tract morphology, vocal tract morphology and body size, body size and craniofacial structures, it is intuitive to infer an association between formant frequencies and craniofacial structures and to assume that that association help to explain the distinctive acoustic properties of patients with dentofacial anomalies. This association includes variations in the length and shape of the vocal tract in these patients, and to the inherent link between vocal tract morphology and formant position and dispersion [41]. Although the current literature lacks consensus on vocal tract length in patients with different types of occlusion, numerous authors argue that variations in acoustic properties in patients with class III malocclusion in comparison to subjects with class I occlusion are associated with variations in vocal tract dimension and variations in hyoid bone position. In the study by Viegas et al., the high F1, F2, and F3 in patients with class III malocclusion were attributed to the high positioned hyoid bone [17]. This was in agreement with the study by Abu Alhajia and Al-Khateeb, who also showed that "the hyoid bone was closer to the mandible vertically and to C3 horizontally in patients with class III malocclusion in comparison to patients with class I occlusion" [42]. The study of Xue et al. also showed higher value for F1 /u/ in patients with class III malocclusion, in comparison to their cohort with normal occlusion [12]. However, the difference in F1/u/ value between the two groups was not attributed to the high-positioned hyoid bone but to the inability of class III malocclusion patients to protrude their lips during the production of the vowel /u/ [12]. It is important to note that although the authors proved that patients with class III malocclusion had significantly longer oral length and non-significant shorter pharyngeal length in comparison with the control group, the total vocal tract length was not statistically significant between the two groups [12].

Acoustic Implications of Dentofacial Anomalies in Wind Instrument Players

Sound production in wind instrumentalists involves three components: a generator, an oscillator, and a resonator. Breathing is the energizer that makes the reed oscillate within the mouthpiece, producing a tone that amplifies within the body of the musical instrument. The musical instrument acts as a resonator, very similar to the resonating cavities in phonation [43]. Numerous authors have investigated the laryngeal biomechanics of wind instrumentalists and shown engagement of the glottis and supraglottis during playing [44–46]. The vocal folds help regulate the airflow to the mouthpiece by controlling the glottic aperture, whereas the supraglottis help modulate the music tone. A constrictive pattern, often referred to as "lateral laryngeal tension" [44] or "supraglottic adduction" [45], is often seen as a sign of strain or difficulty in performance. Hence, it is possible that anatomic variations in vocal tract anatomy associated with dentofacial anomalies might impact the laryngeal behavior of wind instrumentalists and carry significant acoustic implications on their performance. Similar to singers who exhibit variations in vocal tract length across different vocal registers, and who learn how to modulate the length of the vocal tract by lifting or lowering the laryngeal framework during transition between various registers [7], wind instrumentalists also rely heavily on vocal tract to regulate the musical tone. Lengthening or shortening of the vocal tract in patients with malocclusion may present a challenge to wind instrumentalists with malocclusion, a challenge that may facilitate or hinder musical performance depending on the musical instrument.

Variations in vocal tract shape, particularly in its oral division also, are important wind instrumentalists with dentofacial anomalies. A narrow dental arch and/or constricted maxilla may lead to changes in the acoustic properties of the musical tone by modulating the airstream prior to its entry into the mouthpiece. This is analogous to the well-known correlation between voice classification and shape of the palate described among singers, and the known impact of palatal configuration on formant frequencies [7, 47, 48]. In 2013, Lammert et al. investigated the interplay between vocal tract morphology and acoustic inter-subject variability and demonstrated that palatal configuration impacts the position of the lowest three formants. With an increase in palatal concavity, there is an increase in F1 and a decrease in F2 and F3. Similarly, palatal anteriority, which refers to the position of the apex of the dome anteroposteriorly, had a substantial impact on the second and third formants [48]. In addition to these acoustic implications associated with palatal morphology, wind instrumentalists with dentofacial anomalies may also suffer from difficulties in embouchure such as mal-fitting of the mouthpiece due to crowding or irregular anterior teeth. This may lead to excessive tension that extends beyond the orofacial complex to the laryngopharyngeal complex. Excessive laryngeal and/or pharyngeal tension may be added to the list of well-known disorders associated with wind instrument playing, such as orofacial dystonia, velopharyngeal insufficiency, and reduced tongue agility and flexibility. As described by Weikert and Schlömicher-Thier, the vocal tract does not act only as a conduit for the airstream to the mouthpiece, but also as a regulator of that airflow [45]. The excessive laryngeal tension associated with oropharyngeal tension may interfere with laryngeal behavior and jeopardize performance in wind instrumentalists. This is similar to variations in laryngeal biomechanics and tension seen across the different styles of singing [49–51]. Opera singers, for instance, display a funnel-shaped vocal tract aperture, whereas often jazz singers have more laryngeal muscle constrictions. However, it has not been established whether this difference is due to the musical style or to the extent of training of the performers studied. A disturbance in this laryngeal biomechanical behavior secondary to excessive laryngeal tension may have significant acoustic implications for both singers and wind instrumentalists. Additionally, the associated increase in laryngeal and pharyngeal pressure in wind instrumentalists with dentofacial anomalies may increase the risk of laryngeal pathologies such as laryngocele or pharyngocele, commonly encountered in brass players. Kahane et al. performed videofluoroscopic and laryngeal examination on double-reed woodwind instrument players (four and three, respectively), and noted expansion of the pharyngeal cavity to various degrees with alterations in pressure, pitch, and intensity. The study was conducted on three musicians who were asked to perform different musical passages and scales. It is worth noting that the level of training, which is an important variable to consider in the interpretation of the results, was not reported [52].

In summary, dentofacial anomalies impact the shape and length of the upper airway space in wind instrumentalists. As a result, both anatomic and functional disorders may emerge. Given the known role of the larynx in music tone initiation and modulation, variations in vocal tract morphology should be considered in the work-up of wind instrumentalists with difficulty in performance. Similar issues occur in singers and other high-performance voice professionals.

References

1. Titze IR. Nonlinear source–filter coupling in phonation: theory. J Acoust Soc Am. 2008;123(5):2733–49.
2. Collins SA. Men's voices and women's choices. Anim Behav. 2000;60(6):773–80.
3. González J. Formant frequencies and body size of speaker: a weak relationship in adult humans. J Phon. 2004;32(2):277–87.
4. Rendall D, Kollias S, Ney C, Lloyd P. Pitch (F0) and formant profiles of human vowels and vowel-like baboon grunts: the role of vocalizer body size and voice-acoustic allometry. J Acoust Soc Am. 2005;117(2):944–55.
5. Evans S, Neave N, Wakelin D. Relationships between vocal characteristics and body size and shape in human males: an evolutionary explanation for a deep male voice. Biol Psychol. 2006;72(2):160–3.
6. Pisanski K, Jones BC, Fink B, et al. Voice parameters predict sex-specific body morphology in men and women. Animal Behav. 2016;112:13–22.
7. Roers F, Mürbe D, Sundberg J. Voice classification and vocal tract of singers: a study of x-ray images and morphology. J Acoust Soc Am. 2009;125(1):503–12.
8. Hamdan A, Sataloff RT, Hawkshaw MJ. Obesity, body size and voice. In: Hamdan AL, Sataloff RT, Hawkshaw MJ. Obesity and voice. San Diego: Plural Publishing; 2019. p. 115–30.
9. Sataloff RT. Clinical anatomy and physiology of the voice. In: Sataloff RT. Professional voice: the science and art of clinical care. San Diego: Plural Publishing; 2017. p. 157–96.
10. Bowers J, Tobey EA, Shaye R. An acoustic-speech study of patients who received orthognathic surgery. Am J Orthod. 1985;88(5):373–9.
11. Lee AS, Whitehill TL, Ciocca V, Samman N. Acoustic and perceptual analysis of the sibilant sound /s/ before and after orthognathic surgery. J Oral Maxillofac Surg. 2002;60(4):364–72.
12. Niemi M, Laaksonen JP, Peltomäki T, Kurimo J, Aaltonen O, Happonen RP. Acoustic comparison of vowel sounds produced before and after orthognathic surgery for mandibular advancement. J Oral Maxillofac Surg. 2006;64(6):910–6.
13. Xue SA, Lam CW, Whitehill TL, Samman N. Effects of class III malocclusion on young male adults' vocal tract development: a pilot study. J Oral Maxillofac Surg. 2011;69(3):845–52.

14. Mishima K, Moritani N, Nakano H, Matsushita A, Iida S, Ueyama Y. Voice characteristics before versus after mandibular setback surgery in patients with mandibular prognathism using nonlinear dynamics and conventional acoustic analyses. J Craniomaxillofac Surg. 2012;41(8):706–9.
15. Macari AT, Karam IA, Tabri D, Sarieddine D, Hamdan AL. Formants frequency and dispersion in relation to the length and projection of the upper and lower jaws. J Voice. 2015;29(1):83–90.
16. Hamdan AL, Khandakji M, Macari AT. Maxillary arch dimensions associated with acoustic parameters in prepubertal children. Angle Orthod. 2018;88(4):410–5.
17. Viegas F, Viegas D, Guimarães GS, Ritto F, Simões-Zenari M, Nemr K. Acoustic analysis of voice and speech in men with skeletal class III malocclusion: a pilot study. Folia Phoniatr Logop. 2020;7:1–9.
18. Fitch WT, Giedd J. Morphology and development of the human vocal tract: a study using magnetic resonance imaging. J Acoust Soc Am. 1999;106(3):1511–22.
19. Sataloff RT. Endocrine function. In: Sataloff RT. Professional voice: the science and art of clinical care. 4th ed. San Diego: Plural Publishing; 2017. p. 665–71.
20. Sundberg J. Vocal tract resonance. In: Sataloff RT. Professional voice: the science and art of clinical care. 4th ed. San Diego: Plural Publishing; 2017. p. 309–28.
21. Fant G. A note on vocal tract size factors and non-uniform F-pattern scalings. Speech Transmission Laboratory Quarterly Progress and Status Report. 1966;1:22–30.
22. Cleveland TF. Acoustic properties of voice timbre types and their influence on voice classification. J Acoust Soc Am. 1977;61(6):1622–9.
23. Dmitriev L, Kiselev A. Relationship between the formant structure of different types of singing voices and the dimensions of supraglottic cavities. Folia Phoniatr (Basel). 1979;31(4):238–41.
24. Sulter AM, Miller DG, Wolf RF, Schutte HK, Wit HP, Mooyaart EL. On the relation between the dimensions and resonance characteristics of the vocal tract: a study with MRI. Magn Reson Imaging. 1992;10(3):365–73.
25. Shelton KE, Woodson H, Gay S, Suratt PM. Pharyngeal fat in obstructive sleep apnea. Am Rev Respir Dis. 1993;148(2):462–6.
26. Mortimore IL, Marshall I, Wraith PK, Sellar RJ, Douglas NJ. Neck and total body fat deposition in nonobese and obese patients with sleep apnea compared with that in control subjects. Am J Respir Crit Care Med. 1998;157(1):280–3.
27. Horner RL, Mohiaddin RH, Lowell DG, et al. Sites and sizes of fat deposits around the pharynx in obese patients with obstructive sleep apnoea and weight matched controls. Eur Respir J. 1989;2(7):613–22.
28. Shen CM, Soong WJ, Jeng MJ, et al. Nasopharyngeal tract length measurement in infants. Acta Paediatr Taiwan. 2002;43(2):82–5.
29. Rose GJ. A cross-sectional study of the relationship of facial areas with several body dimensions. Angle Orthod. 1960;20:6–13.
30. Burstone CJ. Process of maturation and growth prediction. Am J Orthod. 1963;49:907–19.
31. Johnston FE, Hufham HP, Moreschi AF, Terry GP. Skeletal maturation and cephalofacial development. Angle Orthod. 1965;35:1–11.
32. Bambha JK. Longitudinal cephalometric roentgenographic study of face and cranium in relation to body height. J Am Dent Assoc. 1961;63(6):776–99.
33. Hunter CJ. The correlation of facial growth with body height and skeletal maturation at adolescence. Angle Orthod. 1966;36(1):44–54.
34. Bishara SE, Jamison JE, Peterson LC, DeKock WH. Longitudinal changes in standing height and mandibular parameters between the ages of 8 and 17 years. Am J Orthod. 1981;80(2):115–35.
35. Introna F Jr, Di Vella G, Petrachi S. Determination of height in life using multiple regression of skull parameters. Boll Soc Ital Biol Sper. 1993;69(3):153–60.
36. Chiba M, Terazawa K. Estimation of stature from somatometry of skull. Forensic Sci Int. 1998;97(2–3):87–92.
37. Cozza P, Stirpe G, Condó R, Donatelli M. Craniofacial and body growth: cross-sectional anthropometric study on children during prepuberal period. Eur J Pedtiatr Dent. 2005;6(2):90–6.
38. Krishan K, Kumar R. Determination of stature from cephalo-facial dimensions in a North Indian population. Legal Med. 2007;9(3):128–33.
39. Ryan I, Bidmos MA. Skeletal height reconstruction from measurements of the skull in indigenous South Africans. Forensic Sci Int. 2007;167(1):16–21.
40. Krishan K. Estimation of stature from cephalo-facial anthropometry in north Indian population. Forensic Sci Int. 2008;181(1–3):52.e1–6.
41. Sundberg J. The singer's formant revisited. STL-QPSR. 1995;36(2–3):83–96.
42. Abu Alhajia ES, Al-Khateeb SN. Uvulo-glosso-pharyngeal dimensions in different anteroposterior skeletal patterns. Angle Orthod. 2005;75(6):1012–8.
43. Trollinger VL, Sataloff RT. Respiratory behaviors and vocal tract issues in wind instrumentalists. In: Sataloff RT. Professional voice: the science and art of clinical care. 4th ed. San Diego: Plural Publishing; 2017. p. 1017–28.
44. Eckley CA. Glottic configuration in wind instrument players. Rev Bras Otorrinolaingol. 2006;72(1):45–7.
45. Weikert M, Schlömicher-Thier J. Laryngeal movements in saxophone playing: video-endoscopic investigations with saxophone players: a pilot study. J Voice. 1999;13(2):265–73.
46. Mukai S. Laryngeal control while playing wind instrument. Nihon Jibiinkoka Gakkai Kaiho. 1989;92(2):260–70.
47. Marunick MT, Menaldi CJ. Maxillary dental arch form related to voice classification: a pilot study. J Voice. 2000;14(1):82–91.

48. Lammert A, Proctor M, Narayanan S. Interspeaker variability in hard palate morphology and vowel production. J Speech Lang Hear Res. 2013;56(6):S1924–33.
49. King AI, Ashby J, Nelson C. Laryngeal function in wind instrumentalists: the woodwinds. J Voice. 1988;1(4):365–7.
50. Koufman JA, Radomski T, Johari GM, Russel GB, Pillsbury DC. Laryngeal biomechanics of the singing voice. Otolaryngol Head Neck Surg. 1996;115(6):527–37.
51. Hamdan AL, Sibai A, Moukarbel RV, Deeb R. Laryngeal biomechanics in middle eastern singing. J Voice. 2006;20(4):579–84.
52. Kahane JC, Beckford NS, Chorna LB, Teachey JC, McClelland DK. Videofluoroscopic and laryngoscopic evaluation of the upper airway and larynx of professional bassoon players. J Voice. 2006;20(2):297–307.

Part III

Impact of Orthodontic Treatment and Orthognathic Surgery on Voice and Wind Instrument Performance: The Role of Pedagogy, Speech and Singing Therapy

10 Orthodontic and Orthognathic Surgery Procedures

Anthony T. Macari

The orthodontist combines biological knowledge (i.e., bone apposition and resorption) with the art of mechanics and is considered a biomechanical scientist. Accordingly, and if biology and physiological processes are determined well, technical applications of mechanics have undergone constant changes in efforts to achieve optimal underlying biological responses. Of course, biological processes remain under intensive study especially to decipher the molecular basis of bone turnover and the link between the different layers of the periodontium during the orthodontic treatment. Orthodontic appliances transmit compression on one side of the tooth all the way to the root and tension on the opposing side. This compression and tension coupling results in bone resorption and later bone apposition, allowing the tooth to move in the arch.

The determination of the optimal amount and duration of force, along with the design of orthodontic appliances, have evolved greatly in the last century. A variety of orthodontic appliances may be used for the same objectives. In general, orthodontic appliances are divided under two main categories:

1. Removable appliances: They can be inserted and removed by the patient or patient's guardian, in the case of children. The forces applied on the teeth are intermittent because of removal of the appliance for a set period of time, such as when eating or playing sports.
2. Fixed appliances: One of the greatest advances in orthodontics was the invention of "braces" which are attachments bonded on the surface of the teeth. Over the years, these appliances underwent major changes in design, objective, and application to evolve into the current 3D, straight-wire, fixed appliances. Additional progress in manufacturing, including customized 3D printing, is taking place [1]. The interface between "braces" and the archwires inserted in them is a pivotal mechanical advance that improves ease and efficiency of tooth movement.

Orthodontic Appliances

Removable Appliances

Since its inception as the first dental specialty, orthodontics has embraced biomechanics as a keystone of its science. Originally, tooth movement was achieved by applying forces on the teeth through appliances that could be removed by the patient.

A main advantage of removable appliances is the reduction in treatment of chairside time because they are fabricated in an orthodontic laboratory. In addition, removable appliances can be removed by the patient as needed (e.g., social or sporting events, and sometimes eating). Consequently, new designs and materials have

A.-L. Hamdan et al., *Dentofacial Anomalies*, https://doi.org/10.1007/978-3-030-69109-7_10

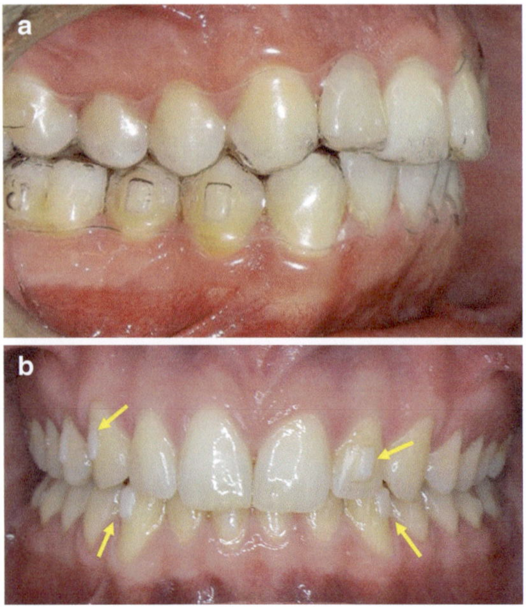

Fig. 10.1 (**a**) Clear aligners inserted on upper and lower teeth for orthodontic treatment. (**b**) Arrows pointing at accessory attachments bonded on the surface of the teeth for better control of tooth movement induced by clear aligners

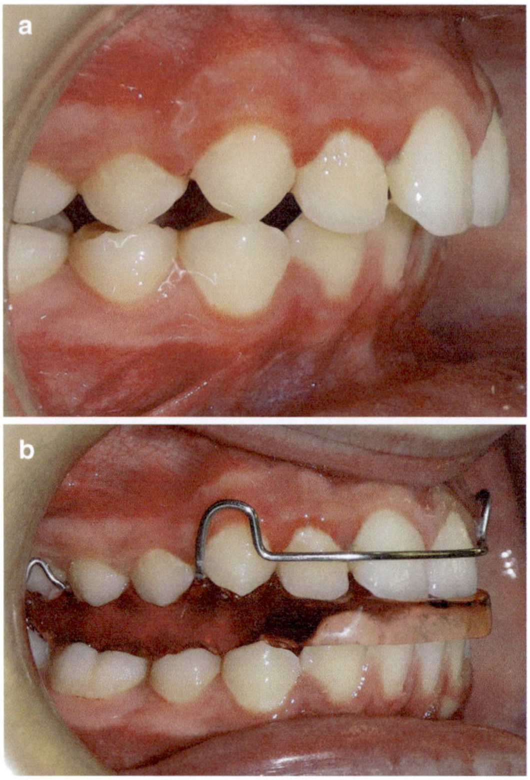

Fig. 10.2 (**a**) Class II malocclusion with increased anterior overjet in an 11-year-old girl. (**b**) Functional appliance inserted in the mouth to enhance differential growth of the mandible by positioning it forward

regularly been introduced for fabrication of removable appliances to enhance aesthetic appearance and patient tolerance. Nevertheless, two disadvantages of the removable appliances remain:

1. Patient compliance is needed to achieve the goal of treatment [2]. Many studies investigated the association between compliance and success rate [3, 4].
2. It is difficult to treat complex malocclusions with removable appliances because of the difficulty of creating two-point contacts on the teeth. Thus, to counteract this limitation, orthodontists introduced "accessories," attachments on the teeth to ensure effective control on tooth movement (Fig. 10.1a, b).

Because of these drawbacks, most of removable appliances are used in growing children in phase one of treatment. In this phase, orthodontists target the growth potential/direction of the jaws and attempt to enhance differential growth of the jaws (this approach is discussed in another section of this chapter).

In general, removable appliances are divided into two categories:

- Intraoral: Intraoral appliances include a set of so-called functional appliances (Fig. 10.2a, b). They include other appliances such as expanders and retainers. Clear aligners are also removable appliances, mostly used in adults.
- Extraoral: Extraoral removable appliances have been used for more than a century. Headgear (Fig. 10.3a) and face masks (Fig. 10.3b) are the most commonly used external appliances to correct class II and class III malocclusions, respectively.

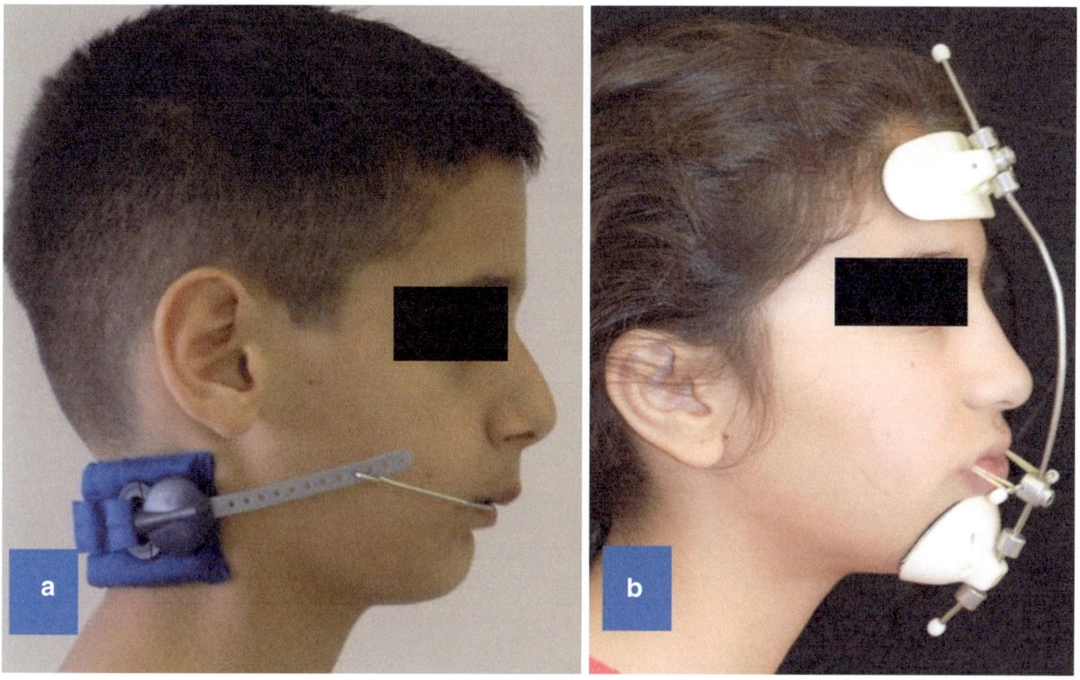

Fig. 10.3 Extraoral appliances. (**a**) Headgear (cervical) to enhance differential growth of a retrognathic mandible and correct class II malocclusion in an 11-year-old boy. (**b**) Face mask to advance the maxilla and correct class III malocclusion in a 10-year-old girl

Fixed Appliances

The orthodontic fixed appliances, commonly known as brackets or braces, underwent major design modifications to reach their contemporary form. Edward Angle, who introduced classification of malocclusion and was known as the father of contemporary orthodontics, also had a major impact on the practice of orthodontics through the creation of fixed orthodontic appliances [5]. Originally, the E-arch ("E" stands for Expansion) designed by Angle [5] included bands only on molars and a heavy archwire extended around all the other teeth, with which all teeth were bonded to the E-arch for alignment through tipping of the crowns. Later, Angle tried to maximize tooth movement and counteract the tipping effect by inserting bands on all teeth by using a vertical tube. He soldered pins to the archwire that was positioned in the tubes, and named it the Pin and Tube Appliance. The Ribbon Arch came later as a modification of the Pin and Tube Fixture. Angle modified the tube by providing a vertical slot behind it to insert the archwire. It was more successful at positioning the teeth. However, little control on the root's movement was achieved. Finally, and to overcome the limitations of the Ribbon Arch, Angle "tipped" the tube 90 degrees so that he could insert the wire horizontally instead of vertically and created the famous Edgewise Bracket. This design was advantageous because it allowed twisting of the archwire and creation of force that could torque the roots of the teeth. The Edgewise design is still used widely by orthodontists, although it was subjected to further development through the insertion of tip, angulation, and torque information in the braces to facilitate daily practice. The latter design is known as a Straightwire Appliance [6] because the practitioner does not necessarily perform additional bends in the archwires.

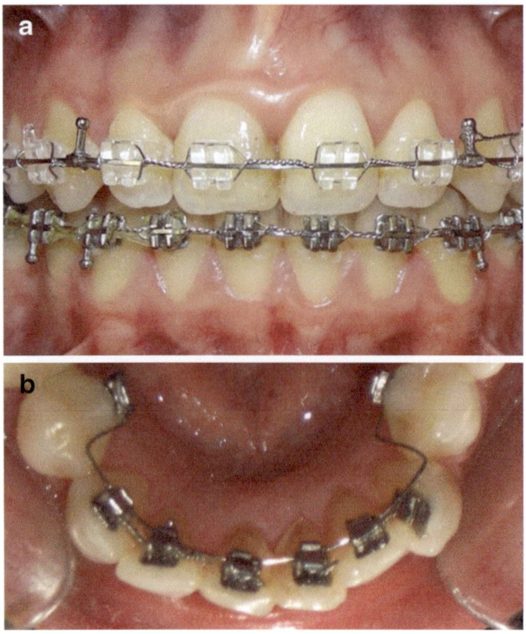

Fig. 10.4 "Aesthetic" appliances. (**a**) Intraoral photograph showing the difference between ceramic brackets on maxillary teeth versus metallic brackets on mandibular teeth. (**b**) Lingual brackets bonded on the inner surface of the teeth

The main advantage of fixed appliances is the great control that the orthodontist has on tooth movement in all three dimensions. This advance in design facilitated completion of orthodontic treatment with long-term stability, unlike removable appliances.

Given the increase number of adults seeking orthodontic treatment, orthodontists and the orthodontic industry developed ceramic braces (Fig. 10.4a) with a similar design to the metal brackets. The ceramic braces are better aesthetically and show less during talking and smiling without undermining treatment efficacy or time. In an effort to hide orthodontic appliances totally behind-the-teeth, lingual braces (Fig. 10.4b) were introduced a few decades ago. Lingual braces gained popularity despite difficulty in attaching and managing the appliances. However, patient intolerance at the beginning of treatment also was reported [7, 8].

Orthodontic Treatment in the Prepubertal Period (Primary and Mixed Dentition)

A common age for orthodontic treatment coincides with the transition from mixed to full permanent dentitions. Most malocclusion can be treated during this period of a child's growth and development. However, some other problems may need earlier intervention when primary or early mixed dentition is present. These treatments are described as preventive or interceptive. They target both dental and skeletal malocclusion. Preventive treatment aims at stopping the transformation of malocclusions into a complex status, whereas interceptive treatment aims at early intervention to manage malocclusions that otherwise will be very difficult to manage at later growth stages. The interceptive approach is considered a first phase of treatment because it generally is followed by a second phase at a later stage of dental and skeletal maturation.

Problems that need to be addressed in primary or mixed dentition can be divided in dentoalveolar and skeletal problems.

Dentoalveolar (Non-skeletal) Problems

Lack of Space or Crowding

A common problem in early mixed dentition is lack of space, or crowding. Arch circumference discrepancy (ACD) is calculated by subtracting the available space on the arch and the required space (defined as the addition of the mesio-distal diameter of all teeth). An early diagnosis of crowding entails overcoming the difficulty in estimating the width of non-erupted permanent teeth. Orthodontists have developed many methods to accomplish this assessment [9, 10].

There are two major causes of lack of space in early mixed dentition. One is interference with the eruption path of permanent teeth, preventing them from coming into the arch at the predeter-

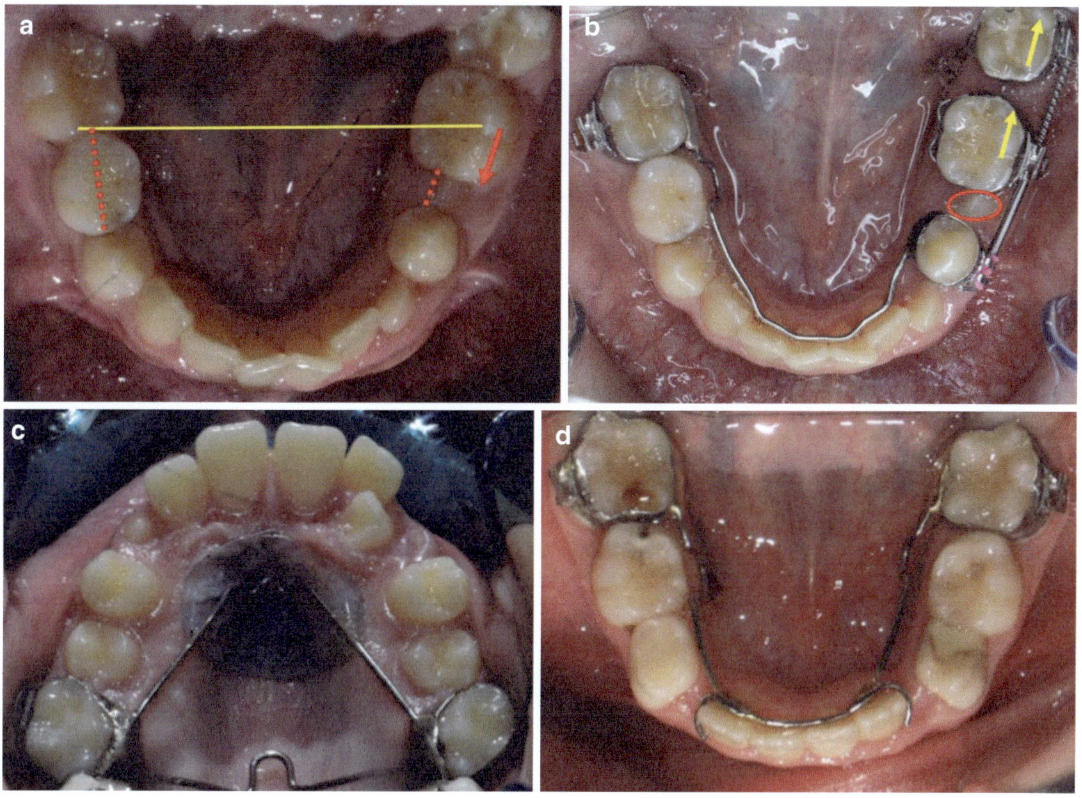

Fig. 10.5 (**a**, **b**) Mandibular arch views of a 10-year-old boy (**a**) Early loss of second primary molar on the left side induces a mesial shift of the left permanent first molar—6 (red arrow) and closure of the space needed for the eruption of the successor second premolar. (**b**) Regaining the space by distalizing the first and second permanent molars—6&7 (yellow arrows). (**c**) Transpalatal Nance appliance in a 10-year-old girl, acting as a "passive" space maintainer to hold the leeway space shown in red arrows on both sides. (**d**) Lower lingual holding arch or space maintainer to maintain the leeway space (differential space between second primary molars (E) and permanent second premolars) in the mandibular arch of an 8-year-old girl

mined time. This abnormality can induce drift in the adjacent teeth into the space of the non-erupted tooth and create lack of space (Fig. 10.5a). In this case, regaining space through an "active" orthodontic procedure is required (Fig. 10.5b). Another cause of crowding is the required space being larger than the available one. It is important that this problem be recognized early to be able to save the so-called Leeway space. Leeway space is the positive difference in space between the width of the primary molars (the second primary molars) and the successor, permanent second premolars. On average, the leeway space in the mandibular arch is 2.5 mm on each side, and 2 mm in the maxillary arch. A total of around 5 mm can be gained if the leeway space is saved. When needed, a lower lingual holding arch or a "space maintainer" is inserted in the lower arch and an equivalent Nance Button in the maxillary arch (Fig. 10.5c). This procedure is a passive method to gain space and prevent future crowding in the arches (Fig. 10.5d).

Problems in the Eruption of Teeth

Problems in the eruption of teeth can be divided into two components: intrinsic as they relate to the primary teeth themselves, and extrinsic including problems of the surrounding tissues either in the bones or the gingiva.

On average, permanent teeth erupt when their roots are around 2/3 formed. At this point, roots of the primary teeth are almost fully resorbed,

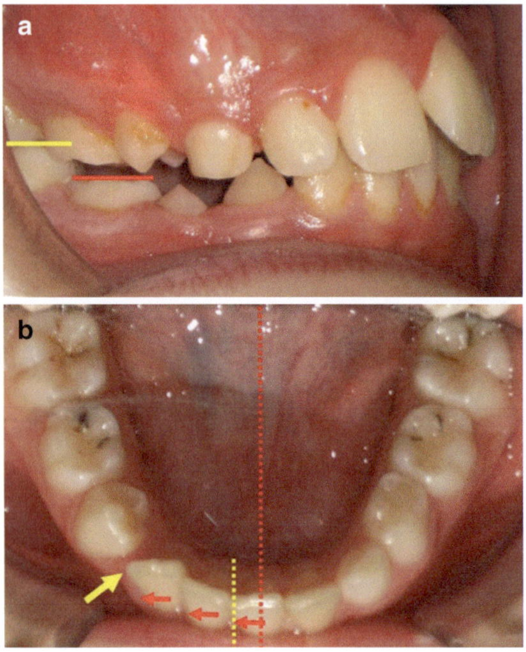

Fig. 10.6 (**a**) Ankylosed second primary tooth on a 12-year-old boy. Notice the step between the permanent first molar occlusal surface (yellow) and that of the primary second molar (red) indicating an ankylosed primary tooth. (**b**) Drifting of the permanent incisors to the right as a response to early loss of a primary canine (yellow arrow) in an 8-year-old boy. The red line indicates the midline of the arch, and the yellow line is where the midline of the teeth had shifted to

and the tooth may fallout spontaneously. Deviation from this balanced process may include ankylosis of the primary tooth or fusing of the roots and the bone. The root of the primary tooth that is ankylosed fails to provide the place for the permanent tooth and can cause impaction. An early diagnosis and timely intervention for this problem are important. Usually in the case of ankylosed primary tooth, a step with the adjacent teeth is present along with a typical sound upon percussion on the occlusal surface of the ankylosed tooth (Fig. 10.6a).

An over-retained primary tooth may induce deviation in the path of eruption of the permanent tooth underneath. When it occurs, over-retention of mandibular primary incisors will induce lingual eruption of the permanent incisors. In addition, early loss of primary teeth can cause space problems. The premature loss or extraction of a mandibular primary canine can result in shift of the incisors toward the extraction side and induce midline deviation and loss of the space necessary for the eruption of the permanent canine teeth (Fig. 10.6b). An "active" phase of orthodontic treatment is required to restore the lost space and facilitate the spontaneous eruption of the canine. If this opportunity for early intervention is missed, the permanent tooth may get impacted in the bone, which will complicate substantially the problem and the solution.

The presence of an obstacle in the eruption path of permanent teeth may lead to failure of eruption and later to space problem. Supernumerary teeth [11] constitute the most common obstacle to the normal eruption of teeth. Early diagnosis and removal will permit the eruption and avoid impaction of permanent teeth. Other than supernumerary teeth, trauma to primary teeth can cause delay in eruption or cause impaction of the permanent teeth. Trauma to the face and to the front teeth is common in childhood. Its effect can extend from a simple fracture of the crown to a full exfoliation of the primary tooth. However, in both cases, orthodontists and pediatric dentists must evaluate the position of the unerupted permanent teeth buds and consider intervening, if necessary (Fig. 10.7).

Another dentoalveolar problem necessitating attention early in childhood is the presence of crossbite. Crossbite is present when the occlusion between maxillary and mandibular teeth in reversed and can occur with either a single tooth or with multiple teeth in the posterior or anterior regions (Fig. 10.7). When it is from dental origins, crossbite is caused by interference on one or more teeth upon closing the jaw. In this case, simple grinding of the interference point can help resolving the problem. In more severe crossbite, skeletal expansion of the maxillary arch may be needed, as discussed below.

Finally, children may develop "bad" oral habits that, when persistent, can cause both dentoalveolar and skeletal malocclusion [12, 13]. Thumb sucking is one of the bad oral habits, and if persistent at the time of eruption of the permanent incisors, it can induce anterior open bite and flaring of the maxillary incisors (Fig. 10.7). As much

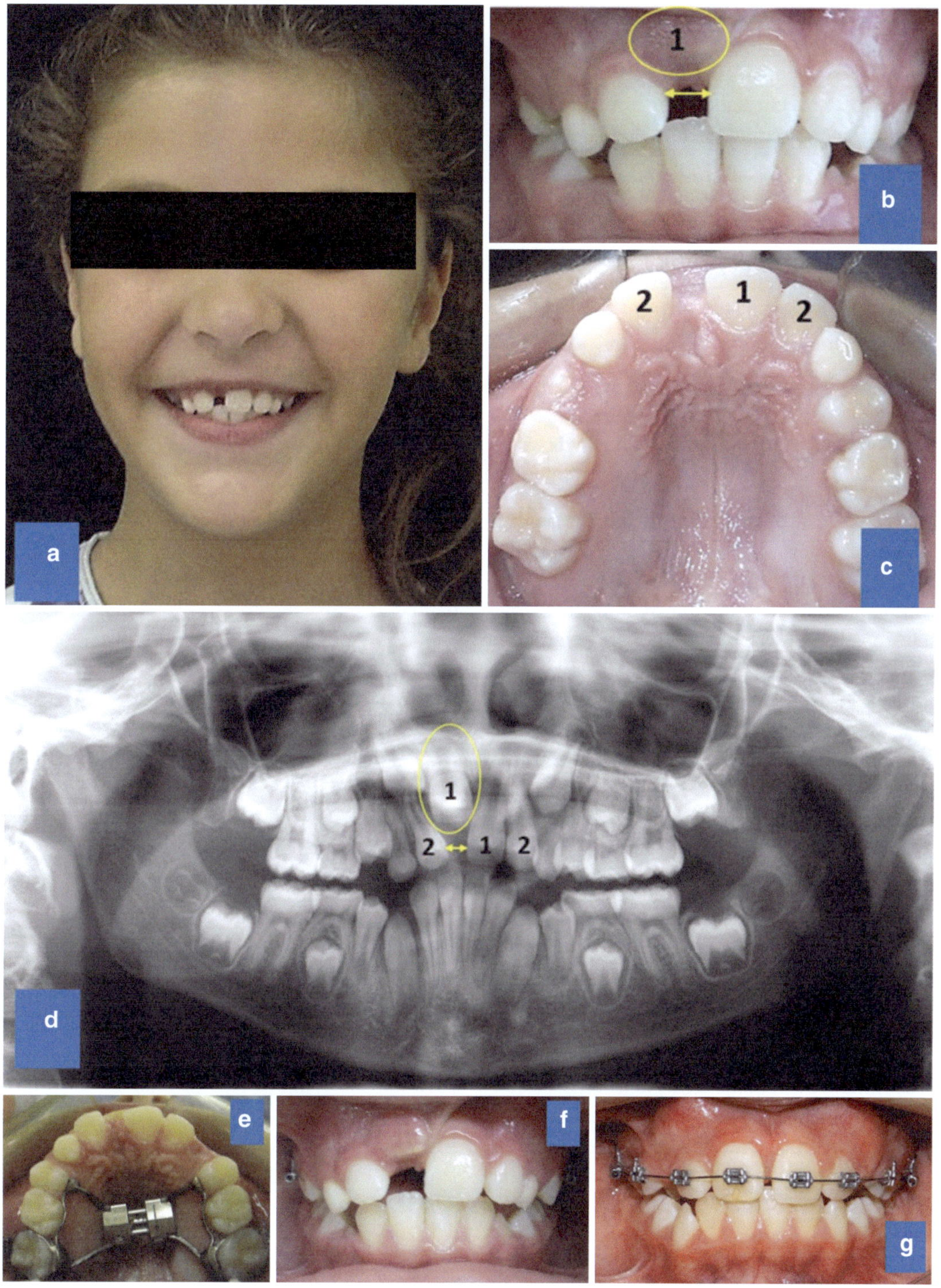

Fig. 10.7 (**a**) Extraoral photograph of a 7-year-old girl showing the asymmetric smile because of the impacted maxillary right central incisor (1) following an earlier trauma to the primary dentition. (**b**, **c**) Intraoral photograph showing lack of space for the eruption of the maxillary right 1. (**d**) Panoramic radiograph of the same patient indicating the impaction position of the maxillary right 1. (**e**) Maxillary expansion to regain space for the impacted maxillary right 1. (**f**) Crown of the impacted tooth starting to show under the gingiva. (**g**) Orthodontic fixed appliances to align the impacted tooth after it started to erupt

as it is possible for a thumb sucking habit to resolve on its own, orthodontists must intervene to stop the bad habits from causing further damage to the teeth and occlusion. A common appliance to treat thumb sucking is the habit breaker appliance (or a tongue crib appliance). This appliance will instantly inhibit the child from sucking his/her thumb (Fig. 10.7). In addition, tongue thrust is a "bad" oral habit and may cause anterior open bite and excess spacing among the incisors. Similar to the treatment of thumb sucking, insertion of a tongue crib helps stop the habit and correct the open bite.

Skeletal Problems

When a skeletal abnormality in the face exists, optimal solutions involve treatment during the active growth period. The potential of orthodontic/orthopedic treatment to correct skeletal malocclusions is well established [14, 15]. Initiation of growth modification through an orthopedic approach is mandatory before the growth spurt. Thus, it is important to decide on the timing of treatment by evaluating bone maturation and weighing the severity of the malocclusion in the transverse, vertical, and sagittal dimensions.

Timing of Treatment

The optimal time of treatment has been subjected to extensive investigation [16]. Over the years, orthodontists experienced a change of thought about when to attempt correcting malocclusion through growth modification, between early and late mixed dentitions. The optimal timing to initiate orthopedic treatment remains controversial, and the practitioner faces this dilemma daily. However, and in few instances, there is general agreement on starting treatment earlier than the "usual" orthodontic age [17]. A severe skeletal malocclusion whether class II or class III is a clear indication for early treatment. Not only functional, but also the psychological status of the child is to be considered primary when screening for malocclusions. The American Association of Orthodontists recommends that every child should be checked by the age of 7 years by an orthodontist, because the eruption of the first molars and incisors at around 7–8 years of age constitutes a cornerstone in the development of the dentition. Consequently, orthodontists would be able to evaluate the presence of, and predict, any potential for malocclusion.

Maxillary Constriction

The correction of maxillary constriction, which is a skeletal problem in the transverse dimension, is made possible because of the presence of the mid-palatal suture. It connects the two maxillary and palatine bones, and it starts to interdigitate by early adolescence. Its bone bridging will be completed by the late teens [18]. Thus, splitting the palate is possible in childhood and, to a certain extent, in early adolescence. Thereafter, that treatment option may be lost. A narrow maxilla is characterized by a deep palatal vault and accompanied usually by crossbite of the teeth. The expansion can be performed with different appliances. The most commonly used hardware is the bonded fixed jack screw (Fig. 10.8). Maxillary expansion may alter the position of the palatal rugae and affect a few voice parameters briefly [19, 20].

Class II Malocclusion

Epidemiological studies have shown that around 23% of children, 15% of adolescents and 13% of adults have an increased overjet of >5 mm [21, 22]. Accordingly, in an orthodontic practice, the majority of patients exhibit class II malocclusion. While dentoalveolar abnormalities may be the sole cause, the presence of skeletal discrepancies between the maxilla and the mandible is more prevalent in class II malocclusions. This highlights the importance of treating this malocclusion prior to growth cessation.

Mandibular retrognathism is the main feature of class II skeletal malocclusion. The treatment of deficient mandibular projection requires orthodontic and orthopedic approaches. Historically, the two main appliances used in the treatment of class II malocclusion are functional appliances and headgear. Many randomized clinical trials have investigated the differences between these

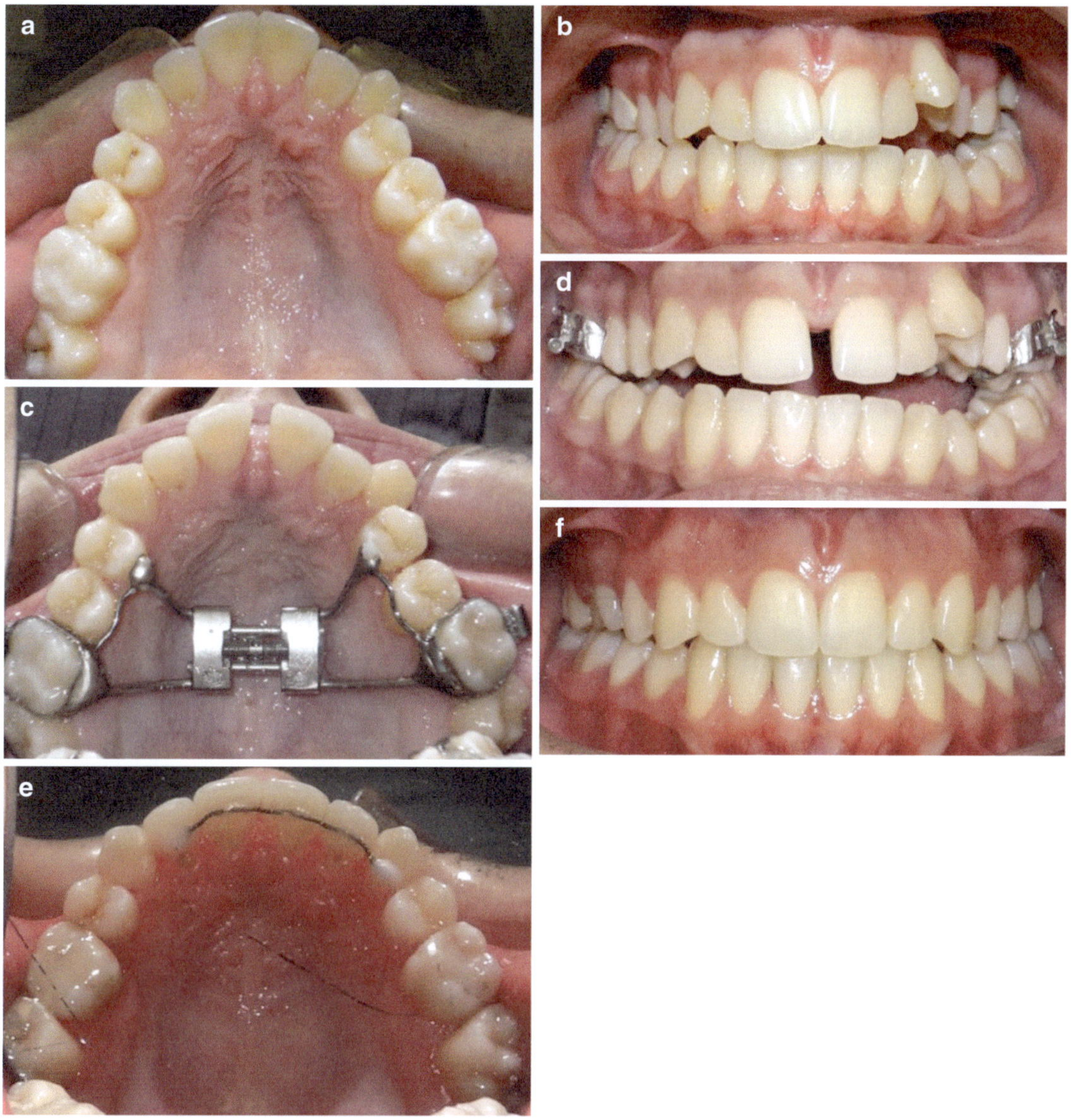

Fig. 10.8 (**a**) Pre-treatment intraoral photographs of a 14-year-old girl showing maxillary constriction. (**b**) Unilateral crossbite on the left side. (**c**) Palatal expander with jackscrew inserted to widen the maxillary arch. (**d**) Intraoral frontal view showing the split of the mid-palatal suture indicating success of the expansion procedure. (**e**) Post-treatment maxillary arch view showing a wider arch in comparison to pre-treatment. (**f**) Frontal view showing correction of the crossbite. Note that maxillary expansion was followed by an orthodontic treatment with fixed appliances (braces)

two appliances in the treatment of class II malocclusion and concluded that no major differences exist in their efficacy in affecting differential growth of the mandible.

It remains controversial whether the orthopedic correction of the mandibular retrognathism entails redirecting of the growth vector or increasing in the potential of mandibular growth. However, the treatment of class II malocclusion in prepubertal stages generally is efficient in reducing skeletal and dentoalveolar discrepancies (Fig. 10.9) [23].

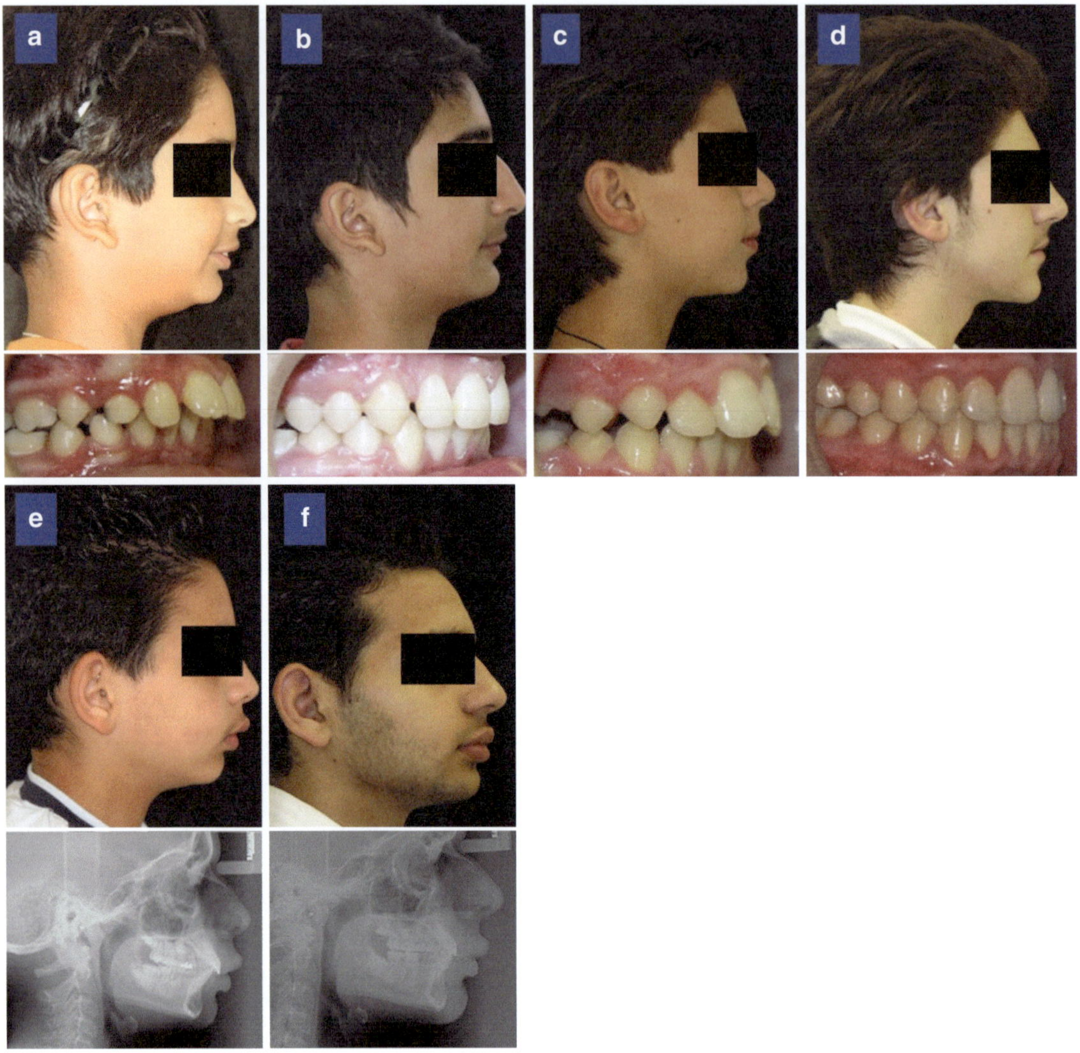

Fig. 10.9 (**a**) Pre-treatment profile and intraoral view of a 10-year-old boy with mandibular retrognathism and class II malocclusion. (**b**) Post-treatment profile and lateral intraoral view of the same patient treated with a functional appliance as a first phase followed by fixed orthodontic appliances. Note the enhancement of the mandibular projection in the profile along with correction to class I occlusion. (**c**) Pre-treatment record of an 11-year-old boy with class II malocclusion and slightly retruded chin. (**d**) Post-treatment record of the same patient treated with headgear and showing correction to class I occlusion and enhancement of chin projection in the face. (**e**) Pre-treatment record of a 10-year-old boy showing the extent of the class II skeletal discrepancy on the lateral cephalogram. (**f**) Post-treatment record of the same patient treated with head gear to enhance differential growth of the mandible. Normalization of the inclination of the anterior teeth also was achieved

Class III Malocclusion

Class III malocclusion is less prevalent than class II malocclusion. It ranges between 1% and 5% in certain populations. Class III is usually caused by either maxillary retrognathism or mandibular prognathism and is the most commonly inherited malocclusion. Its genetic etiology is characterized by polygenic influence and is transmitted within families as an autosomal dominant trait [24].

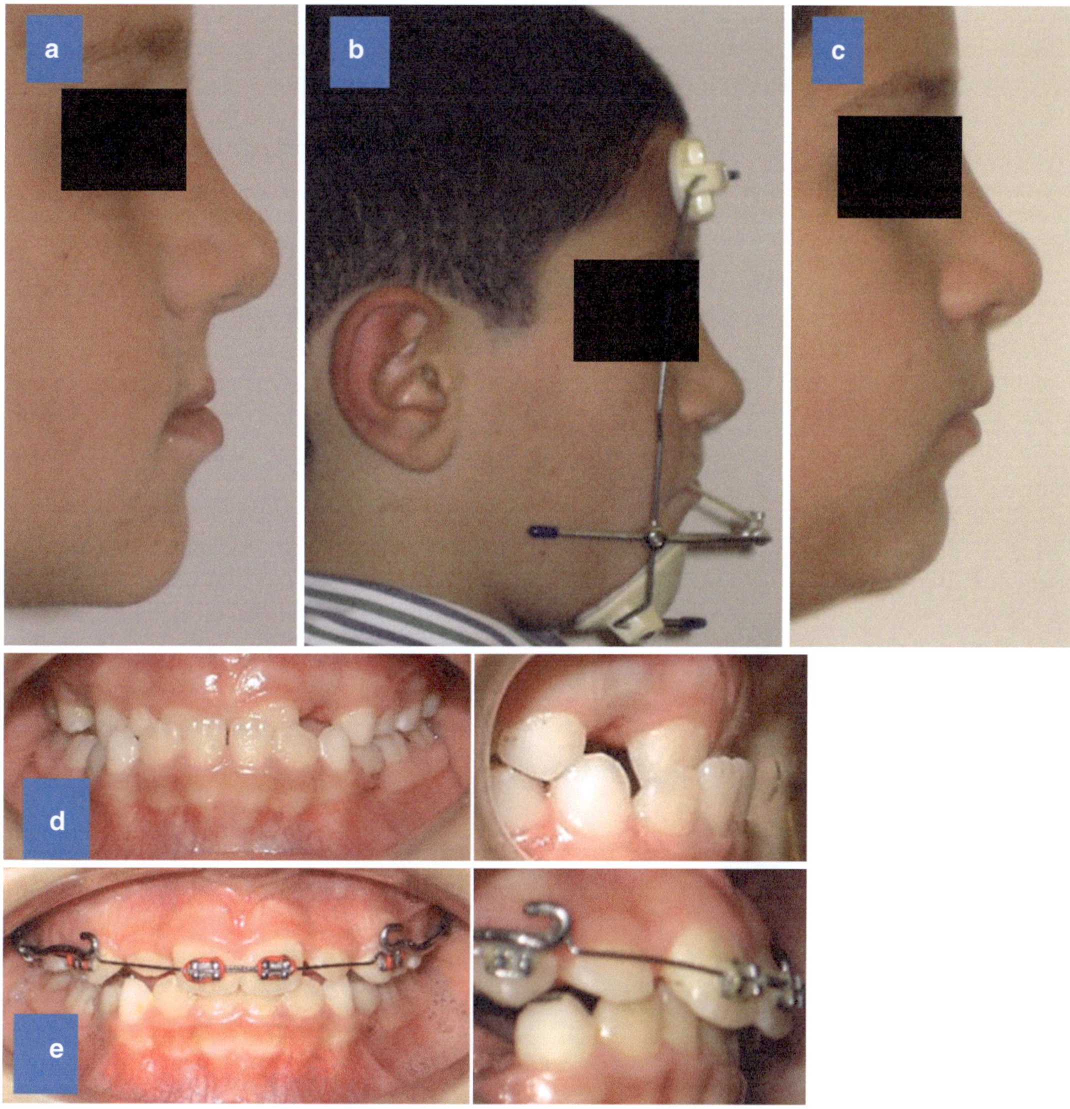

Fig. 10.10 (**a**) Pre-treatment profile view of an 8-year-old boy with forward position of the chin and forward step between the lips indicating a class III malocclusion. (**b**) Profile during treatment view showing the face mask appliance used to correct the class III malocclusion. (**c**) Post-treatment profile view 4 months after face mask therapy. Note the correction of the chin position and the step between the lips. (**d**) Pre-treatment intraoral photographs of the same patient showing the anterior crossbite, characteristic of the class III malocclusion. (**e**) Intraoral photographs 4 months after start of the face mask therapy showing correction of the anterior crossbite

The treatment of class III malocclusion in prepubertal stages targets correction of the underlying skeletal discrepancy. Enhancement of the maxillary growth is the major component of class III orthopedic treatment. Face mask appliance (or reverse-headgear) is the appliance of choice used by orthodontists (Fig. 10.10).

Orthodontic Treatment in Adolescents and Adults (Permanent Dentition)

The number of adult subjects seeking orthodontic treatment has been increasing steadily over the years [25]. Although orthodontic intervention for aesthetic reasons remain a main objective, adult patients may seek treatment as part of a multidisciplinary approach to enhance both function and longevity of the dentition.

Comprehensive Orthodontic Treatment

When skeletal discrepancy between the jaws is mild, orthodontic compensation of the dentoalveolar processes may be enough to satisfy both aesthetic and functional objectives. Conventional orthodontic treatment is efficient in correcting class II, class III, and vertical malocclusions to normal neutrocclusion in adults (Figs. 10.11 and 10.12). In these instances, orthodontists commonly use fixed appliances bonded to all permanent teeth.

In few instances, orthodontic treatment in adults may necessitate extraction of teeth to create space to accommodate the remaining ones, to optimize overjet and overbite, and to correct class II or class III malocclusions. Setting anchorage for tooth movement is considered a key to a successful outcome. The introduction of temporary skeletal anchorage devices (STADs) two decades ago was a major technical advance in orthodontics. STADs are used on daily basis by practitioners to achieve solid anchorage and thus decrease duration of treatment [26].

Orthodontists' skills have been challenged particularly by treatment of malocclusions that include vertical discrepancies [27]. Anterior open bite (AOB), one of the manifestations of vertical discrepancy, is a condition in which the anterior teeth (incisors) do not overlap when the jaws are closed. Depending on the ethnic background, the prevalence of AOB can reach up to 11% of the population and 17% of orthodontic patients [28]. Functional and genetic problems have been shown to be etiologic factors of open bite [29, 30]. Treatment modalities in adult subjects exhibiting open bite may include extractions of teeth to help close the bite, mini-implants to intrude posterior teeth, and orthognathic surgery [31].

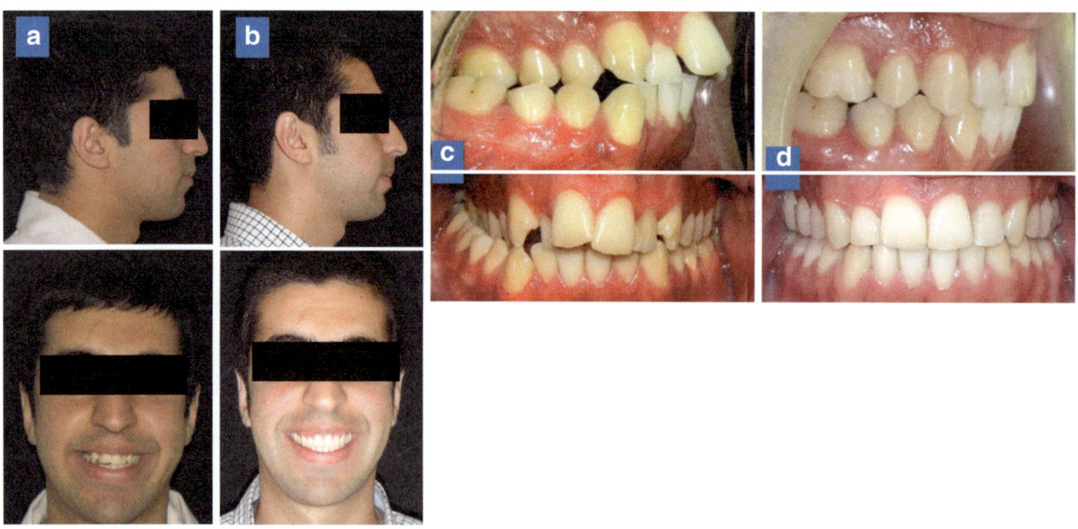

Fig. 10.11 (**a**) Pre-treatment profile and smile views of a 26-year-male with slight chin retrusion. (**b**) Post-treatment profile and smile views showing correction of the smile with no changes in the profile outline. (**c**) Intraoral photographs of the same patient showing class II malocclusion with an increased overjet and unilateral crossbite on the right side. (**d**) Post-treatment intraoral photographs of correction of the class II malocclusion by extraction of two maxillary premolars (one on each side) and correction of the unilateral crossbite. Had this patient been treated during the active growth period, the treatment approach would have entailed mid-palatal suture split by palatal expansion, followed by enhancement of mandibular differential growth with head gear or a functional appliance to correct the class II malocclusion

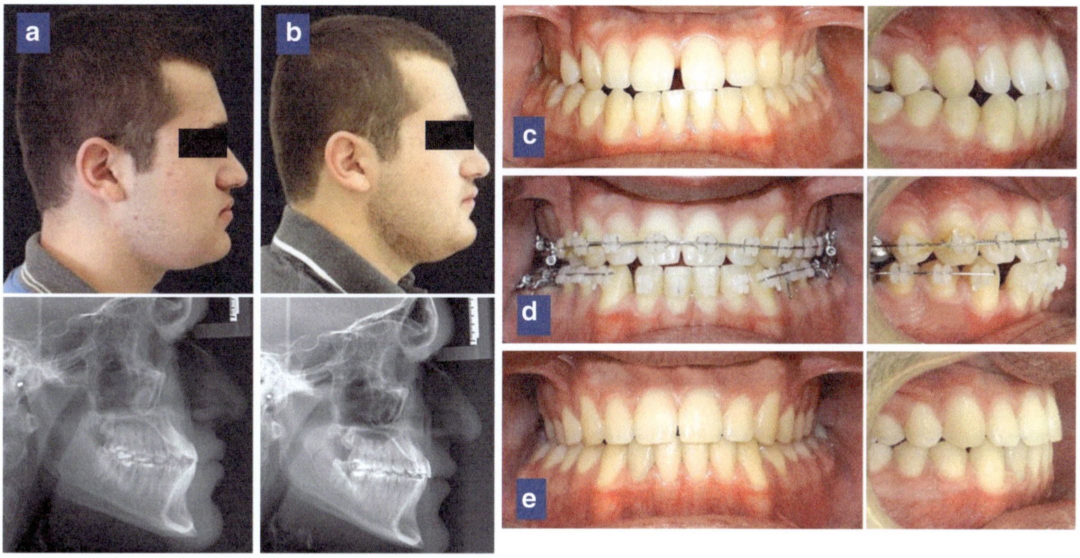

Fig. 10.12 (**a**) Pre-treatment profile view and lateral cephalometric radiograph of a 22-year-old male subject with a strong chin and mandibular prognathism indicating a class III malocclusion. (**b**) Post-treatment profile view showing no changes in comparison to the pre-treatment profile. However, dentoalveolar changes are shown clearly on the lateral cephalometric radiograph. (**c**) Pre-treatment intraoral photographs of the same patient showing the class III malocclusion with anterior edge to edge relationship (reduced overjet). (**d**) Intraoral photographs during treatment intraoral photographs with fixed appliances. (**e**) Post-treatment intraoral photographs showing the correction of the class III malocclusion to class I or neutrocclusion

Regardless of the treatment modality, long-term stability has been the ultimate goal, including when combined orthodontic and orthognathic surgery was required [32].

Adjunctive Orthodontic Procedures

A percentage of adult patients needs to be treated orthodontically as part of a multidisciplinary approach to achieve specific aims ranging from simple space re-opening for tooth implant replacement to total oral rehabilitation. Given the increased number of adult patients asking for orthodontic treatment, dealing with compromised periodontium, bone loss, and mutilated dentition is common.

In compromised periodontium, bone loss may be generalized or localized in the maxilla and/or the mandible. Prior to initiation of orthodontic treatment, inflammation-free periodontium should be established. This process may result in reduced but healthy periodontium with bone level below average norms but with no inflammation. Tooth movement should be well controlled not only to prevent further bone loss, but also to enhance bone formation, if possible. Uprighting tipped molars by orthodontic treatment enhances the surrounding bone levels (Fig. 10.13). Extraction of periodontally compromised teeth may substitute a more routinely convenient extraction of other teeth to enhance bony and soft tissues standings (Fig. 10.14). Extrusion of fractured teeth may be performed at a controlled rate to create new bone and enhance prosthetic correction. Intrusion of teeth may be necessary to open enough space for crown replacement.

Combined Orthodontic and Orthognathic Procedures

For adult patients whose dentofacial problems are severe and cannot be treated with dentoalveolar compensation, a combination of orthodontic treatment and orthognathic surgery is necessary

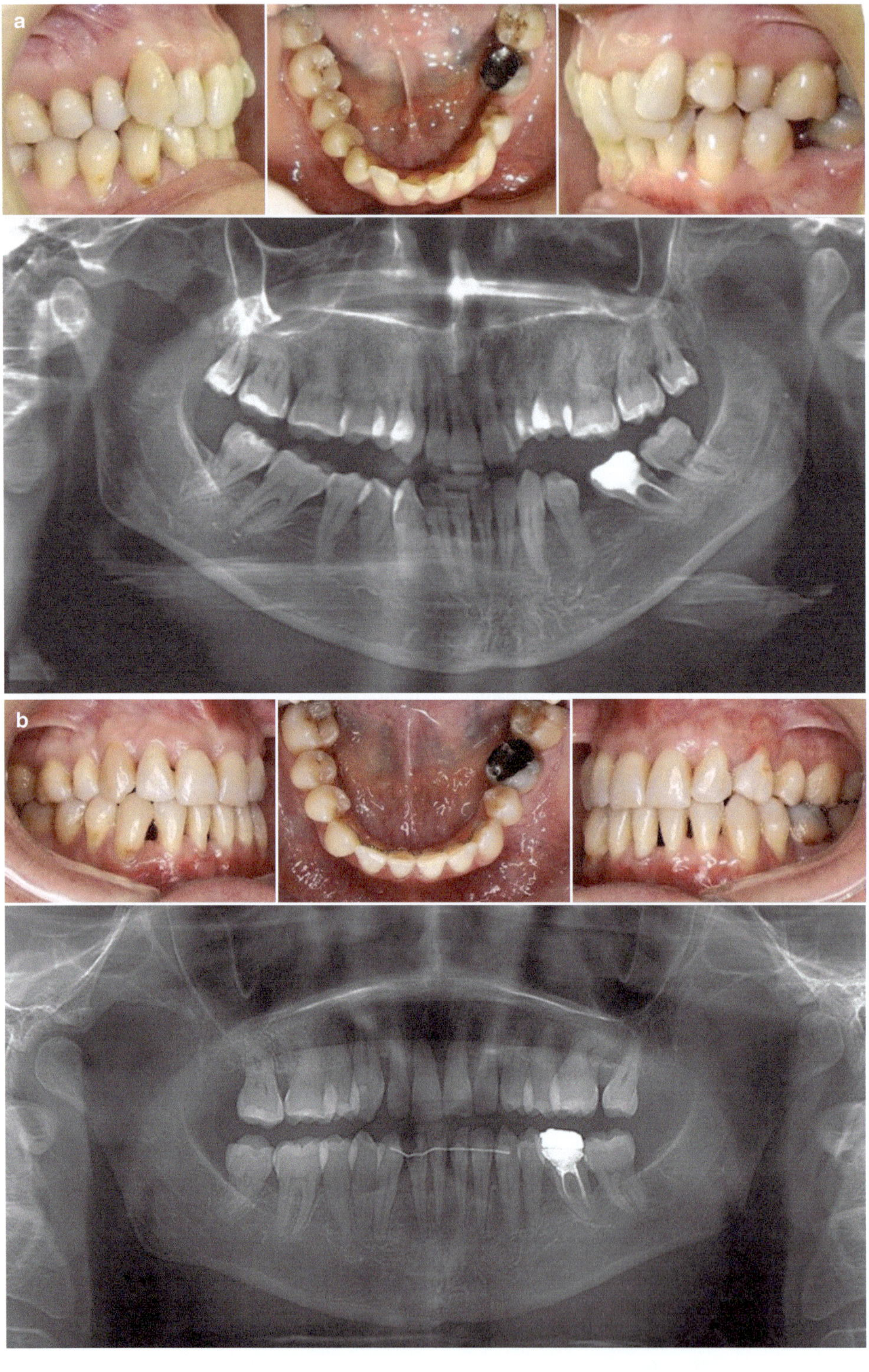

Fig. 10.13 (**a**) Pre-treatment intraoral views and panoramic radiograph of a 42-year-old woman, showing mutilated dentition with compromised periodontium and angular bone loss (red arrows) following mesial crown tipping of mandibular second molars. (**b**) Post-treatment intraoral views and panoramic radiograph indicating enhancement of the periodontium following uprighting of the mandibular second molars by eliminating the angular bone loss (green arrows)

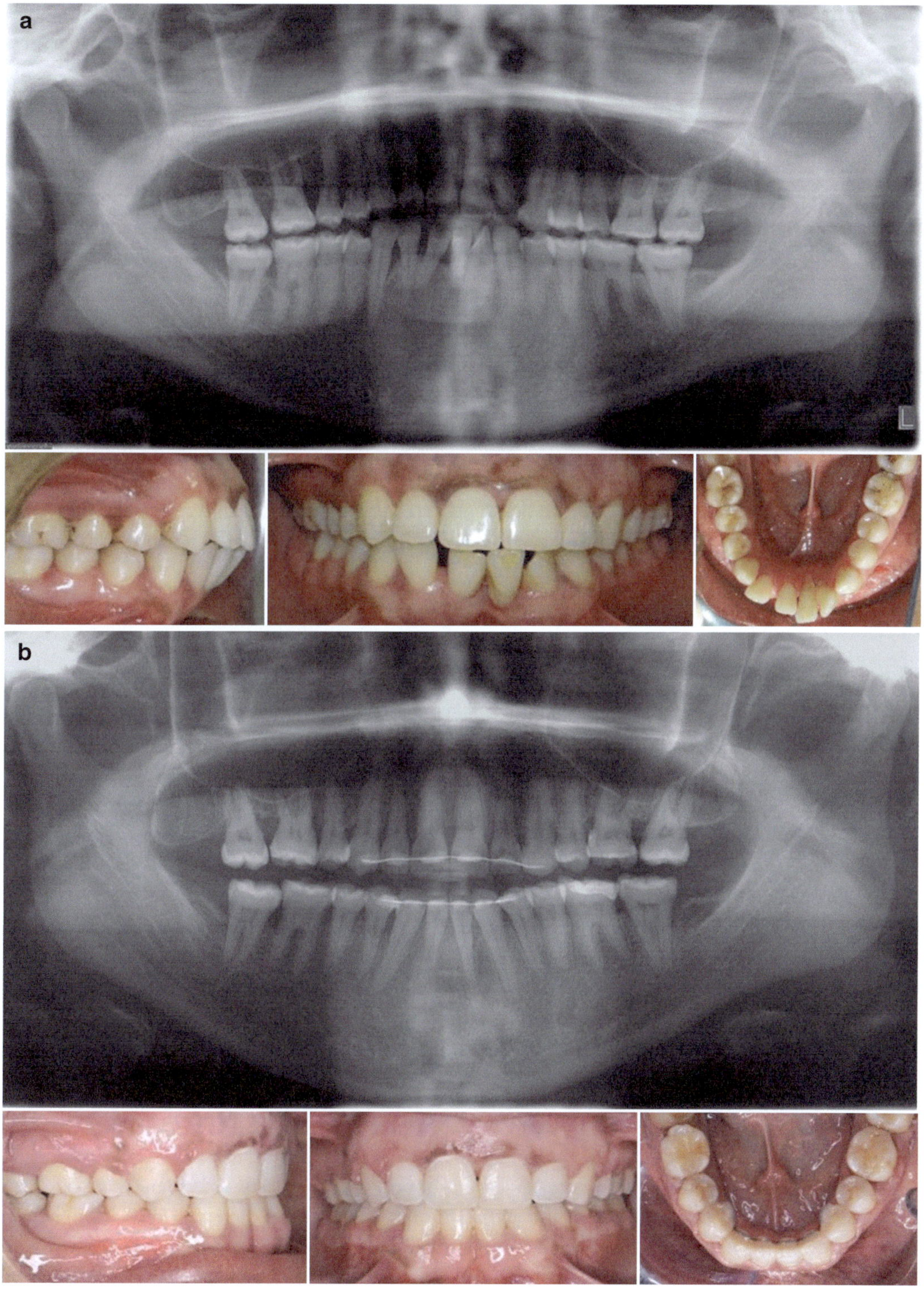

Fig. 10.14 (**a**) Pre-treatment panoramic radiograph and intraoral views a 36-year-old woman, showing severe bone loss of mandibular central incisors (red circle). (**b**) Post-treatment panoramic radiograph and intraoral views indicating enhancement of the periodontium at the level of the mandibular anterior region (green circle) following the extraction of the mandibular central incisors and closure of the spaces

to realign the underlying skeletal structures (i.e., maxilla and mandible) in the correct position. With the increase in treatment demand for adults, surgery has become routine to achieve both aesthetic and functional objectives.

Orthognathic surgery can be performed on the maxilla, the mandible, and the symphysis. Over the years, original surgical cuts of the jaws were modified to facilitate movement of the skeleton and long-term stability. The most common osteotomies for the maxilla are LeFort 1 and 2, and bilateral or unilateral sagittal split is most common for the mandible. Recently, combining soft (lips) and hard (jaws) tissue modification in one surgery to enhance aesthetic outcome has been reported [33]. In addition, genioplasty is performed to reduce or increase the height of the chin, and to advance the symphysis for better projection of the chin in the face. Moreover, it can compensate for deficient chin soft tissue thickness particularly in patients with present hyperdivergent long face [34].

During the last two decades, orthognathic surgery has enjoyed important advances in diagnosis and treatment approaches. The introduction of simulation programs facilitated the prediction of outcome and enhanced patients' confidence about treatment. Other advances included the introduction of plates and screws, which made it easy to stabilize the jaws without impairing post-surgical jaw function. In addition, relying on piezo surgery to cut the bone decreased the risk of nerve injury and post-surgical numbness of the lips [35, 36].

It is unlikely for one dimension of the face to be at fault solely. In general, adult patients necessitate combined orthodontic and orthognathic surgery approaches to address connection between vertical and sagittal skeletal problems. Thus, the importance of accurate diagnosis and surgical planning cannot be overemphasized. Decompensation or "normalization" of the teeth prior to surgery is crucial to allow optimal surgical movement of the jaw.

In young adults, evaluation of any remaining growth potential is important prior to any surgical correction. On average, girls may be subjected to orthognathic surgery at 16–17 years of age, and boys not until 18–19 years of age. However, and in some malocclusions in which more growth is expected in one or both jaws, growth has to be assessed through longitudinal superimpositions of two consecutive lateral cephalometric radiographs before finalizing treatment recommendations.

Anteroposterior Dimension

Whether class II or class III malocclusions, skeletal discrepancies must be identified in order to decide whether one or both jaws are at fault. In class II malocclusions, mandibular advancement is required most often, with or without genioplasty. It is very rare to set back the upper jaw to correct a "skeletal" class II malocclusion. However, in class III malocclusion, orthognathic surgery usually entails advancement of the maxilla. In a few instances, double jaw surgery is needed to ensure optimal results with long-term stability (Figs. 10.15 and 10.16).

Vertical Dimension

A decreased lower facial height with a flat mandibular plane and deep overbite is usually accompanied by a low smile line and less than full height of teeth showing upon smiling. This feature gives the appearance of an older person. In this case, down fracture of the maxilla is needed to restore maxillary height and, consequently, a normal smile line. Normalization of the dimension of the lower face height induces a more youthful appearance and enhances occlusal function (Fig. 10.17).

An increased lower face height (more than 55% of total face height) is characterized by lip incompetency at rest and muscle strain to close the lips, along with increased gingival display upon smiling. When it is difficult or impossible to bridge the gap of the open bite through tooth movement only, surgery is ideal to reposition the maxilla upward. The maxillary impaction will be followed by mandibular autorotation that enhances chin projection in the face.

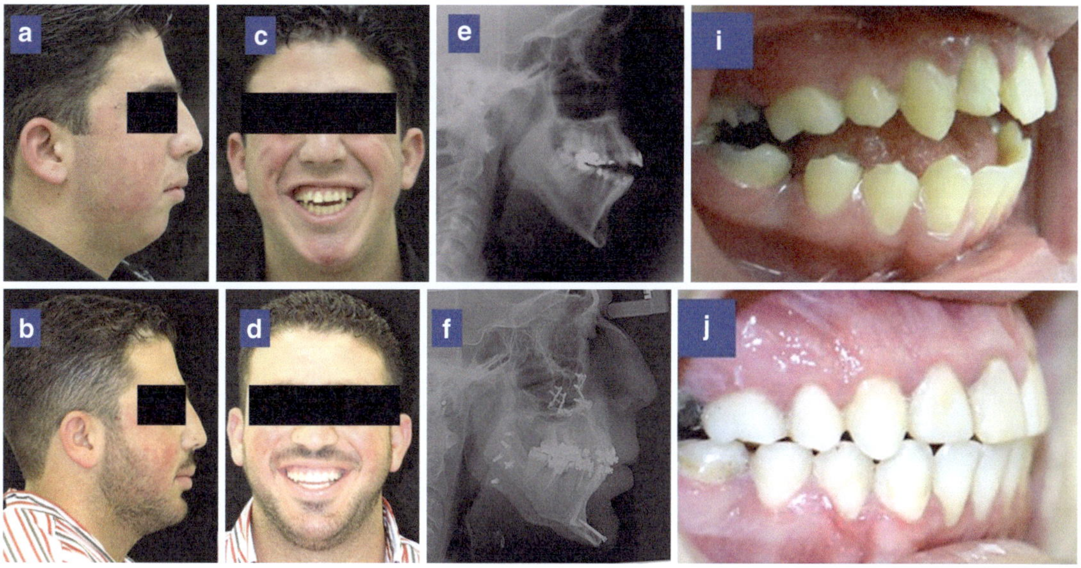

Fig. 10.15 (**a**) Pre-treatment facial profile of a 22-year-old man showing mandibular retrognathism and increased lower facial height. (**b**) Post-treatment facial profile with harmonious features following combined orthodontic and orthognathic surgery treatment with LeFort 1 maxillary impaction and mandibular bilateral sagittal split osteotomy (BSSO) advancement with genioplasty. (**c**, **d**) Pre- and post- surgical smile views. Note the balance between the lips and the teeth along with the restoration of normal proportions of the face. (**e**, **f**) Pre- and post-surgical lateral cephalometric images showing the surgical screws and plates and the correction of the skeletal discrepancy between the jaws. (**i**, **j**) Pre- and post-orthodontic/ orthognathic surgery treatment intraoral views showing the correction of the class II malocclusion and the severe open bite

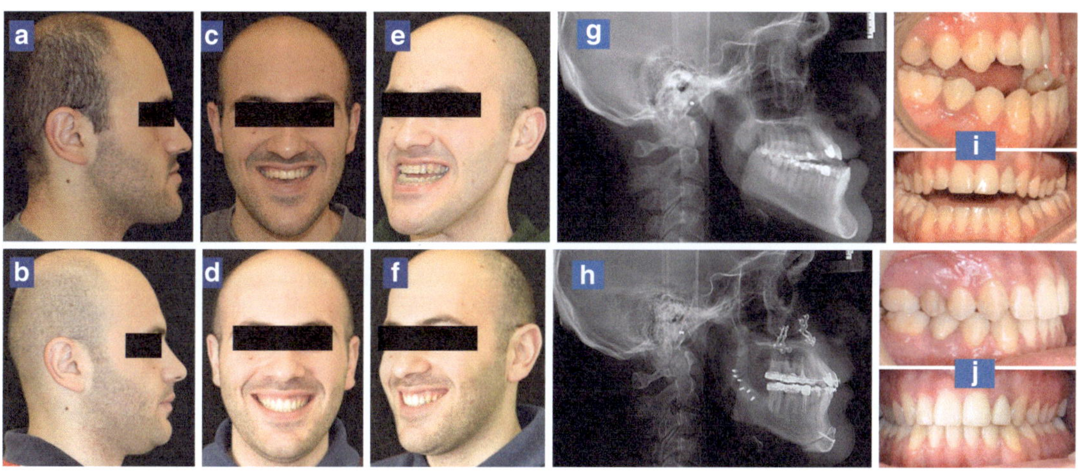

Fig. 10.16 (**a**) Pre-treatment facial profile of a 26-year-old man showing the mandibular prognathism and maxillary retrognathism. (**b**) Post-treatment facial profile with harmonious features following combined orthodontic and orthognathic surgery treatment with LeFort 1 maxillary advancement and mandibular BSSO with genioplasty. (**c**, **d**) Pre- and post-surgical smile views. Note the balance between the lips and the teeth along with the restoration of normal proportions of the face. (**e**, **f**) Pre- and post-surgical oblique smile views (**g**, **h**) Pre- and post-surgical lateral cephalometric showing the surgical screws and plates and correction of the skeletal discrepancy between the jaws. (**i**, **j**) Pre- and post-orthodontic/ orthognathic surgery treatment intraoral views showing the extent of the dental malocclusion correction through the orthognathic surgery movements

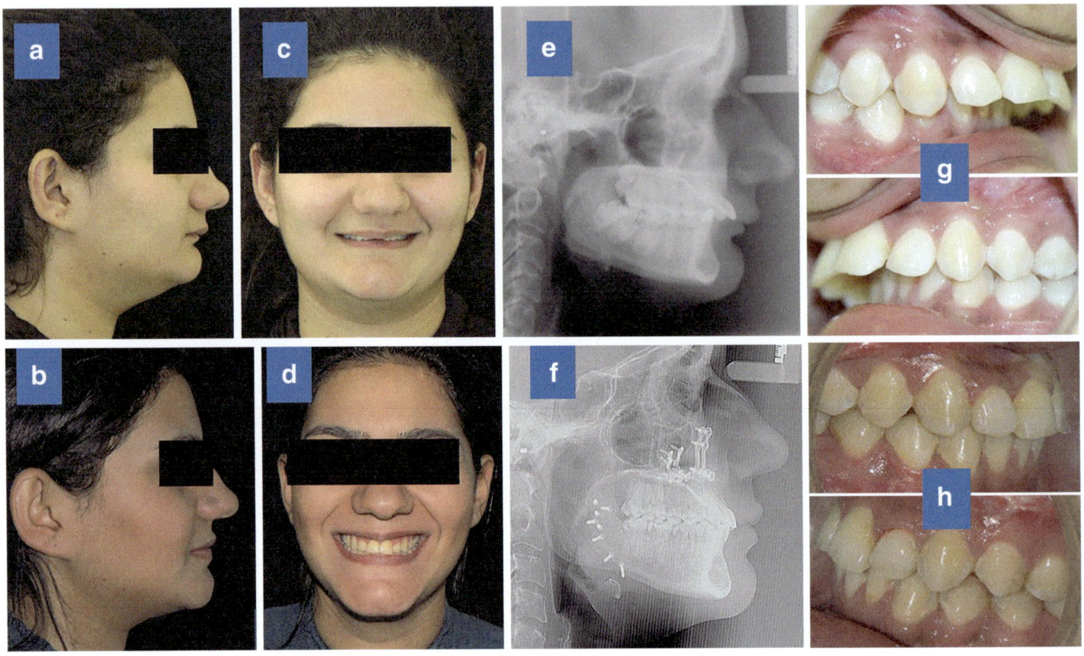

Fig. 10.17 (**a**) Pre-treatment facial profile of a 22-year-old female subject showing a decreased lower facial height and a retruded chin, indicating presence of skeletal discrepancy in both vertical and sagittal planes. (**b**) Post-treatment facial profile with harmonious features following combined orthodontic and orthognathic surgery treatment with LeFort 1 maxillary downward movement and mandibular BSSO with genioplasty. Restoration of the vertical height and normal vertical proportion of the lower face is shown well. (**c**, **d**) Pre- and post-surgical smile views. Note the amount of teeth showing post-surgically in comparison to hidden teeth at smile during pre-treatment smile. (**e**, **f**) Pre- and post-surgical lateral cephalometric images showing the surgical screws and plates and the correction of the skeletal discrepancy between the jaws. (**g**, **h**) Pre- and post-orthodontic/orthognathic surgery treatment intraoral views showing the extent of the dental malocclusion correction through the orthognathic surgery movements

Transverse Dimension

Non-surgical rapid maxillary expansion (RME) may work on young adult patients, but it is not consistent. Therefore, split of the mid-palatal suture often is required in addition to non-surgical expansion. Thus, two-part maxillary treatment may be ideal to correct maxillary constriction in adults. In addition, surgically assisted rapid palatal expansion (SARPE) is also valuable in cases of narrow maxilla. In SARPE, the surgeon performs maxillary LeFort 1 osteotomy cuts, which will allow more predictable palatal widening with the jackscrew expansion appliance [37, 38].

Summary

This chapter provides an overview of orthodontic and related interventions for dentofacial anomalies. As noted in other chapters, the treatments themselves may alter voice or instrumental performance including not just surgery but even braces. The new dentofacial structure also has the potential to affect resonance, articulation, embouchure, and other aspects of performance. In some cases, changes may be for the better, but they also may impair performance, and it often is impossible to predict the effects of treatment on performance. Hence, performers must be informed comprehensively about potential risks and benefits before treatment is initiated, and orthodontists should be aware of performance requirements and modified interventions when reasonable and necessary.

References

1. Krey KF, Darkazanly N, Kühnert R, Ruge S. 3D-printed orthodontic brackets - proof of concept. Int J Comput Dent. 2016;19(4):351–62.
2. Proffit WR, Fields HW, Sarver DM. Treatment in preadolescent children. In: Proffit WR, Fields HW, Sarver DM, editors. Contemporary orthodontics. 6th ed. St. Louis: Mosby; 2019. p. 356–402.
3. Arreghini A, Trigila S, Lombardo L, Siciliani G. Objective assessment of compliance with intra- and extraoral removable appliances. Angle Orthod. 2017;87(1):88–95.
4. Charavet C, Le Gall M, Albert A, Bruwier A, Leroy S. Patient compliance and orthodontic treatment efficacy of Planas functional appliances with TheraMon microsensors. Angle Orthod. 2019;89(1):117–22.
5. Proffit WR, Fields HW, Sarver DM. Biomechanics, mechanics, and contemporary orthodontic appliances. In: Proffit WR, Fields HW, Sarver DM, editors. Contemporary orthodontics. 6th ed. St. Louis: Mosby; 2019. p. 248–356.
6. Castro IO, Frazão Gribel B, Alencar AHG, Valladares-Neto J, Estrela C. Evaluation of crown inclination and angulation after orthodontic treatment using digital models: comparison to the prescription of the brackets used. J Orofac Orthop. 2018;79(4):227–34.
7. Hohoff A, Fillion D, Stamm T, Goder G, Sauerland C, Ehmer U. Oral comfort, function and hygiene in patients with lingual brackets. A prospective longitudinal study. J Orofac Orthop. 2003;64(5):359–71.
8. Hohoff A, Stamm T, Goder G, Sauerland C, Ehmer U, Seifert E. Comparison of 3 bonded lingual appliances by auditive analysis and subjective assessment. Am J Orthod Dentofac Orthop. 2003;124(6):737–45.
9. Tanaka MM, Jonston LE. The prediction of size of unerrupted canines and premolars in contemporary orthodontic population. J Am Dent Assoc. 1974;88:798–801.
10. Moyers RE. Handbook of orthodontics. 3rd ed. Chicago: Yearbook Medical Publishers; 1988. p. 369–79.
11. Mossaz J, Suter VG, Katsaros C. Bornstein MM. Supernumerary teeth in the maxilla and mandible-an interdisciplinary challenge. Part 1: epidemiology, etiology, classification and associated complications. Swiss Dent J. 2016;126(2):131–49.
12. Rijpstra C, Lisson JA. Etiology of anterior open bite: a review. J Orofac Orthop. 2016;77(4):281–6.
13. Borrie FR, Bearn DR, Innes NP, Iheozor-Ejiofor Z. Interventions for the cessation of non-nutritive sucking habits in children. Cochrane Database Syst Rev. 2015;(3):CD008694.
14. Ghafari JG. Early treatment. Interview with Joseph George Ghafari by Anthony A. Gianelly. Prog Orthod. 2007;8(1):174–90.
15. Ghafari J. Timing the early treatment of class II, division 1 malocclusion--clinical and research considerations. Clin Orthod Res. 1998;1(2):118–29.
16. Ghafari J, King GJ, Tulloch JF. Early treatment of class II, division 1 malocclusion--comparison of alternative treatment modalities. Clin Orthod Res. 1998;1(2):107–17.
17. Thiruvenkatachari B, Harrison J, Worthington H, O'Brien K. Early orthodontic treatment for class II malocclusion reduces the chance of incisal trauma: results of a Cochrane systematic review. Am J Orthod Dentofac Orthop. 2015;148(1):47–59.
18. Melsen B. Palatal growth studied on human autopsy material. A histologic microradiographic study. Am J Orthod. 1975;68(1):42–54.
19. Macari AT, Ziade G, Khandakji M, Tamim H, Hamdan AL. Effect of rapid maxillary expansion on voice. J Voice. 2016;30(6):760.e1–6.
20. Saadeh M, Macari A, Haddad R, Ghafari J. Instability of palatal rugae following rapid maxillary expansion. Eur J Orthod. 2017;39(5):474–81.
21. Ghafari J, Shofer FS, Jacobsson-Hunt U, Markowitz DL, Laster LL. Headgear versus function regulator in the early treatment of class II, division 1 malocclusion: a randomized clinical trial. Am J Orthod Dentofac Orthop. 1998;113(1):51–61.
22. Phan KL, Bendeus M, Hägg U, Hansen K, Rabie AB. Comparison of the headgear activator and Herbst appliance--effects and post-treatment changes. Eur J Orthod. 2006 Dec;28(6):594–604.
23. Ghafari JG, Macari AT. Component analysis of class ii, division 1 discloses limitations for transfer to class I phenotype. Semin Orthod. 2014;20(4):253–71.
24. Genno PG, Nemer GM, Zein Eddine SB, Macari AT, Ghafari JG. Three novel genes tied to mandibular prognathism in eastern Mediterranean families. Am J Orthod Dentofac Orthop. 2019;156(1):104–112.e3.
25. Proffit WR, Fields HW, Sarver DM. The orthodontic problem. In: Proffit WR, Fields HW, Sarver DM, editors. Contemporary orthodontics. 6th ed. St. Louis: Mosby; 2019. p. 2–140.
26. Antoszewska-Smith J, Sarul M, Łyczek J, Konopka T, Kawala B. Effectiveness of orthodontic miniscrew implants in anchorage reinforcement during en-masse retraction: a systematic review and meta-analysis. Am J Orthod Dentofac Orthop. 2017;151(3):440–55.

27. Cangialosi T. Skeletal morphologic features of anterior open bite. Am J Orthod. 1984;85:28–36.
28. Ng CS, Wong WK, Hagg U. Orthodontic treatment of anterior open bite. Int J Paediatr Dent. 2008;18:78–83.
29. Proffit WR, Ackerman JL. Diagnosis and treatment planning in orthodontics. In: Graber TM, Vanarsdall RL, editors. Orthodontics. Current principles and techniques. 2nd ed. St Louis: Mosby- Yearbook Inc.; 1994. p. 1–95.
30. Watson WG. A computerized appraisal of the high-pull face-bow. Am J Orthod. 1972;62:561–79.
31. Aras I, Tuncer AV. Comparison of anterior and posterior mini-implant-assisted maxillary incisor intrusion: root resorption and treatment efficiency. Angle Orthod. 2016;86(5):746–52.
32. Solano-Hernández B, Antonarakis GS, Scolozzi P, Kiliaridis S. Combined orthodontic and orthognathic surgical treatment for the correction of skeletal anterior open-bite malocclusion: a systematic review on vertical stability. J Oral Maxillofac Surg. 2013;71:98–109.
33. Macari AT, Abou Chebel N. Upper lip shortening combined with lefort 1 maxillary intrusion: a novel approach to correct the long face syndrome. Eur J Plast Surg. 2014;37(4):245–50.
34. Macari AT, Hanna AE. Comparisons of soft tissue chin thickness in adult patients with various mandibular divergence patterns. Angle Orthod. 2014;84(4):708–14.
35. Landes CA, Stübinger S, Rieger J, Williger B, Ha TK, Sader R. Critical evaluation of piezoelectric osteotomy in orthognathic surgery: operative technique, blood loss, time requirement, nerve and vessel integrity. J Oral Maxillofac Surg. 2008;66(4):657–74.
36. Pagotto LEC, de Santana Santos T, de Vasconcellos SJA, Santos JS, Martins-Filho PRS. Piezoelectric versus conventional techniques for orthognathic surgery: systematic review and meta-analysis. J Craniomaxillofac Surg. 2017;45(10):1607–13.
37. de Gijt JP, Gül A, Tjoa ST, Wolvius EB, van der Wal KG, Koudstaal MJ. Follow up of surgically-assisted rapid maxillary expansion after 6.5 years: skeletal and dental effects. Br J Oral Maxillofac Surg. 2017;55(1):56–60.
38. Northway WM, Meade JB Jr. Surgically assisted rapid maxillary expansion: a comparison of technique, response, and stability. Angle Orthod. 1997;67(4):309–20.

11 Orthodontic Treatment and Voice and Wind Instrument Performance

Introduction

Orthodontic therapy with or without adjunctive orthognathic surgery is the mainstay treatment modality for dentofacial anomalies. The main purpose of treatment is to enhance facial balance through restoration of soft tissue, dental, and skeletal symmetries. Traditionally, orthodontic therapy is performed prior to surgical intervention, although "surgery first" has emerged as a viable alternative with similar outcome in terms of functionality and aesthetics. Both models, the conventional "intermediate surgery" and "surgery first," achieve comparable stability of facial skeletal structures [1]. Despite recent advances in technology and reform in the management of patients with dentofacial anomalies, orthodontic treatment in the form of internal and/or external appliances may impair short- and long-term quality of life of affected patients. Potential complications include periodontal diseases leading to gingival recession, embrasures and gingivitis, pain often resulting in cessation of therapy, dental root resorption particularly in patients with hormonal deficiencies and alcoholism, tooth devitalization, and enamel decalcification [2–6].

The effects of orthodontic treatment on articulation and voice is a topic of thorough discussion in the literature. Given that treatment-induced morphologic changes are limited to the oral and pharyngeal divisions of the vocal tract, the focus has been on nasalance and on variations in low formant frequencies. Indirect effects of treatment on voice secondary to pain during the course of therapy and/or disorders in the temporomandibular joint, also has been deliberated with emphasis on patients' tolerance of and adaptability to treatment [7–10].

This chapter reviews the risks of orthodontic treatment on voice and discusses the direct and indirect mechanisms by which treatment can affect patients' acoustic properties during and after therapy. Physicians need to be aware of the impact of orthodontic therapy on voice while trying to meet patients' expectations. This information is invaluable in developing a management strategy that considers vocal needs with importance equal to that of facial aesthetic and functional impairment. This is particularly true in professional voice users and wind instrumentalists whose performance may be at jeopardy during treatment and afterward.

Effect of Orthodontic Treatment on Voice

The vocal tract is a main component of the phonatory apparatus. Its length and configuration play an important role in defining the position and interspace of formant frequencies [11]. A change in these preferred harmonics, secondary to alteration in behavioral patterns and/or vocal tract anatomy, can lead to change in voice quality. Orthodontic treatment, with or without orthognathic surgery, affects voice by alterating both.

A.-L. Hamdan et al., *Dentofacial Anomalies*, https://doi.org/10.1007/978-3-030-69109-7_11

Articulatory and dentofacial anatomic changes occur during the course of therapy and afterward. The configuration of the oropharyngeal division of the vocal tract is affected most.

There are numerous reports in the literature on the effect of orthodontic treatment on voice, with emphasis on maxillary distraction and/or the use of external and internal devices during the course of therapy. The voice measures reported most are nasalance and formant frequencies. In 2001, Guyette et al. studied the long-term impact of maxillary distraction osteogenesis on velopharyngeal function and articulation in 18 patients with maxillary dysplasia and showed an increase in hyper-nasality in 16.7% of the cases. Moreover, there was a decrease in hyponasality in three out of four patients [12]. In 2004, Satoh et al. investigated the impact of maxillary distraction on the morphology and function of the velopharynx using radiologic imaging, nasal endoscopy and perceptual voice evaluation in nine patients with repaired cleft palate [13]. The authors showed an increase in the mean pharyngeal depth by 2.9 mm (4.6 mm preoperatively vs. to 7.5 mm postoperatively), mild increase in velar length, and worsening of hyper-nasality following treatment in one patient. The pharyngeal depth was measured as the distance between the most-posterior pharyngeal wall at the intersection with the palatal plane, and the most-posterior maxillary point [13]. In 2007, Chanchareonsook et al. investigated velopharyngeal function and quality of speech in 22 patients with maxillary hypoplasia who underwent either Le Fort I distraction osteogenesis or conventional Le Fort I osteotomy. Using nasal-endoscopy, the authors showed worsening of velopharyngeal function in almost one third of the cases. With respect to nasal emission, resonance, and nasalance, the majority of patients had no change after therapy [14]. In 2008, Pereira et al. investigated the effect of distraction osteogenesis on nasalance score, articulation errors, and velopharyngeal function in seven patients with craniofacial disostosis. Four patients were rated hyper-nasal following surgery, whereas three were rated as hyponasal, and three had an oral tone preoperatively. Moreover, there was a positive increase in the mean percentage of correct consonants (59.7% preoperatively vs. 63.7% postoperatively), and an increase in the mean nasalance score from 18.4% to 40.2% [15]. In 2010, Chua et al. compared the effect of distraction osteogenesis vs. conventional orthognathic surgery in cleft lip and palate patients and showed no correlation between the extent of maxillary advancement and nasalance [16]. Their results were in agreement with a previous study in 2008 by the same authors, also showing no significant difference in the effect of either modality on nasalance [17]. In 2010, De Felippe et al. evaluated the impact of various types of palatal expanders on speech and reported alteration in speech in 89.4% of cases. Moreover, 93.9%, 90.2%, and 67.9% reported oral discomfort, difficulty in chewing, and swallowing, respectively [18]. In 2011, Stevens et al. examined the effect of rapid maxillary expansion (RME) on speech perturbation and low formant frequencies by analyzing three sentences, the vowel formants for /i/, and the fricative spectra for /s/ and /i/. The authors reported deterioration in speech acceptability during therapy together with an increase in F1/i/ and a decrease in F2/i/. Both speech acceptability and formant frequencies returned to normal following treatment. The study included 22 patients whose voices were rated by 10 listeners during and after treatment [19]. In 2016, Macari et al. investigated the impact of RME on voice in 14 patients and reported lowering of F1/ɑ/ and F2/ɑ/ in 11 and 10 patients out of the 14, respectively. The authors emphasized the need to alert patients, particularly professional voice users, to the potential change in voice quality following therapy [20]. In 2017, Yurttadur et al. evaluated the effect of RME on voice in 20 patients with bilateral maxillary crossbite, in comparison with 20 controls. The acoustic variables used for analysis were F1, F2, F3, and F4, in addition to shimmer and jitter. Despite the presence of a decrease in F1 and F2 and an increase in F3 following removal of the appliances, the authors found no statistically significant difference in formant frequencies between the two groups before or after treatment [21]. In 2017, Biondi et al. reported mild impairment in phonetic habits following rapid maxillary expansion (RME) in 35 patients treated with banded two-arm Hyrax or banded four-arm Hyrax. The results indicated lowering of F1/i/ and an increase in F2/i/ and F3/i/. Moreover, there was a change in the acoustics of fricative consonants but not palatal consonants. The authors confirmed the impact of RME on the acoustic characteristics of treated patients, although the effect was mild [22]. In 2018, Bilgiç et al. investigated the effect of RME on voice in 30 patients with maxillary crossbite and reported a decrease in maximum F0 and cycle-to-cycle variation in frequency (jitter) and an increase in cycle-to-cycle variation in intensity (shimmer). Moreover, using coronal computed tomography, the authors showed an association between change in voice quality and nasal width [23]. In 2019, Singh et al. studied the effect of RME on voice in patients with and without cleft lip/palate. The voice measurements were taken before treatment, 0.8 month and 3 months during treatment, and 6 months after treatment. The authors reported significant differences in F0 3 months after treatment in the non-cleft group [24].

In summary, the impact of rapid maxillary expansion and/or distraction on voice is controversial. In the presence of acoustic changes, patients almost invariably develop adaptive articulatory behavior that masks the adverse consequences of treatment. The adaption is mainly in the position of the tongue, in terms of height and length, which compensates for the change in intraoral volume. Further discussion is presented in another section of this chapter.

The effect of various retaining devices on voice during the course of orthodontic treatment and following their removal also has been discussed thoroughly in the literature [25]. In 2012, Kayikci et al. investigated the effect of Hawley retainers on formant frequencies of vowels and consonants and reported significant changes after treatment in the first three formants for the vowel /i/ [26]. There was an increase in F1/i/ and a decrease in F2/i/ and F3/i/. Moreover, there were significant speech disturbances particularly for the consonants [s] and [z]. In 2017, Atik et al. investigated the articulatory-acoustic changes and the temporal-acoustic pattern of 25 subjects with class I and II malocclusion following treatment with one of two retaining devices (Essix or Hawley). The retainers were used 24 hours a day for 6 days a week, and the assessment was made at different points in time up to 3 months. All three formants F1, F2, and F3 were affected in both groups. The vowel /α/ was affected the most in the Hawley group, while the vowel /e/ was affected the most in the Essix group. The vowel /u/ was affected in both groups. In the Hawley group, there was a decrease in F1/u/ when the upper retainer was used (397.22 Hz to 382.94 Hz), a decrease in F2/α/ value when both upper and lower retainers were used, and an increase in F3/u/ when the lower retainer was used (3.014 Hz to 3.253 Hz). In the Essix group, there was an increase in the value of F2 /e/ when either the upper retainer or both retainers were used, and a decrease in F2/u/ when both retainers were used (995.79 Hz to 943.36 Hz). Moreover, there was a significant difference in the voice onset time (VOT) of the sound [d] between the two groups. With the use of a maxillary retainer in the Hawley group, there was a significant shortening of the VOT from 8.19 msecond to −31.81 msecond. In conclusion, the authors alluded to the extended time needed for speech adaptation in patients wearing removable retainers [27].

How Orthodontic Treatment Can Affect Voice?

Orthodontic treatment can have a direct effect on voice by inducing anatomic changes in the oral and pharyngeal divisions of the vocal tract. The sites affected most commonly are the palate/velopharynx, oropharynx, and hypopharynx. Other anatomical sites that may be affected are the nasal cavities, nasal septum, and nasopharynx. Orthodontic treatment also may have an indirect effect on voice by causing or exacerbating temporomandibular joint disorders and by inflicting pain that sometimes leads to cessation of therapy.

A summary of the direct and indirect mechanisms by which orthodontic treatment can impact voice is presented below.

Direct Impact of Orthodontic Treatment on Voice

Effect of Orthodontic Treatment on the Morphology of the Palate and Velopharyngeal Function

The shape of the palate is determined by its length, width, height of its dome, and the position and angularity of its apex [28]. Maxillary expansion/protraction and/or the use of fixed or removable appliances in orthodontic treatment lead to change in the configuration of the palate. In 2008, De Felippe et al. reported short-term increase in palatal area and inter-molar distance, and long-term increase in the mean palatal volume in 38 patients treated with RME in comparison to a control group [29]. A year later, the same authors showed substantial long-term changes in the volume and surface area of the palate following RME in larger group of patients ($n = 25$), whose volumetric measures were taken using three-dimensional morphometric analysis [30]. These results were in agreement with many reports that consistently indicated an increase in the mid-palatal suture during and/or after maxillary expansion. In 2010, Ballanti et al. reported an increase in the transverse dimension and a decrease in the anteroposterior dimension of the mid-palate suture following RME. Most of the increase in the transverse dimension seen at the end of treatment regressed partially following the retention period [31]. Similarly, in 2013, Bazargani et al. reviewed the literature on the impact of RME on facial sutures and reported an increase in mid-palatal suture accounting for 20–50% of the total screw expansion [32]. In 2015, Liu et al. corroborated the results of Bazargani et al. and demonstrated an expansion of the mid-palatal suture that accounted for 12–52.5% of the total screw expansion during treatment. The authors also reported re-calcification of the mid-palatal suture on long-term follow-up [33]. In 2015, Celikoglu et al. investigated the effect of maxillary protraction on soft and hard tissues in a group of 32 patients with class III malocclusion, 16 of whom wore the mini maxillary protractor, and 16 of whom were treated with facemask and RME. In both groups, there was anterior displacement of the maxilla with rotation of the palatal plane. This latter change was more evident in the group treated with mini maxillary protractor [34]. In 2019, Bruder et al. investigated palatal area following RME in 14 patients treated with Hyrax expander. Using cone-beam computed tomography, the authors demonstrated an increase in the palatal surface area by 9.27% and an increase in its width by 9.71%. Both palatal dimensions decreased non-significantly 6 months after treatment [35].

The changes in the volume and surface area of the palate described in the above reports often come at a cost, namely, velopharyngeal dysfunction. Elevation of the velum is one of the mandates for proper velopharyngeal function, in addition to anterior movement of the posterior pharyngeal wall and medial movement of the lateral pharyngeal walls. Alteration in velopharyngeal function following orthodontic treatment, often referred to as velopharyngeal insufficiency, can be secondary to treatment-induced anatomic changes in the nasopharynx and/or treatment-induced changes in the morphology of the palate as indicated in the previous section. Patients with velopharyngeal dysfunction will complain of nasal emission, the passage of airflow into the nasal cavity during the production of resonant vowels or high-pressure consonants. The effect will vary with the status of velopharyngeal function before treatment and with the type of orthodontic therapy. Patients with a narrow velopharyngeal port tend to improve following maxillary protraction, whereas patients with pre-existing velopharyngeal incompetence often worsen. Velopharyngeal insufficiency can be problematic for singers and disabling for wind instrumentalists.

In summary, orthodontic therapy affects the morphology of the palate and velopharyngeal function. Affected patients complain of hypernasality and increased nasalance. In many instances, the acoustic changes are hardly perceived in real speech due to adaptation in lingual articulation [28]. Velopharyngeal insufficiency may be problematic for voice professionals and especially for wind instrumentalists. Conservative therapy and at times surgical intervention can be offered with promising results.

Effect of Orthodontic Treatment on Airway Space Dimensions

In the interpretation of acoustic changes in patients undergoing orthodontic treatment, it is important to consider the shape of the airway space, particularly the oropharynx and nasopharynx. In 2002, Hiyama et al. investigated the effect of maxillary protraction on the upper airway in 25 patients with class III malocclusion and showed enlargement of the superior upper airway that was commensurate with the forward growth of the maxilla [36]. In 2004, Satoh et al. reported an increase in the pharyngeal depth (at the velopharyngeal level) in nine patients undergoing maxillary expansion. Although the pharyngeal depth was not proportional to the extent of advancement, the changes in nasopharyngeal dimensions were associated with speech deterioration following treatment [13]. In 2006, Sayınsu et al. investigated nasopharyngeal dimensions in 19 patients with class III malocclusion who underwent maxillary expansion combined with protraction and showed an increase in these dimensions. The patients were assessed using cephalometric measures before and after treatment for 6.78 +/− 0.93 months, and there was an increase in the nasopharyngeal airway measurements (PNS-ad1, PNS-ad2) of 2.71 +/−3.35 and 3.03+/−2.37, respectively [37]. "Ad1, the point where posterior nasal spine (PNS)-basin (Ba) line intersects the posterior pharyngeal wall; ad2 is the point where a line perpendicular to sella (S)-Ba plane passing through PNS intersects the posterior pharyngeal wall" [37]. In 2008, Oktay et al. investigated the pharyngeal space dimensions in 20 patients with class III malocclusion treated with maxillary protraction appliances and reported an increase in the pharyngeal area and width. The changes in upper airway dimensions were commensurate with the treatment-induced sagittal growth of the maxilla. The authors concluded that maxillary protraction appliances on the shape and volume of the upper airway [38]. That same year, Kilinc et al. examined the impact of RME and protraction headgear therapy on the upper airway dimensions, particularly the nasopharyngeal space. Using cephalometric radiographs, the authors showed an increase in the nasopharyngeal and oropharyngeal dimensions in parallel with the forward movement of the maxilla and limited movement of the mandible [39]. In 2009, Mucedero et al. investigated the effect of maxillary expansion in two groups of patients, 22 treated with face mask and bite block, and 17 treated with RME and facemask. Using cephalometric images, the authors demonstrated an increase in the sagittal pharyngeal dimensions in comparison to a control group with class III malocclusion. However, the increase was nonsignificant [40]. In 2011, Lee et al. substantiated the correlation between maxillary forward displacement, inhibition of forward growth of the mandible, and the increase in nasopharyngeal dimensions. The study was conducted on 20 patients with class III malocclusion who underwent maxillary protraction and were analyzed using cephalometric radiographs [41]. In 2012, Aloufi et al. studied the impact of RME on the upper and lower airway in 30 patients with maxillary constriction and reported sagittal enlargement of the upper airway by a mean of 1.3 mm in comparison to only 0.5 mm in the control group. The study, conducted using cephalometric analysis, confirmed the impact of RME on the upper pharyngeal airway [42]. In 2014, Li et al. investigated the changes in the upper airway in patients with class II division I malocclusion who underwent twin block therapy. Using cone-beam computed tomography, the authors showed enlargement of the nasopharynx, oropharynx, and hypopharynx, with alteration in the shape of the nasopharynx and oropharynx. Moreover, there was anterior movement of the hyoid bone following treatment [43]. Similarly, in 2014, El and Palomo studied the three-dimensional changes in the oropharyngeal airway of patients treated with RME vs. conventional orthodontic treatment and demonstrated an increase in airway dimensions following treatment. However, the volumetric changes of the oropharyngeal airway were non-significant in patients treated with RME [44]. In 2014, Pamporakis et al. assessed alterations in the pharyngeal airway space in 22 patients treated with RME and facemask. Using cone-beam computed tomography, the authors reported an increase in pharyngeal airway volume in comparison to a control group, but the increase was non-significant [45]. In 2015, Chen et al. evaluated upper airway morphologic changes in patients with class III malocclusion who underwent RME and protraction headgear and demonstrated a significant increase in the volume and cross-sectional area of the upper airway, but no significant difference was noted in the hypopharynx [46]. In 2018, Isidor et al. studied three-dimensional changes of the upper airway in 20 patients with class II malocclusion and reported enlargement of total airway volume following treatment with functional appliances. In comparison to the control group with class I occlusion, only enlargement at the level of the oropharynx was significantly different [47]. In 2019, Thereza-Bussolaro et al. investigated the effect of orthodontic treatment on the oropharyngeal airway space using either intermaxillary elastics or a Forsus fatigue resistance device in 29 patients with class II malocclusion. The authors showed an increase in the oropharyngeal airway dimensions in both subgroups, more in male subjects under the age of 14 years [48]. In 2019, Abdalla et al. compared the pharyngeal airway in 26 children undergoing RME vs. a control group. Using cone-beam computed tomography, the authors showed a greater but not significant increase in upper airway volume and its minimal cross-sectional area in the treated group [49]. In 2020, Zhao et al. investigated the effect of maxillary skeletal expansion on the upper airway using three-dimensional finite element models. The authors demonstrated a positive improvement in the upper airway cross-sectional areas mostly at the level of the oropharynx, by 40.65% [50].

In summary, orthodontic treatment leads to significant changes in the volume and cross-sectional area of the upper airway at various levels. These alterations are secondary to treatment-induced changes in the position of the upper and lower jaw, and soft tissue structures. Given the well-known interplay between vocal tract morphology and voice quality, it seems clear that treatment-induced changes in the airway space dimensions can impact voice [11] and are discussed in further detail in Chap. 6.

Effect of Orthodontic Treatment on the Position of the Tongue

In agreement with the above reports on changes in airway space dimensions following orthodontic treatment, numerous studies associated these changes with variation in the position of the tongue. Orthodontic treatment can affect the position of the tongue both in terms of height and length [51–54]. In the study by Atik et al., the increase in F2/e/ in the Essix group reflected a forward change in position of the tongue, whereas the decrease in the value of F2/a/ in the Hawley group was associated with a lower and more backward position of the tongue [27]. In 2013, Iwasaki et al. investigated the impact of RME on the pharyngeal intraoral airway in 28 patients using cone-beam computed tomography and reported elevation in the position of the tongue in association with enlargement of the pharyngeal airway. Following treatment, there was a decrease in intraoral airway volume from 1212.9 mm^3 to 279.7 mm^3 [52]. Similarly, in the study by Aras et al. on upper airway changes in patients undergoing mandibular advancement, the authors reported an increase in tongue height in the subgroup of patients treated by stepwise mandibular advancement [53]. This is in agreement with the study by Brown et al. that proved elongation of the tongue in the anteroposterior dimension and widening of the oropharyngeal space during treatment with mandibular advancement. Their study was performed on 30 subjects with hypopnea/apnea who were assessed using dynamic magnetic resonance imaging [54].

Effect of Orthodontic Treatment on the Nasal Cavity

Orthodontic treatment also may cause changes in the anatomy of the nasal cavity and its structures. The dimensions of the nasal passages have been studied primarily in the context of patients with crossbites and maxillary constriction who are undergoing treatment. The consensus is that treatment, depending on age and maturity, usually leads to enlargement of the nasal space with or without improvement in nasal breathing [55–59]. In 2008, De Felippe et al. studied the effect of RME on the nasal cavity and airway resistance using radiologic imaging and acoustic rhinometry. The study was conducted on 38 patients who were evaluated during treatment, following removal of the expander, and 9–12 months afterward. The authors reported an increase in the minimal cross-sectional area and mean nasal cavity volume following treatment. The volumetric changes in the nasal cavity were still present on long-term follow-up and were associated with breathing enhancement in almost two-thirds of the cases [30]. In 2009, De Felippe et al. investigated the effect of RME on the nasal cavity in 25 patients using acoustic rhinometry. The authors reported an increase in the volume of the nasal cavity and minimal cross-sectional area during treatment and 1 year following treatment. Similarly, there was a decrease in nasal airway resistance that stabilized following removal of the expander [29]. These results were supported in 2010 by Sökücü et al. in their study on 30 subjects with posterior crossbites, constricted maxilla, or maxillary transverse discrepancies. The authors showed an increase in the minimal cross-sectional area and nasal volume in both subgroups, those treated with the rapid maxillary expander and those treated with the fan-type rapid maxillary expander [60]. In 2013, Bazargani et al. reviewed the literature on the effect of RME on facial structures and showed an increase in nasal cavity dimensions that accounted for 17–33% of the screw expansion in total [32]. In 2014, El and Palomo evaluated the nasal passage in 35 patients treated with RME and showed a twofold enlargement in the mean nasal passage space in comparison to those managed with comprehensive orthodontic treatment [44]. Last but not least, in the study in 2020 by Zhao et al., using computational fluid dynamics analysis, the authors showed an increase in the nasal cavity area by an average of 7.42% following rapid skeletal maxillary expansion. This was accompanied by a decrease in nasal and pharyngeal airflow pressure in the range of 11.34–23.68% [50].

In summary, maxillary expansion causes an increase in the nasal cavity dimensions (area and volume) and passages leading to a decrease in nasal resistance. The long-term impact on breathing is controversial given the unpredictability of growth of facial structures. Given the importance of nasal breathing in phonation and wind instrument performance, and its well-known role in humidifying and regulating airflow temperature, it is reasonable to speculate that changes in nasal breathing have sequelae on phonation and wind instrument performance [61]. Future investigations on the phonatory threshold pressure and other parameters, before and after maxillary expansion, are warranted.

Indirect Effect of Orthodontic Treatment on Voice

Orthodontic treatment also may have an indirect effect on voice by inducing or exacerbating temporomandibular joint (TMJ) dysfunction. There is strong evidence to substantiate a link between disorders of the TMJ and orthodontic treatment, although the cause-effect relationship remains controversial [62–69]. When present, TMJ disorders often are associated with an array of symptoms that adversely impacts voice. In a large patient population study of 4528 patients with TMJ disorders, Cooper and Kleinberg reported pain as the most common symptom in 96.1%, followed by headache and ear discomfort in 79.3% and 82.4% of cases, respectively [70]. The symptoms and signs may fluctuate and may originate either from the temporomandibular joint, and/or its surrounding muscles and dentition [8]. It is also important to keep in mind the high prevalence of TMJ disorders in patients with genetic predisposition, particularly in elderly [8, 71]. In a study by Camacho et al. investigating 200 elderly subjects, the authors reported temporomandibular disorders in 61% of the cases, 17.5% of whom were moderate to severe [72]. The TMJ is important in phonation and especially in professional voice users during voice performance [73]. In cases of dysfunction, patients may complain of a contracted vocal range and inability to reach the high notes. Other associated vocal symptoms include excessive tension in neck musculature and surrounding structures. The muscle tension can extend to the laryngeal muscles leading to voice dysfunction and muscle tension dysphonia. Despite the adverse effect of orthodontic treatment on TMJ, patients and particularly professional voice users should not be discouraged from undergoing therapy. Though the management strategy of TMJ disorders is not the topic of this chapter, it is important to know that several treatment modalities such as self-education, physical/manual therapy, and use of occlusal splints can be offered to affected patients with promising results. Further information on the management of TMJ disorders can be found in the literature.

Pain is also a major concern in patients undergoing orthodontic treatment [74–82]. The importance of considering pain in the overall evaluation and treatment of patients undergoing therapy cannot be overemphasized. In a review by Pacheco-Pereira et al. on factors associated with patients' satisfaction following orthodontic treatment, the authors reported pain level, in addition to the duration of therapy, as major contributing factors [77]. Other factors associated with patients' dissatisfaction were the associated functional impairment and not being informed about the risks of treatment. The intensity and frequency of pain are related to gender in addition to the type of orthodontic treatment and the extent of force applied to dentition [74–76]. In a study by Feldmann et al. on the impact of various orthodontic anchoring techniques on pain and jaw function, the authors reported an increase in pain intensity on the second day following treatment, which regressed on the seventh day [75]. In another systemic review by Monk et al. on the effectiveness of pharmacologic intervention for pain relief in patients undergoing orthodontic treatment, the authors highlighted the need for and effectiveness of analgesics in the treatment of symptomatic patients [76]. In rare cases, the associated pain may be so severe that it can lead to cessation of therapy.

Pain is particularly important in professional voice users and instrumentalists whose vocal performance ability might be in jeopardy. Pain can lead to dysphonia. In a study by Ramos et al. on 74 adults, the authors demonstrated a correlation between musculoskeletal pain and voice-related quality of life. In the subgroup with vocal complaints (n-34), there was significantly higher intensity of pain in the neck, larynx, and submandibular region [78]. In another investigation by Silverio et al. on muscular pain in dysphonic women, the authors reported higher intensity and frequency of pain in the laryngeal area, neck and upper back in dysphonic women compared with women with no dysphonia or vocal complaints [79]. Similarly, Korn et al. described vocal loading and overuse, in addition to stress and anxiety, as risk factors for throat pain [80]. Conversely, locoregional pain may predispose to dysphonia and be the first manifesting symptom. In an epidemiologic study by Cohen on self-reported impact of dysphonia, the authors showed that neck pain is a risk factor for dysphonia, as are gastroesophageal reflux disease, allergy, and depression. The study included 789 patients, one third of whom almost (29%) had had dysphonia [81]. O'Rourke et al. showed that hyoid bone tenderness may be an early sign of laryngeal dysfunction. There was a significant association between neck pain, dysphonia, and hyoid tenderness. The study was performed on 94 patients with or without hyoid tenderness [82].

Orthodontic Treatment in Wind Instrumentalists with Dentofacial Anomalies

The adverse effect of dentofacial anomalies on wind instrument playing is well-supported in the literature [83–85]. Lovius and Huggins conducted a survey on the association between dentition, oral health, and performance in wind instrumentalists and concluded that sound dentition with minimal occlusion abnormality is an asset to musicians who aim at high standard of performance. The study group included 20 musicians, half of whom had class II or III malocclusion, and 6 had either gingival or periodontal diseases [85]. In a systematic review of the literature that included four studies, van der Weijden showed that tooth irregularities have an adverse effect on embouchure and performance in wind instrumentalists. Having an open bite or extreme spacing of the anterior dentition were disadvantageous to musicians [86]. Similarly, in a study by Kula et al. on 70 trumpet players, the authors showed a significant association between various performance skills such as flexibility and endurance, and arch widths and incisors' inclination and rotation. Dental parameters were assessed using three-dimensional cone-beam computed tomography [84].

With normal occlusion being important for performance of many instruments, the role of orthodontic treatment in wind instrumentalists who have trouble while playing requires careful scrutiny. Phillips reported a 12-year-old boy who experienced embouchure discomfort with painful indentation of the upper lip secondary to an anteriorly positioned upper left incisor. Orthodontic treatment with premolar extraction helped mitigate the embouchure discomfort [87]. Van Der Weijden et al. reported a case of a horn player who suffered from lower lip pain during playing attributed to a protruding lower front tooth. The patient also complained of upper lip irritation secondary to crowding of his upper teeth, which also affected the onset of tones during performance. The patient underwent orthodontic treatment using fixed appliances and improved markedly afterward [88]. Such reports lead us to conclude that orthodontic treatment may assist in reducing embouchure discomfort often experienced by musicians with extreme anterior spacing or teeth crowding [83]. Similarly, maxillary expansion may have a favorable effect in wind instrumentalists with constricted maxilla, given the significant positive correlation between maxillary inter-canine and inter-molar width and performance [84]. Although these reports substantiate the long-term benefit of orthodontic treatment, wind instrumentalists may endure short-term discomfort with major effects on their daily performance. Raney conducted a survey on the effect of orthodontic appliances on wind instrumentalists' performance using a questionnaire that consisted of questions such as: How braces affect your playing? How long did it take you to adjust? What aids have you used to help you adjust? The majority of students (86%) reported adverse effects of braces, and woodwind players adjusted more quickly than brass players. Some of the aids used to help adjust were the use of wax and/or folded tape [89].

While analyzing the impact of orthodontic treatment on performance in wind instrumentalists, it is also important to consider the choice of wind instrument as an important variable that affects treatment outcome. There are few reports in the literature geared toward the belief that there is a "proper" instrument based on the dentofacial physical set-up of the player, and hence choosing the "wrong" or "improper instrument" may lead to adverse consequences in musicians with dentofacial anomalies. For instance, in the review by Van der Weijden et al., the authors reported that a wide jaw is better than a small jaw for a trumpet player [86]. Similarly, few studies have advocated that the wrong choice of wind instrument may also deter the outcome of orthodontic treatment. The aforementioned speculation is based on the concept that force exerted using wind instruments exceeds by far the force needed to tilt the position of a tooth. Hence, playing a wind instrument may assist in worsening or rectifying a pre-existing malocclusion and in attaining the proper movement of dentition [90, 91]. Pang investigated the impact of wind instrument playing on the anterior tooth position in 76 students who were evaluated before the initiation of playing and 6 months after. Despite the relatively short period of playing, the authors showed a reduction in overjet, mostly in those who played the class A instruments "cup-shaped mouthpieces made of metal which vary in size and in the depth and width of the brim" [92]. Similarly, Herman showed that cup-shaped mouthpieces can decrease the extent of overjet and overbite, whereas single-reed mouthpieces can increase overjet and overbite. The authors argued in favor of proper instrument selection as an aid to orthodontic treatment [91]. Despite the above reports, factors such as the "oneness with the instrument" and the personal inclination toward playing a specific wind instrument must be considered in deciding what to play, irrespective of one's dentofacial configuration. Moreover, the individual level of adaptability and tolerance argue against changing the type of instrument secondary to orthodontic treatment. Students and musicians can learn how to work around the challenges of internal and external orthodontic appliances, and thus keep playing their own instrument. The mouth and orofacial structures will reconfigure the way to adjust and perform despite the anatomic changes. This topic will be covered in detail in Chap. 4.

In summary, wind instrumentalists undergoing orthodontic treatment need special attention. The choice of instrument can deter the benefits of orthodontic treatment and worsen pre-existing orofacial associated problems. It is also important to note that musicians may not be aware of when treatment should be initiated and the benefits or adverse effects of treatment. Van der Weijdein reported that "A talented musician does not know what orthodontic treatment will bring him/her, but knows that during the time of treatment, exercise with playing the instrument will be less intense" [88]. That being stated, the treatment of wind instrument players should be a priority and should be initiated as early as possible in order not to jeopardize their performance ambitions.

References

1. Yang L, Xiao YD, Liang YJ, Wang X, Li JY, Liao GQ. Does the surgery-first approach produce better outcomes in orthognathic surgery? A systematic review and meta-analysis. J Oral Maxillofac Surg. 2017;75(11):2422–9.
2. von Bohl M, Ren Y, Fudalej PS, Kuijpers-Jagtman AM. Pulpal reactions to orthodontic force application in humans: a systematic review. J Endod. 2012;38(11):1463–9.
3. Zachrisson BU. Tooth movements in the periodontally compromised patient. In: Lindhe J, Lang N, Karring T, editors. Clinical periodontology and implant dentistry. Copenhagen/Munksgaard: Wiley-Blackwell; 2008. p. 1271.
4. Weltman B, Vig KWL, Fields HW, Shanker S, Kaizar EE. Root resorption associated with orthodontic tooth movement: a systematic review. Am J Orthod Dentofac Orthop. 2010;137(4):462–76.
5. Javed F, Al-Kheraif AA, Romanos EB, Romanos GE. Influence of orthodontic forces on human dental pulp: a systematic review. Arch Oral Biol. 2015;60(2):347–56.
6. Chatterjee R, Kleinberg I. Effect of orthodontic band placement on the chemical composition of human incisor tooth plaque. Arch Oral Biol. 1979;24(2):97–100.
7. Christensen L, Luther F. Adults seeking orthodontic treatment: expectations, periodontal and TMD issues. Br Dent J. 2015;218(3):111–7.
8. Okeson JP. Evolution of occlusion and temporomandibular disorder in orthodontics: past, present, and future. Am J Orthod Dentofac Orthop. 2015;147(5):S216–23.
9. Oliver RG, Knapman YM. Attitudes to orthodontic treatment. Br J Orthod. 1985;12(4):179–88.
10. Sergl HG, Klages U, Zentner A. Functional and social discomfort during orthodontic treatment–effects on compliance and prediction of patients' adaptation by personality variables. Eur J Orthod. 2000;22(3):307–15.
11. Sundberg J. Vocal tract resonance. In: Sataloff RT. Professional voice: the science and art of clinical care. 4th ed. San Diego: Plural Publishing; 2017. p. 309–28.
12. Guyette TW, Polley JW, Figueroa A, Smith BE. Changes in speech following maxillary distraction osteogenesis. Cleft Palate Craniofac J. 2001;38(3):199–205.
13. Satoh K, Nagata J, Shomura K, et al. Morphological evaluation of changes in velopharyngeal function following maxillary distraction in patients with repaired cleft palate during mixed dentition. Cleft Palate Craniofac J. 2004;41(4):355–63.
14. Chanchareonsook N, Whitehill TL, Samman N. Speech outcome and velopharyngeal function in cleft palate: comparison of Le Fort I maxillary osteotomy and distraction osteogenesis—early results. Cleft Palate Craniofac J. 2007;44(1):23–32.
15. Pereira V, Sell D, Ponniah A, Evans R, Dunaway D. Midface osteotomy versus distraction: the effect on speech, nasality, and velopharyngeal function in craniofacial dysostosis. Cleft Palate Craniofac J. 2008;45(4):353–63.
16. Chua HD, Whitehill TL, Samman N, Cheung LK. Maxillary distraction versus orthognathic surgery in cleft lip and palate patients: effects on speech and velopharyngeal function. Int J Oral Maxillofac Surg. 2010;39(7):633–40.
17. Cheung LK, Chua HD. Distraction or orthognathic surgery for cleft lip and palate patients: which is better? Ann R Australas Coll Dent Surg. 2008;19:133–5.
18. De Felippe NL, Da Silveira AC, Viana G, Smith B. Influence of palatal expanders on oral comfort, speech, and mastication. Am J Orthod Dentofac Orthop. 2010;137(1):48–53.
19. Stevens K, Bressmann T, Gong SG, Tompson BD. Impact of a rapid palatal expander on speech

articulation. Am J Orthod Dentofac Orthop. 2011;140(2):67–75.
20. Macari AT, Ziade G, Khandakji M, Tamim H, Hamdan AL. Effect of rapid maxillary expansion on voice. J Voice. 2016;30(6):760.e1–6.
21. Yurttadur G, Bascıftcı FA, Ozturk K. The effects of rapid maxillary expansion on voice function. Angle Orthod. 2017;87(1):49–55.
22. Biondi E, Bandini A, Lombardo L, Orlandi S, Siciliani G, Manfredi C. Phonetic analysis during treatment with rapid maxillary expander. Orthod Craniofac Res. 2017;20(1):21–9.
23. Bilgiç F, Damlar İ, Sürmelioğlu Ö, Sözer ÖA, Tatlı U. Relationship between voice function and skeletal effects of rapid maxillary expansion. Angle Orthod. 2018;88(2):202–7.
24. Singh H, Maurya RK, Sharma P, Kapoor P, Mittal T, Atri M. Effects of maxillary expansion on hearing and voice function in non-cleft lip palate and cleft lip palate patients with transverse maxillary deficiency: a multicentric randomized controlled trial. Braz J Otorhinolaryngol. 2019; pii: S1808-8694(19)30121-1
25. Moyer N. What to know before you get a retainer. Healthline website. Updated May 29, 2018. Accessed 15 April 2020. https://www.healthline.com/health/retainer-types.
26. Kayikci ME, Akan S, Ciger S, Ozkan S. Effects of Hawley retainers on consonants and formant frequencies of vowels. Angle Orthod. 2012;82(1):14–21.
27. Atik E, Aydınlı FE, Kulak Kayıkçı ME, Ciğer S. Comparing the effects of Essix and Hawley retainers on the acoustics of speech. Eur J Orthod. 2017;39(4):440–5.
28. Lammert A, Proctor M, Narayanan S. Interspeaker variability in hard palate morphology and vowel production. J Speech Lang Hear Res. 2013;56(6):S1924–33.
29. De Felippe NL, Da Silveira AC, Viana G, Kusnoto B, Smith B, Evans CA. Relationship between rapid maxillary expansion and nasal cavity size and airway resistance: short-and long-term effects. Am J Orthod Dentofac Orthop. 2008;134(3):370–82.
30. De Felippe NL, Bhushan N, Da Silveira AC, Viana G, Smith B. Long-term effects of orthodontic therapy on the maxillary dental arch and nasal cavity. Am J Orthod Dentofac Orthop. 2009;136(4):490.e1–8.
31. Ballanti F, Lione R, Baccetti T, Franchi L, Cozza P. Treatment and posttreatment skeletal effects of rapid maxillary expansion investigated with low-dose computed tomography in growing subjects. Am J Orthod Dentofac Orthop. 2010;138(3):311–7.
32. Bazargani F, Feldmann I, Bondemark L. Three-dimensional analysis of effects of rapid maxillary expansion on facial sutures and bones: a systematic review. Angle Orthod. 2013;83(6):1074–82.
33. Liu S, Xu T, Zou W. Effects of rapid maxillary expansion on the midpalatal suture: a systematic review. Eur J Orthod. 2015;37(6):651–5.
34. Celikoglu M, Yavuz I, Unal T, Oktay H, Erdem A. Comparison of the soft and hard tissue effects of two different protraction mechanisms in class III patients: a randomized clinical trial. Clin Oral Investig. 2015;19(8):2115–22.
35. Bruder C, Ortolani CL, de Lima TA, Artese F, Faltin K Jr. Evaluation of palate area before and after rapid maxillary expansion, using cone-beam computed tomography. Dental Press J Orthod. 2019;24(5):40–5.
36. Hiyama S, Suda N, Ishii-Suzuki M, et al. Effects of maxillary protraction on craniofacial structures and upper-airway dimension. Angle Orthod. 2002;72(1):43–7.
37. Sayınsu K, Isik F, Arun T. Sagittal airway dimensions following maxillary protraction: a pilot study. Eur J Orthod. 2006;28(2):184–9.
38. Oktay H, Ulukaya E. Maxillary protraction appliance effect on the size of the upper airway passage. Angle Orthod. 2008;78(2):209–14.
39. Kilinc AS, Arslan SG, Kama JD, Özer T, Dari O. Effects on the sagittal pharyngeal dimensions of protraction and rapid palatal expansion in class III malocclusion subjects. Eur J Orthod. 2008;30(1):61–6.
40. Mucedero M, Baccetti T, Franchi L, Cozza P. Effects of maxillary protraction with or without expansion on the sagittal pharyngeal dimensions in class III subjects. Am J Orthod Dentofac Orthop. 2009;135(6):777–81.
41. Lee JW, Park KH, Kim SH, Park YG, Kim SJ. Correlation between skeletal changes by maxillary protraction and upper airway dimensions. Angle Orthod. 2011;81(3):426–32.
42. Aloufi F, Preston CB, Zawawi KH. Changes in the upper and lower pharyngeal airway spaces associated with rapid maxillary expansion. ISRN Dent. 2012;2012:290964.
43. Li L, Liu H, Cheng H, et al. CBCT evaluation of the upper airway morphological changes in growing patients of class II division 1 malocclusion with mandibular retrusion using twin block appliance: a comparative research. PLoS One. 2014;9(4):e94378.
44. El H, Palomo JM. Three-dimensional evaluation of upper airway following rapid maxillary expansion: a CBCT study. Angle Orthod. 2014;84(2):265–73.
45. Pamporakis P, Nevzatoğlu Ş, Küçükkeleş N. Three-dimensional alterations in pharyngeal airway and maxillary sinus volumes in class III maxillary deficiency subjects undergoing orthopedic facemask treatment. Angle Orthod. 2014;84(4):701–7.
46. Chen X, Liu D, Liu J, et al. Three-dimensional evaluation of the upper airway morphological changes in growing patients with skeletal class III malocclusion treated by protraction headgear and rapid palatal expansion: a comparative research. PLoS One. 2015;10(8):1–13.
47. Isidor S, Di Carlo G, Cornelis MA, Isidor F, Cattaneo PM. Three-dimensional evaluation of changes in upper airway volume in growing skeletal class II patients following mandibular advancement treatment with functional orthopedic appliances. Angle Orthod. 2018;88(5):552–9.
48. Thereza-Bussolaro C, Oh HS, Lagravère M, Flores-Mir C. Pharyngeal dimensional changes in class II malocclusion treatment when using Forsus® or inter-

maxillary elastics–an exploratory study. Int Orthod. 2019;17(4):667–77.
49. Abdalla Y, Brown L, Sonnesen L. Effects of rapid maxillary expansion on upper airway volume: a three-dimensional cone-beam computed tomography study. Angle Orthod. 2019;89(6):917–23.
50. Zhao T, Zhang X, Ngan P, et al. Effects of maxillary skeletal expansion on upper airway airflow: a computational fluid dynamics analysis. J Craniofac Surg. 2020;31(1):e6–10.
51. Ladefoged P, editor. Phonetic data analysis: an introduction to fieldwork and instrumental techniques. Malden: Wiley-Blackwell; 2003.
52. Iwasaki T, Saitoh I, Takemoto Y, et al. Tongue posture improvement and pharyngeal airway enlargement as secondary effects of rapid maxillary expansion: a cone-beam computed tomography study. Am J Orthod Dentofac Orthop. 2013;143(2):235–45.
53. Aras I, Pasaoglu A, Olmez S, Unal I, Aras A. Upper airway changes following single-step or stepwise advancement using the Functional Mandibular Advancer. J Orofac Orthop. 2016;77(6):454–62.
54. Brown EC, Cheng S, McKenzie DK, Butler JE, Gandevia SC, Bilston LE. Tongue and lateral upper airway movement with mandibular advancement. Sleep. 2013;36(3):397–404.
55. Doruk C, Bicakci AA, Basciftci FA, Agar U, Babacan H. A comparison of the effects of rapid maxillary expansion and fan-type rapid maxillary expansion on dentofacial structures. Angle Orthod. 2004;74:184–94.
56. Basciftci FA, Mutlu N, Karaman AI, Malkoc S, Kucukkolbasi H. Does the timing and method of rapid maxillary expansion have an effect on the changes in nasal dimensions? Angle Orthod. 2002;72(2):118–23.
57. Cross DL, McDonald JP. Effect of rapid maxillary expansion on skeletal, dental, and nasal structures: a postero-anterior cephalometric study. Eur J Orthod. 2000;22(5):519–28.
58. Neeley WW 2nd, Edgin WA, Gonzales DA. A review of the effects of expansion of the nasal base on nasal airflow and resistance. J Oral Maxillofac Surg. 2007;65(6):1174–9.
59. Ramires T, Maia RA, Barone JR. Nasal cavity changes and the respiratory standard after maxillary expansion. Braz J Otorhinolaryngol. 2008;74(5):763–9.
60. Sökücü O, Doruk C, Uysal Öİ. Comparison of the effects of RME and fan-type RME on nasal airway by using acoustic rhinometry. Angle Orthod. 2010;80(5):870–5.
61. Hamdan AL, Barazi A, Tabri D, Khneisser G, Sinno S, Ashkar J, Hussari A. The effect of snoring on voice: a controlled study of 30 subjects. ENT J. 2012;91(1):28–33.
62. Okeson JP, editor. Management of temporomandibular disorders and occlusion. 7th ed. St Louis: Mosby; 2013. p. 164.
63. McNamara JA Jr. Orthodontic treatment and temporomandibular disorders. Oral Surg Oral Med Oral Pathol Oral Radiol Endod. 1997;83(1):107.
64. Reynders RM. Orthodontics and temporomandibular disorders: a review of the literature (1966-1988). Am J Orthod Dentofac Orthop. 1990;97(6):463–71.
65. McNamara JA Jr, Seligman DA, Okeson JP. Occlusion, orthodontic treatment, and temporomandibular disorders: a review. J Orofac Pain. 1995;9(1):73–90.
66. Kim M-R, Graber TM, Viana MA. Orthodontics and temporomandibular disorder: a meta-analysis. Am J Orthod Dentofac Orthop. 2002;121(5):438–46.
67. Luther F. TMD and occlusion part I. Damned if we do? Occlusion: the interface of dentistry and orthodontics. Br Dent J. 2007;202(1):38–9.
68. Luther F, Layton S, McDonald F. Orthodontics for treating temporomandibular joint (TMJ) disorders. Cochrane Database Syst Rev. 2010;7(7):CD006541.
69. Michelotti A, Iodice G. The role of orthodontics in temporomandibular disorders. J Oral Rehabil. 2010;37(6):411–29.
70. Cooper BC, Kleinberg I. Examination of a large patient population for the presence of symptoms and signs of temporomandibular disorders. Cranio. 2007;25(2):114–26.
71. Slade GD, Diatchenko L, Ohrbach R, Maixner W. Orthodontic treatment, genetic factors, and risk of temporomandibular disorder. Semin Orthod. 2008;14(2):146–56.
72. Camacho JG, Oltramari-Navarro PV, Navarro RD, et al. Signs and symptoms of temporomandibular disorders in the elderly. Codas. 2014;26(1):76–80.
73. Rose B, Horman M, Sataloff RT. Voice therapy. In: Sataloff RT. Professional voice: the science and art of clinical care. 4th ed. San Diego: Plural Publishing; 2017. p. 1171–94.
74. Ferreira CL, da Silva MA, de Felício CM. Signs and symptoms of temporomandibular disorders in women and men. Codas. 2016;28(1):17–21.
75. Feldmann I, List T, Bondemark L. Orthodontic anchoring techniques and its influence on pain, discomfort, and jaw function—a randomized controlled trial. Eur J Orthod. 2012;34(1):102–8.
76. Monk AB, Harrison JE, Worthington HV, Teague A. Pharmacological interventions for pain relief during orthodontic treatment. Cochrane Database Syst Rev. 2017;11(11):CD003976.
77. Pachêco-Pereira C, Pereira JR, Dick BD, Perez A, Flores-Mir C. Factors associated with patient and parent satisfaction after orthodontic treatment: a systematic review. Am J Orthod Dentofac Orthop. 2015;148(4):652–9.
78. Ramos AC, Floro RL, Ribeiro VV, Brasolotto AG, Silverio KC. Musculoskeletal pain and voice-related quality of life in dysphonic and non-dysphonic subjects. J Voice. 2018;32(3):307–13.
79. Silverio KC, Siqueira LT, Lauris JR, Brasolotto AG. Muscleskeletal pain in dysphonic women. Codas. 2014;26(5):374–81.

80. Korn GP, de Lima Pontes AA, Abranches D, de Lima Pontes PA. Vocal tract discomfort and risk factors in university teachers. J Voice. 2016;30(4):507e1–8.
81. Cohen SM. Self-reported impact of dysphonia in a primary care population: an epidemiological study. Laryngoscope. 2010;120(10):2022–32.
82. O'Rourke C, Attique S, Rehman AU, Saunders J, Fenton JE. Hyoid bone tenderness as a clinical indicator of laryngeal pathology. J Voice. 2014;28(6):835–7.
83. Cheney EA. Adaptation to embouchure as a function of dentofacial complex. Am J Orthod. 1949;35(6):440–56.
84. Kula K, Cilingir HZ, Eckert G, Dagg J, Ghoneima A. The association of malocclusion and trumpet performance. Angle Orthod. 2016;86(1):108–14.
85. Lovius BB, Huggins DG. Orthodontics and the wind instrumentalist. J Dent. 1973;2(2):65–8.
86. van der Weijden FN, Kuitert RB, Berkhout FRU, van der Weijden GA. Influence of tooth position on wind instrumentalists' performance and embouchure comfort: a systematic review. J Orofac Orthop. 2018;79(3):205–18.
87. Phillips WH. Orthodontics and embouchure. A case report. Br Dent J. 1972;132:501–2.
88. van der Weijden F, Berkhout FR, Lobbezoo F. Improvement of embouchure after correction of irregular front teeth: the case of a professional French horn player. Br Dent J. 2019;226(4):261–4.
89. Raney NA. The effects of orthodontic appliances on wind-instrument players. J Clin Orthod. 2006;40(6):384.
90. Proffit WR. The biological basis of orthodontic therapy. In: Rudolph P, editor. Contemporary orthodontics. 3rd ed. St. Louis: Mosby; 2000. p. 296–325.
91. Herman E. Influence of musical instruments on tooth positions. Am J Orthod. 1981;80(2):145–55.
92. Pang A. Relation of musical wind instruments to malocclusion. J Am Dent Assoc. 1976;92(3):565–70.

12 Orthognathic Surgery: Effects on Voice and Wind Instrument Performance

Introduction

Dentofacial structures constitute a major component of the vocal tract. Surgery-induced anatomic changes affect voice by redefining the boundaries of that component. This consensus is based on the well-known link between vocal tract morphology and voice quality, and it is well supported by numerous studies on the impact of oropharyngeal surgery on voice [1–12]. Behrman et al. studied the acoustic properties of 44 patients following upper airway surgery and reported significant changes postoperatively. The amplitude of the first formant (A1) was used as an acoustic descriptor of vowels, and nasal murmur (P0) and nasal peak formant (P1n) were used as acoustic descriptors of the nasal consonants. Though there were no postoperative changes in the voice handicap index (VHI), the A1-P1n distance on the spectrum of nasal consonants "m" and "n," and nasalized vowels, increased significantly [7]. These results concurred with previous studies asserting that surgically induced structural changes in the oral cavity can lead to articulatory and voice changes. Nakai et al. in their perceptual and acoustic study on the effect of uvulopalatoplasty on voice demonstrated significant changes in the first and second formants 21–50 days following surgery [4]. Similarly, Murry and Bone evaluated voice and speech of four patients before and after uvulopalatoplasty, and showed lowering of the second formant for nine vowels in all four patients, together with a decrease in fundamental frequency in one. In addition, there was a decrease in the time needed to read the passage suggesting changes in respiratory parameters [3]. The effect of tonsillectomy on voice has also been investigated by numerous authors [7–12]. In 2010, Lundeborg et al. investigated the impact of tonsillectomy on voice in 67 children with adenotonsillar hypertrophy in comparison to 56 children matched according to age and gender. Acoustic analysis was performed on 3 sustained vowels and 14 words. The F2 /i/, and F3 for vowels /i/ and /u/ were found to be lower in patients with adenotonsillar hypertrophy in comparison to controls. Following surgery, there was a significant increase in F3/α/ and F3/u/. Moreover, there was a decrease in the perturbation measures and noise-to-harmonic ratio, which decreased in the study group after surgery but remained higher than in the control group [11]. Heffernan and Rafferty conducted a similar study on 26 adults who had their voices analyzed before and twice following tonsillectomy. The authors described an increase in the first formant by 58.6% (308.3 Hz vs. 744.4 Hz), but no change in F2 and F3 was noted. Moreover, the authors reported accentuation of the fourth formant, which had not been observed in the study group preoperatively. The authors attributed alterations in formant frequencies to changes in resonance secondary to an increase in the cross-sectional area of the oral cavity. Additional causes of change in formants' position are scarring at the

A.-L. Hamdan et al., *Dentofacial Anomalies*, https://doi.org/10.1007/978-3-030-69109-7_12

surgical site between the base of tongue and palate, and/or subsequent velopharyngeal dysfunction [12].

Orthognathic surgery, which aims at restructuring the dentofacial skeleton, can have an impact on voice. Changes in the length, width, and/or volume of the oropharyngeal division of the vocal tract are inevitable. Given the paramount role of vocal tract in voice resonance, surgery-induced changes in its anatomic configuration inadvertently lead to alteration in its resonant characteristics. This chapter reviews the impact of orthognathic surgery on voice and discusses the pathophysiology of voice changes. This chapter also addresses surgery-induced variations in the shape of the upper airway, as well as the position of the palate, hyoid bone, and tongue in the context of voice changes. This information is particularly important to professional voice users and wind instrument players.

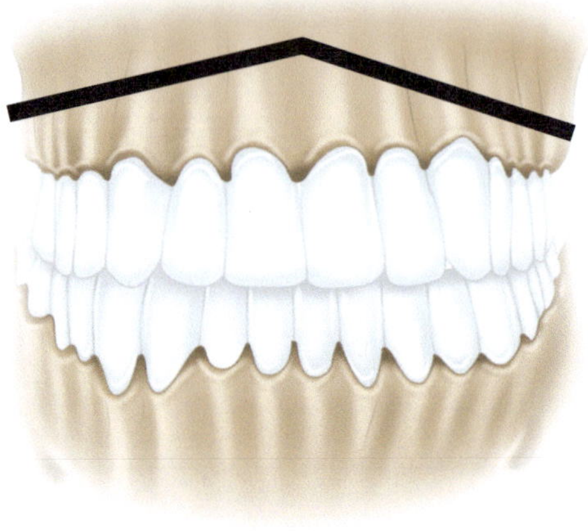

Fig. 12.1 Maxillary osteotomy Le Fort I. Surgical cuts are made above the root of the maxillary teeth, and above the anterior nasal spine. Variation on the routine cuts include lowering the anterior surgical cut below anterior nasal spine to avoid widening of the nose base especially in maxillary advancement and impaction. (Credit: Macari and Abou Chebel [97])

Effect of Orthognathic Surgery on Voice

Orthognathic surgery consists primarily of surgery that is performed on the maxilla and mandible to correct dento-maxillofacial asymmetries, congenital abnormalities, and skeletal angle deformities [13–16]. In cases of skeletal angle deformities and malocclusion, which is the focus of this chapter, maxillary surgery consists primarily of Le Fort 1 osteotomy and segmental osteotomy (Figs. 12.1, 12.2, and 12.3), whereas mandibular surgery incorporates bilateral sagittal split osteotomy, segmental osteotomy, and osseus genioplasty (Figs. 12.4 and 12.5) [13]. Complications following orthognathic surgery are numerous with the most common being cranial nerve injury and/or alteration in sensitivity [14–18]. Based on a large review by Jędrzejewski et al., nerve injury occurs in almost one out of two patients, and the inferior alveolar nerve is affected most commonly. Temporomandibular joint disorders and hemorrhage are second and third in order, occurring in 13.64% and 9.09% of cases, respectively. Less commonly reported complications include infection, malocclusion,

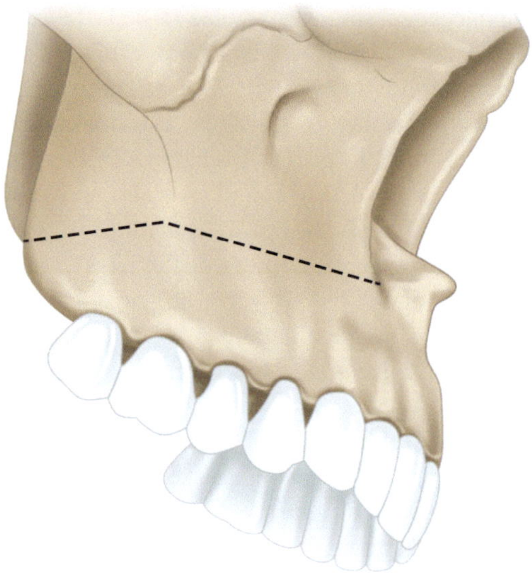

Fig. 12.2 Le Fort I osteotomy showing the posterior limit of the osteotomy reaching the level of the pterygomaxillary junction

eustachian tube dysfunction, and dental complications [19–23].

The impact of orthognathic surgery on articulation has been investigated thoroughly. Reports

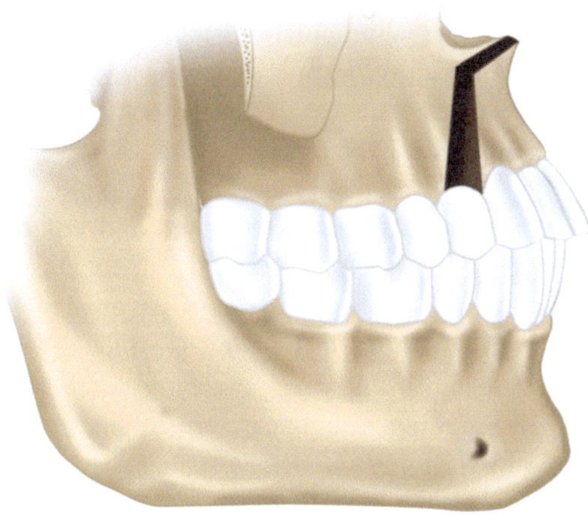

Fig. 12.3 Anterior segmental osteotomy performed for anterior movement of the maxilla. The most commonly performed anterior segmental osteotomy is named "Wassmund" segmental

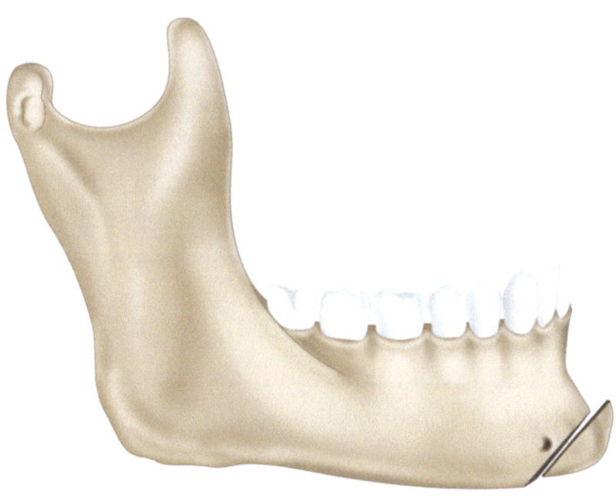

Fig. 12.4 Mandibular genioplasty. Surgery performed on the symphysis to advance, elongate, or reduce the chin projection in the face. Surgical cuts are usually done below the mental foramen to avoid any injury to the nerve

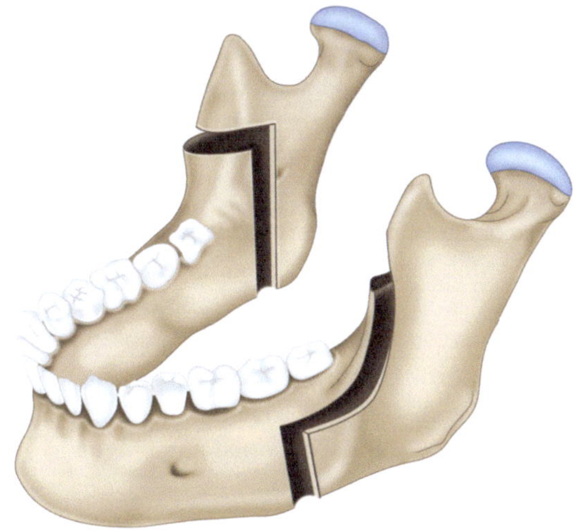

Fig. 12.5 Bilateral sagittal split osteotomy. The bilateral sagittal split osteotomy (BSSO) includes surgical cuts within the thickness of the ramus toward the mandibular corpus. It is commonly used in to advance or set back the mandible

on the effects of orthognathic surgery on voice are not as numerous despite the well-known impact of these surgeries on vocal tract anatomy. The phonatory changes most discussed commonly relate to nasality and velopharyngeal function. The results of these studies vary with the premorbid condition of the study group and the type of surgery performed. In 1984, Dalston and Vig investigated the impact of orthognathic surgery on nasality, nasal-oral acoustic coupling, and nasal resistance in 40 adult females who had their voices rated by three experienced speech-language pathologists before and after surgery. The results showed that nasal resistance and nasal-oral acoustic coupling differed significantly postoperatively [24]. In 1985, Bowers et al. investigated the effect of orthognathic surgery on voice by analyzing the formant frequencies for vowels /e/, /α/, and /u/ before and after surgery. The study included three patients with class II Division I malocclusion who underwent mandibular advancement with or without posterior maxillary impaction, and two patients with class III malocclusion who underwent mandibular setback with or without maxillary advancement or impaction. There was a significant shift in F2/e/, and non-significant shift in F2/α/ and F2/u/ following surgery. Notably, the postoperative changes in F2 for the aforementioned vowels were not appreciated perceptually, suggesting that a compensatory articulatory behavior had masked the effect of surgery on voice [25]. In 1986, Ruscello et al. studied the speech characteristics of 20 patients with different skeletal anomalies before and after orthognathic surgery. Using a self-report questionnaire, the authors showed no significant changes. Notably that preexisting articulatory errors were present in 60%

of the cases, but they had no adverse effect on speech intelligibility [26]. In 1989, Kummer et al. evaluated 16 patients who had setback of the mandible and advancement of the maxilla (Le Fort I) and noted postoperative changes in nasal resonance and/or nasal emission in two out of eight patients without cleft palate. Velopharyngeal dysfunction also was observed in nine patients in the study group [27]. In 1990, Vallino studied the effect of orthognathic surgery on voice and resonance over the course of 1 year in a group of 34 patients with severe skeletal malocclusions. Although the authors reported improvement in articulatory errors in the majority of cases, surgery had no detectable effect on voice and resonance [28]. Similarly, Wakumoto et al. in 1996 investigated the impact of osteotomy of the upper and lower jaw on speech and voice using electropalatography and acoustic analysis in three patients with mandibular prognathism and two patients with maxillary protrusion. The results indicated significant alteration in articulation that were sustained 6 months following surgery. In patients with mandibular prognathism who had undergone maxillary osteotomy, there was a shift in the concentration region in the spectral envelope from 5 kHz to 7 kHz. Also, patients with maxillary protrusion who had undergone mandibular osteotomy had a shift in the region of concentration on spectral analysis from 8.5 kHz to 7 kHz [29]. In 2002, Lee et al. investigated the effect of various types of maxillary and mandibular osteotomies on the production of /s/ using perceptual judgment and acoustic analysis in nine patients with class III malocclusion. The results indicated a significant change in noise bandwidth 3 months postoperatively and spectral peak II 1 year after surgery. The mean value of spectral peak I decreased at 3 months and increased approximately 12 months after surgery. Similarly, the mean value of spectral peak II decreased after surgery in the first 3 months but increased again to its presurgical value at 12 months [30]. In 2002, Ward et al. investigated the impact of orthognathic reconstruction on resonance and articulation in two patients with class III malocclusion and three patients with class II division 1 malocclusion, and reported worsening in nasality in three of the five patients. However, there was improvement in articulation, namely, precision and intelligibility, in one patient. The improvement was attributed to enhancement in interlabial pressure [31]. In 2006, Van Lierde et al. studied the impact of bilateral sagittal split osteotomy of the mandible on speech and voice in eight patients with class II malocclusion. Nasalance was assessed using a nasometer and the mirror-fogging test, whereas voice quality was assessed using the perceptual evaluation, namely, grading, roughness, breathiness, asthenia, and straining (GRBAS) scale [32] and the dysphonia severity index. The authors reported no statistically significant difference in any of the nasalance and/or voice parameters comparing before and after treatment. They concluded that bilateral sagittal split osteotomy has no effect on voice. Notably, patients with class II malocclusion had three articulatory disorders pre- and post-surgery, namely, the incorrect production of the trill sound /s/ and /r/ and devoicing of the sound /z/ [33]. In 2006, Chanchareonsook et al. reviewed the literature on the impact of orthognathic surgery and distraction osteogenesis on speech and on velopharyngeal function. The review included 747 cases with craniofacial abnormalities who underwent maxillary advancement. The results failed to draw a consensus on the effect of surgery, with no difference between the two aforementioned surgical techniques, namely, conventional osteotomy vs. distraction, being described. That review did not include any randomized, controlled trial comparing conventional osteotomy with distraction osteogenesis [34]. In 2006, Niemi et al. studied the impact of orthognathic surgery on speech in five patients with dentofacial anomalies and reported short-term changes in the fundamental frequency (F0) in four patients, and long-term changes in only one patient. Moreover, there were changes in vocal tract resonances (F1, F2) in three patients [35]. In 2006, Chanchareonsook et al. investigated velopharyngeal function and speech outcome in 22 patients with maxillary hypoplasia who underwent Le Fort I osteotomy with immediate or gradual distraction of the maxilla. Velopharyngeal insufficiency improved in one third of the cases, remained the same in one third, and deteriorated in one third. With respect to nasal emission and resonance, the majority had no change postoperatively (17 out of 22, and 18 out of 22, respectively) [36]. In 2007, Hassan et al. reviewed the literature on the effect of orthognathic surgery on speech and reported improvement in speech articulation in 8 of the 13 studies included in the review [37]. In 2008, Pereira et al. assessed the impact of mid-face advancement by osteotomy ($n = 8$) on nasality and velopharyngeal function using nasopharyngeal endoscopy and video-fluoroscopy. The authors found mild increase in speech articulation (improvement in mean percentage of consonants correct from 71.6% to 75.5%), and an increase in the mean nasalance score from 16.25% to 19.75% postoperatively. None of the patients was rated as hypernasal following surgery [38]. In 2009, Sari and Kiliç studied the impact of surgical rapid maxillary expansion on vowels in a group of 12 patients with constricted (narrow) maxilla. The authors reported a decrease in F2/i/ and F2/oe/ attributed to alteration in oral cavity volume and configuration [39]. In 2009, Jorge et al. reported change in the F0 in one patient who underwent orthognathic surgery. The authors emphasized on the role of orofacial structures in vocal tract anatomy, and attributed the increase in F0 to change in the position of the hyoid bone [40]. In 2011, McComb et al. investigated the predictors of velopharyngeal insufficiency (VPI) in patients with maxillary intrusion undergoing Le Fort I osteotomy. The authors reported an association between the length of the soft palate and VPI, and they recommended diligent preoperative assessment using cephalometric radiographs and nasopharyngeal endoscopic examination [41]. In 2012, Bordbar et al. investigated the impact of mid-face advancement in 15 patients with syndromic craniofacial deformities. The authors reported worsening in velopharyngeal function in 46.7% of cases and improvement in hyponasality score in 66.7% of cases [42]. Only 4 out of the 15 patients had Le Fort III surgery with bone grafting. In 2013, Mishima et al. investigated the impact of mandibular setback on F0 and the first two formants and reported significant changes in mean first (mLE1s) for /u/ in males and for /o/ in females. Moreover, there was a decrease in F2s for /u/ and /i/ in males. The study was conducted on 16 patients with class III malocclusion who underwent bilateral sagittal split ramus osteotomy [43]. In 2015, Knez Ambrožič et al. investigated the effect of jaw surgery on speech and voice in 15 patients diagnosed with skeletal anterior open bite. The correction included the upper and lower jaw in 13 of the 15 cases. The voice outcome measures included F0, perturbation parameters, and the first two formants F1 and F2 for the vowels /a/, /e/, /i/, /o/, and /u/. The results showed no significant difference in any of the parameters comparing before and after surgery [44].

In conclusion, surgery-induced alteration in the position of the upper and lower jaw does not always lead to detectable change in voice quality. The disparity in the results is attributed to the disparity in the premorbid condition of the patient, the type of surgery performed, and the mode of assessment. When present, voice changes relate mainly to nasality and to the first two formant frequencies. Compensatory phonatory and articulatory behavior may mask voice changes that are not commonly perceived by non-professional listeners.

How Orthognathic Surgery Can Affect Voice?

It is known that vocal tract configuration is determined by the structural boundaries of the laryngopharyngeal complex and by the articulatory behavior of the speaker. In the lack of articulatory compensation, the anatomic boundaries of the upper airway space remain primarily responsible for the acoustic differences across speakers. In this section, the authors review the mechanisms by which orthognathic surgery can affect voice. These include the impact of surgery on the shape of the upper airway space, position of the hyoid bone, nasal cavity, and velopharyngeal function.

Impact of Orthognathic Surgery on the Shape of the Upper Airway Space

There are numerous studies in the literature on the impact of orthognathic surgery on the length, width, and volume of the upper airway [45–56]. Many of these studies include subjects with obstructive sleep apnea (OSA). In 1994, Enacar et al. reported a decrease in hypopharyngeal airway space following mandibular setback surgery. The study was conducted on 15 patients with mandibular prognathism who were examined using lateral cephalometric imaging before and after surgery [46]. Similarly, in 2005, Kawakami et al. showed a significant decrease in the pharyngeal airway with narrowing of the retro-lingual space 1 year following mandibular setback surgery. The investigation included 30 patients who were evaluated with digital lateral cephalograms [47]. In 2010, Hwang et al. studied the impact of mandibular setback via vertical ramus osteotomy, with or without maxillary impaction, and reported significant narrowing of the pharyngeal airway postoperatively. The study group included 60 patients with skeletal class III malocclusion who were examined periodically for up to 1 year following surgery [48]. In 2011, Susarla et al. showed that advancement of the maxilla and mandible by an average of 9.8 and 10.8 mm, respectively, results in a decrease in the upper airway length by around 8.8 mm. The study was conducted on 23 adults who underwent maxilla-mandibular advancement for the treatment of OSA, and the upper airway length was measured as the long axis distance between the horizontal plane at the most superior aspect of the hyoid bone and a horizontal plane at the level of the posterior hard palate. The authors attributed the decrease in upper airway length to the possible increase in the suprahyoid muscles' tension secondary to advancement of the lower jaw [49]. In 2012, Sahoo et al. investigated the extent of airway space increase in 20 class II skeletal malocclusion patients who had bilateral sagittal split ramus osteotomy in addition to orthodontic treatment. The authors reported a ratio of 1:0.35 for mandibular advancement/ increase in posterior airway space, and a ratio of 1:0.34 for mandibular advancement/increase in superior airway space [50]. Similarly, in 2013, Raffaini and Pisani reported an increase in pharyngeal airway space area and volume following maxilla-mandibular advancement surgery by 34% and 56%, respectively. All patients were assessed using cone-beam computed tomography (CBCT) before and after surgery [51]. These results supported the systemic review of Hsieh et al. on the effects of maxillomandibular advancement on the upper airway, which also asserted enlargement in both the anteroposterior and lateral dimensions [52]. In 2014, the same authors investigated 16 patients who underwent maxillomandibular advancement for OSA and described a decrease in the length of the upper airway by 3.1 mm, though there was a significant increase in its volume. The authors attributed the decrease in upper airway length to the increased tension in the suprahyoid muscles secondary to anterior displacement of the hyoid bone. The length of the upper airway was computed using three-dimensional model by adding the sum of the thickness of all the axial slices extending from the velopharynx, oropharynx, to hypopharynx [53]. Similarly, Kim et al. in 2013 investigated the impact of bi-maxillary surgery and mandibular setback on the upper airway volume in patients with mandibular prognathism and reported significant decrease up to 6 months after surgery. The study was performed on 25 skeletal class III subjects who were investigated using cone-beam computed tomography before surgery and 2 and 6 months after [45]. In 2015, de Souza Miranda et al. assessed the impact of median mandibular advancement and counterclockwise rotation of the maxilla-mandibular complex in 23 class II patients and showed an increase in the superior airway space volume and surface area by 10.118 mm^3 and 178 mm^2, respectively [54]. Liu et al. evaluated the dimensions of the upper airway space in 20 patients with maxillary transverse deficiency who had surgically assisted rapid palatal expansion with surgically facilitated orthodontic therapy. The authors showed an increase in both volume and minimum cross-sectional area of the upper airway space [55]. In 2019, Wiedemeyer et al. developed a mathematical model to predict changes in the posterior pharyngeal airway space (PAS) following mandibular advancement. Using two-dimensional lateral cephalographic radiographs on 49 patients with class II malocclusion, the authors showed a strong association between the extent of mandibular advancement and the posterior airway dimensions [56]. That same year, de Souza Pinto et al. evaluated changes in the pharyngeal airspace following orthognathic surgery in 43 skeletal class III patients and 36 skeletal class II patients. The authors showed that both the class II group who underwent maxilla-mandibular advancement and the class III group who underwent maxillary osteotomy and mandibular setback had an increase in the pharyngeal airway space (PAS). In class II patients, the increase in PAS volume and area was significant and was attributed mainly to change in position of the hyoid bone, whereas in class III patients, the increase in PAS area was not significant [57].

In addition to the above reports asserting the impact of orthognathic surgery on the pharyngeal airway space, numerous authors went further to analyze the topographic changes in pharyngeal airway dimensions (nasopharyngeal vs. oropharyngeal vs. hypopharyngeal). In 2011, Jakobsone et al. investigated the impact of maxillary advancement/impaction on the upper airway in 76 patients with class III malocclusion and reported long-lasting widening by 13–21% at the nasopharyngeal level. The increase in airspace noted at the nasopharynx compensated partially for the decrease in the oropharyngeal space following mandibular setback [58]. In 2013, Faria et al. showed that a 1 mm maxilla-mandibular advancement results in 0.76 mm and 1.2 mm increase in the retro-palatal and retro-lingual space, respectively. The study was conducted on 19 patients with obstructive sleep apnea who were evaluated in a standard fashion using cephalometry [59]. Also in 2013, Kochel et al. investigated the effect of mandibular advancement on the posterior airway space in 102 patients with class II dysagnathia. Using CBCT, the authors noted enlargement in the posterior airway space, mostly in the lower one third (45.6%). Furthermore, they stressed on the widening effect of these types of surgery at the narrowest portions of the pharynx [60]. Similarly, Li et al. in 2014 reported a significant decrease in the retro-palatal cross-sectional area and oropharyngeal space volume following maxillary advancement and bilateral sagittal split ramus osteotomy in 29 skeletal class III female patients with mandibular prognathism and maxillary hypoplasia. Moreover, there was a significant decrease postoperatively in the volume of the oropharynx and nasopharynx summed together. The authors attributed this decrease to change in the position of the hyoid bone (backward movement and decrease in the horizontal position) which correlated significantly with changes in oropharyngeal space [61]. In 2016, Kochar et al. quantified the enlargement in pharyngeal airway space using three-dimensional computed tomography in 16 patients with class II malocclusion who had bilateral sagittal split osteotomy. The authors demonstrated that the greatest increase, in both cross-sectional area and volume, was at the oropharynx, followed by the hypopharynx [62]. In 2019, Faur et al. evaluated the effect of orthognathic surgery on the rhino-sinusal airway space in 16 patients who underwent Le Fort I osteotomy. Using individual CBCT examination, the authors demonstrated a significant increase postoperatively in the nasal fossa volume by 3.07 cm^3in patients with class III malocclusion, and a significant decrease in patients with class II malocclusion. Moreover, there was a significant decrease in the rhino-sinus airway space in both subgroups of patients [63]. In 2019, Moscarino et al. also showed significant alterations in nasopharyngeal and oropharyngeal space following orthognathic surgery in patients with moderate skeletal malocclusion type II [64]. In 2019, Hwang et al. investigated the effect of maxillary protraction at various levels of the pharyngeal airway in patients with skeletal class III malocclusion and reported an increase in both the nasopharyngeal and superior oropharyngeal dimensions, but no significant changes were noted in the low oropharyngeal dimensions [65].

The durability of orthognathic surgery-induced volumetric changes in the airway also has been discussed extensively in the literature, with no clear consensus. In 2017, Jiang et al. discussed the long-term effect of orthognathic surgery on the pharyngeal airway space in patients with class II malocclusion. Using Dolphin imaging software, the authors showed a stable increase in the oropharyngeal and hypopharyngeal cross-sectional area in 25 patients who underwent mandibular advancement. The follow-up was for up to 2 years following surgery [66]. Similarly, in 2018 Ristow et al. examined the short-term and long-term effects of mandibular advancement in patients with class II malocclusion. Using CBCT, the authors showed that enlargement in the pharyngeal airway space was sustained even 1 year after surgery. The long-term gain in the airway was attributed to "long-term adaptation" as described by the authors [67]. However, Kochar et al. in 2019 investigated the sustainability of the changes in the pharyngeal airway following bilateral sagittal split osteotomy in patients with class II malocclusion, and showed relapse after 1 year in both minimum and mean cross-sectional area by 7.9% and 12.6%, respectively. The study was conducted on 16 patients using acoustic pharyngometry [68].

In summary, the above studies lead us to conclude that orthognathic surgery results in changes in upper airway dimensions. These include minimal cross-sectional area, width, length and volume. Maxillo-mandibular advancement usually is associated with enlargement of the airway space, whereas mandibular setback surgery usually is associated with narrowing of the airway space. Notably, surgery-induced anatomical changes may regress with time. As the upper airway space delineates the morphology of the vocal tract and plays an important role in wind instrument performance, patients undergoing orthognathic surgery need to be aware of possible alteration in their voice quality and possibly their instrumental tone quality. This is particularly important for professional voice users and wind instrument players.

Impact of Orthognathic Surgery on the Position of the Hyoid Bone and Tongue

Surgery-induced changes in the upper airway space are usually associated with change in the position of the hyoid bone. The displacement of the hyoid bone varies with the type of surgery performed, the site of surgery, and its extent. In the study by Enacar et al. on the effect of mandibular setback on hypopharyngeal airway space, the authors demonstrated an association between the decrease in hypopharyngeal airway space and the downward movement of the hyoid bone and base of tongue [46]. In 2010, Marşan et al. reported an association between mandibular setback (mean of 5.6 ± 0.8 mm) and posteroinferior positioning of the hyoid bone. The study was conducted on 42 class III malocclusion patients who were evaluated using lateral cephalograms [69]. Similarly, Kitahara et al. investigated the impact of two types of mandibular setback surgery on the position of the hyoid bone in 46 women with class III malocclusion. The authors demonstrated a cephalic and frontal movement of the hyoid bone 2 years following bilateral sagittal split ramus osteotomy, and a backward movement following bilateral intraoral vertical ramus osteotomy [70]. In the investigation by Sahoo et al., the increase in the superior and posterior airway space following mandibular advancement was accompanied by a 2.1 ± 2.8 mm anterior and superior movement of the hyoid bone [50]. Similarly, in the study by Faria et al., the cephalometric changes in the pharynx following maxilla-mandibular advancement were attributed partially to the cranio-caudal repositioning of the hyoid bone [59]. In keeping with the above, both investigations by Hsieh et al. concurred the strong link between the changes in the airway measures and elevation or anterior displacement of the hyoid bone [52, 53]. Nevertheless, it is important to note that alteration in the position of the hyoid bone is not always sustainable. Kawakami et al. demonstrated that the downward movement of the hyoid bone secondary to mandibular setback was transient, as the hyoid bone resumed its initial position on late follow-up [47]. Similarly, Hwang et al., in their investigation on the impact of mandibular setback on the pharyngeal space reported inferior and posterior movement of the hyoid bone, which they also found to have relapsed on long-term follow-up [48].

Given the strategic location of the hyoid bone and its important role in modulating the configuration and length of the vocal tract, change in its position, whether transient or permanent, undoubtedly affect the acoustic properties of voice [71]. Macari et al. studied the correlation between formant frequencies and the position of the hyoid bone, and demonstrated a moderate negative correlation between the third and fourth formant of the vowel /α/, and two measurements of the vertical position of the hyoid bone: the distance between the hyoid bone and sella-turcica (H-S), and the distance between the hyoid bone and most anterior point of the third cervical vertebra (H-C3). There was also a negative correlation between the second formant and H-S. Similarly, there was a moderate negative correlation between the third and fourth formants for the vowel /i/ and H-C3. The authors concluded that F4 among the first four formants correlated most with the cephalo-caudal position of the hyoid bone (Fig. 12.6) [72]. Hence, patients undergoing mandibular orthognathic surgery need to be aware of possible alterations in voice quality.

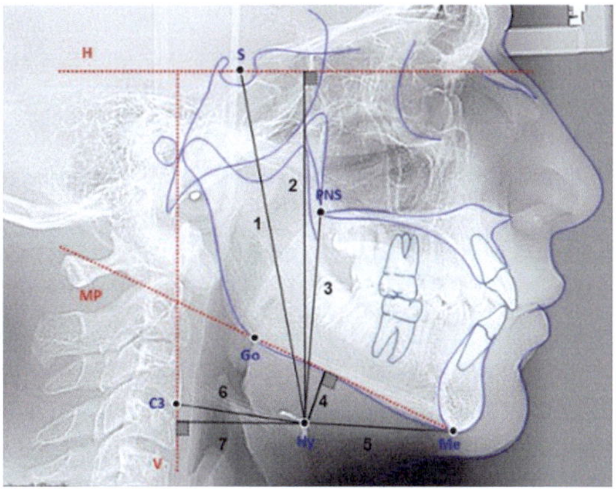

Fig. 12.6 A digitized lateral cephalometric radiograph evaluating hyoid bone position including: (**a**) – Landmarks: Hy: most anterior point of the hyoid; S: midpoint of the sella tursica; posterior nasal spine (PNS): the spine-like projection from the posterosuperior midline of the horizontal plate of the palatine bone; C3: third cervical vertebra; gonion (Go): angle of the mandible (between rhamus and corpus); menton (Me): the most inferior point on the chin; MP: mandibular plane; V: vertebra; H-Horizontal plane; V-Vertical plane (**b**) – Linear measurements: H-S: linear vertical distance from H to S; H-PNS: linear vertical distance from H to PNS; H-C3: linear measure from H to the most anterior point of C3; H-MP: linear vertical distance from H to MP

Impact of Orthognathic Surgery on the Velopharyngeal Function

The potential for improvement or worsening of velopharyngeal function following orthognathic surgery is obvious given the known impact of orthognatic surgery on the nasopharyngeal and oropharyngeal dimensions. Review of the literature shows numerous reports with various results depending on the preoperative velopharyngeal function and the type of surgery performed (conventional Le Fort osteotomies, maxillary advancement, anterior segmental maxillary distraction), and the mode of assessment (perceptual evaluation, nasopharyngoscopy, radiologic imaging, and or aerodynamic measurements). In 2012, Bordbar et al. reported deterioration in velopharyngeal function in syndromic craniofacial patients following mid-face advancement using various surgical techniques, including Le Fort III osteotomies and distraction osteogenesis [42]. The assessment of resonance and articulation was perceptual using GOS.SP.ASS.98 [73]. In the study by Faria et al. published in 2013, the authors showed that a 1 mm advancement of the maxilla results in 0.76 mm increase in the retropalatal space. The study was conducted on 19 patients using cephalometric analysis [59]. In 2013, Kim et al. investigated the impact of bimaxillary surgery on upper airway volume in patients with mandibular prognathism and reported rotation in the palatal plane by 2.04 ± 2.28 degrees with impaction of the maxilla posteriorly. There was also a significant correlation between the position of the palate and the postoperative change in airway volume [45]. Similarly, Karabekmez et al. in 2015 studied changes in velopharyngeal space dimensions following maxillary advancement and showed a significant impact in patients who underwent Le Fort I. There was an increase in velopharyngeal space, specifically the distance between the posterior pharyngeal wall and the posterior nasal spine, and the distance between the posterior pharyngeal wall and the uvula. Although the authors commented on the adverse effect of maxillary surgery on velopharyngeal function, it is important to note that 9 out of the 14 subjects in the study group had cleft lip palate, a premorbid condition known to be associated with VPI [74]. In 2018, Impieri et al. also assessed velopharyngeal dysfunction using cephalometric images in 47 patients who had advancement of the maxilla with or without mandibular setback. The results showed worsening of hypernasality only in those who underwent maxillary advancement. The authors emphasized the adverse effect of this type of orthognathic surgery on velopharyngeal function [75].

In summary, the above studies confirm the effect of orthognathic surgery on velopharyngeal function. As the velopharynx plays a crucial role in adjusting voice resonance, affected patients may have either improvement or worsening of their nasal emission. The presence of preoperative velopharyngeal dysfunction predisposes to deterioration in nasality following maxillary advancement surgery, whereas preoperative hyponasality suggests potential for improvement in nasality following maxillary advancement surgery. Good velopharyngeal function is important for phonation and especially for wind instrumentalists for whom VPI can be career-ending.

Impact of Surgery on the Nasal Cavity

The effect of orthognathic surgery on nasal volume, airflow, and resistance has been investigated by numerous authors [76]. The results vary with the type of skeletal deformity and procedure performed. As early as 1984, Guenthner et al. investigated the impact of maxillary superior movement via Le Fort I osteotomy on nasal airway resistance in 11 patients and reported improvement in nasal resistance. This was attributed to the increase in alar width with subsequent increase in nasal valve angle [77]. Twenty-five years later, Haarmann et al. studied the effect of Le Fort I osteotomy on nasal function and anatomy and reported an increase in the intranasal cross-sectional area with improvement in nasal breathing. Various surgical techniques ranging form sagittal maxillary movement to maxillary impaction were used, in addition to rhinosurgery to alleviate difficulties in nasal breathing when present [78]. In 2010, Seeberger et al. demonstrated an increase in nasal volume in all of 13 patients who underwent surgically assisted rapid palatal expansion. The authors advocated for the added value of this procedure in terms of nasal airway enhancement [79]. Similarly, in 2011 Magnusson et al. investigated the effect of surgically assisted rapid maxillary expansion on nasal cavity and resistance and reported only a transient increase in minimal cross-sectional area and a decrease in nasal resistance (at the 3 months). The study was conducted on 39 patients for whom nasal airway resistance was assessed subjectively using a questionnaire before surgery, 3 months, and 18 months after surgery [80]. In 2012, Pourdanesh et al. evaluated the nasal airway in 25 patients who underwent maxillary impaction and/or advancement. Using rhinomanometry, the results showed a significant decrease in nasal airway resistance commensurate with an increase in nasal airflow by 137 ml/s [81]. In 2015, Gokce et al. investigated the volumetric changes in the nasal cavity volume in 11 patients with skeletal class III anomalies who underwent Le Fort I maxillary distraction osteogenesis. Using a three-dimensional simulation program, the authors demonstrated a significant increase which reflected clinical improvement in sleep quality [82]. In 2015, Marşan et al. investigated the impact of Le Fort I maxillary osteotomy on facial soft tissue in relation to facial bony structures and reported significant changes in both the anteroposterior and superoinferior position of point A, the deepest point on the premaxilla between anterior nasal spine and dental alveolus. The study was performed on 20 patients with class III skeletal deformity and retrognathic maxilla who were evaluated operatively and 1.2–2 years following surgery [83]. In 2016, Kita et al. evaluated the effect of bone trimming at the pyriform aperture inferior edge on nasal breathing in patients undergoing maxillary impaction. The authors advocated this surgical technique which resulted in a decrease in the postoperative pressure effort and an increase in the cross-sectional area of both nasal cavities. Pressure effort was defined as the product of volume flow rate and airway resistance [84]. In 2018, Ha and Han investigated the impact of maxillary impaction with and without advancement on the nasal cavity in 32 patients and reported a decrease in the nasal cavity. Moreover, the volume change ratio (%) and the impaction ratio measured as the impaction volume in relation to the nasal cavity vertical length correlated positively [85]. Zaoui et al. studied the impact of Le Fort I osteotomy on nasal function in 9 patients with skeletal class III malformation and one with skeletal class I occlusion. Using rhinomanometric analysis, the authors demonstrated a significant increase in nasal airway space but no significant changes in relation to flow rates [86].

The nasal septum also is in jeopardy in patients undergoing orthognathic surgery. In 2018, Baeg et al. assessed the effect of Le Fort I osteotomy on the nasal septum and maxillary sinus mucosal lining and reported a decrease in the septal angle postoperatively. The non-significant change in nasal septum was accompanied by a decrease in the maxillary sinus total volume [87]. Atakan et al. studied the impact of Le Fort I advancement and impaction in combination with bilateral sagittal split osteotomy on the nasal cavity in 40 patients. Using cephalometric radiographs, the authors showed a decrease in the heights of the nasal cavities and an increase in nasal cavity width. There was no significant change in nasal septal deviation [88]. Moroi et al. also reported similar results in their study on 40 patients who underwent Le Fort I osteotomy [89]. The impact of orthognathic surgery on the nasal septum ought to be considered in the interpretation of nasal symptoms postoperatively, although the effect is not that significant clinically.

In summary, orthognathic surgery has a significant impact on the nasal cavity and passages. Given the importance of nasal breathing in phonation, and especially double reed instrument performance, enlargement of the nasal width and cavities may have a favorable effect on voice and instrument playing. Moreover, the essential role of nasal breathing for air humidification and filtering cannot be overemphasized. Mouth breathing has been proven to increase the phonatory threshold pressure and precipitate voice fatigue [90, 91].

Effect of Orthognathic Surgery on Wind Instrument Performance

Similar to orthodontic treatment, orthognathic surgery can affect the performance of wind instrumentalists by altering skeletal and non-skeletal dentofacial structures. Surgery-induced changes in occlusion can affect the position of the musical instrument's mouthpiece and can interfere with embouchure. The musician's bite, lip pressure, as well as the use of orofacial muscles need to be adjusted following any change in the dental configuration and/or anatomy of the upper and lower jaw. A saxophone player, for instance, with class III malocclusion who undergoes mandibular setback will lose the customary support of the lower jaw while playing. Similarly, a clarinet player who undergoes mandibular advancement may have to change the type of musical instrument. Hence, musicians will need to reconfigure their embouchure in order to adapt efficiently to the new surgically induced configuration of the orofacial complex. It is important to note that the aforementioned remains speculative, and there are no studies in the literature to support these speculations. The data available have been shared anecdotally among musicians and voice teachers with no clear guidelines or consensus. Hence, wind instrument players need to be assessed individually following surgery and the decision to keep or change the type of instrument remains very personal and contingent on the musician preference and his/her adaptability to the postsurgical results. This field remains embryonic and warrants future investigation.

On another front, changes in the morphology of the palate and maxillary arch can also affect the quality of the musical tone, as discussed in Chap. 11. The association between palatal dome and height and low formant frequencies has been described thoroughly in the literature with emphasis on variations in palatal morphology in singers with different voice classification [92, 93]. The maxillary arch and its width also are linked to the quality of sound in wind instrumentalists [94, 95]. A wider arch is considered a favorable anatomic feature, whereas a narrow maxillary arch with crowding of dentition is unfavorable. Alteration in the width and morphology of the maxilla in patients undergoing maxillary advancement, maxillary distraction, or impaction, may lead to changes in the acoustic properties of the musical sound. Similarly, the role of the vocal tract in modulating the music tone in wind instrumentalists has been documented in the literature [96]. Based on the review presented in the previous section on the impact of orthognathic surgery on upper airway space length and width, it is self-evident that patients who play wind instruments may experience change in musical sound following surgery. Shortening in vocal tract length in patients who undergo mandibular setback may result in elevation in formant frequencies, whereas mandibular advancement surgery may result in elongation of the vocal tract with subsequent lowering of the formant frequencies. Along the same line of thinking, surgery-induced changes in the width and cross-sectional area of the pharyngeal cavity may result in changes in the position and dispersion of the vocal tract formants. Wind instrumentalists need to be alerted that orthognathic surgery for aesthetic or functional reason may deter their musical performance. Patient's counselling and the need for rehabilitation must be included in the management strategy.

References

1. Brosch S, Mathes C, Pirsig W, Verse T. Uvulopalatopharyngoplasty changes in fundamental frequency of the voice: a prospective study. J Laryngol Otol. 2000;114(2):113–8.
2. Coleman RF, Sly DE. Preoperative and postoperative voice analysis of uvulopalatopharyngoplasty patients. Arch Otolaryngol Head Neck Surg. 1991;117(12):1345–9.
3. Murry T, Bone RC. Acoustic characteristics of speech following uvulopalatopharyngoplasty. Laryngoscope. 1989;99(12):1217–9.
4. Nakai K, Sakakura A, Takahashi H, Sadaoka T, Kakitsuba N. Articulation after uvulopalatopharyngoplasty. Eur Arch Otorhinolaryngol. 1996;253:417–20.
5. Rihkanen H, Soini I. Changes in voice characteristics after uvulopalatopharyngoplasty. Eur Arch Otorhinolaryngol. 1992;249(6):322–4.
6. Soldatova L, Mirza N. Long-term voice and swallowing outcomes for oral and oropharyngeal cancer following primary or adjuvant chemoradiation. Ann Otol Rhinol Laryngol. 2019;128(9):802–10.
7. Behrman A, Shikowitz MJ, Dailey S. The effect of upper airway surgery on voice. Otolaryngol Head Neck Surg. 2002;127(1):36–42.
8. Lin P, Gould WJ, Fukazawa T, El-Assuooty A. Acoustic analysis of voice in tonsillectomy. J Voice. 1989;3(1):81–6.
9. Hori Y, Koike Y, Ohyama G, Otsu SY, Abe K. Effects of tonsillectomy on articulation. Acta Otolaryngol Suppl. 1996;523:248–51.
10. Saida H, Hirose H. Acoustic changes in voice after tonsillectomy. Acta Otolaryngol Suppl. 1996;523:239–41.
11. Lundeborg I, Hultcrantz E, Ericsson E, McAllister A. Acoustic and perceptual aspects of vocal function in children with adenotonsillar hypertrophy—effects of surgery. J Voice. 2012;26(4):480–7.
12. Heffernan CB, Rafferty MA. Effect of tonsillectomy on the adult voice. J Voice. 2011;25(4):e207–10.
13. Steinhäuser EW. Historical development of orthognathic surgery. J Craniomaxillofac Surg. 1996;24(4):195–204.
14. Ow A, Cheung LK. Skeletal stability and complications of bilateral sagittal split osteotomies and mandibular distraction osteogenesis: an evidence-based review. J Oral Maxillofac Surg. 2009;67(11):2344–53.
15. Ruiz LP, Lara JC. Facial nerve palsy following bilateral sagittal split ramus osteotomy for setback of the mandible. Int J Oral Maxillofac Surg. 2011;40(8):884–6.
16. Chrcanovic BR, Custódio AL. Optic, oculomotor, abducens, and facial nerve palsies after combined maxillary and mandibular osteotomy: case report. J Oral Maxillofac Surg. 2011;69(6):e234–41.
17. Rai KK, Shivakumar HR, Sonar MD. Transient facial nerve palsy following bilateral sagittal split ramus osteotomy for setback of the mandible: a review of

incidence and management. J Oral Maxillofac Surg. 2008;66(2):373–8.
18. Teerijoki-Oksa T, Jääskeläinen SK, Soukka T, Virtanen A, Forssell H. Subjective sensory symptoms associated with axonal and demyelinating nerve injuries after mandibular sagittal split osteotomy. J Oral Maxillofac Surg. 2011;69(6):e208–13.
19. Jędrzejewski M, Smektała T, Sporniak-Tutak K, Olszewski R. Preoperative, intraoperative, and postoperative complications in orthognathic surgery: a systematic review. Clin Oral Investig. 2015;19(5):969–77.
20. Alpha C, O'Ryan F, da Silva A, Poor D. The incidence of postoperative wound healing problems following sagittal ramus osteotomies stabilized with miniplates and monocortical screws. J Oral Maxillofac Surg. 2006;64(4):659–68.
21. Wong LL, Samman N, Whitehill TL. Are hearing and middle ear statuses at risk in Chinese patients undergoing orthognathic surgery? Clin Otolaryngol Allied Sci. 2002;27(6):480–4.
22. Politis C. Life-threatening haemorrhage after 750 Le Fort I osteotomies and 376 SARPE procedures. Int J Oral Maxillofac Surg. 2012;41(6):702–8.
23. Pereira-Filho VA, Gabrielli MF, Gabrielli MA, et al. Incidence of maxillary sinusitis following Le Fort I osteotomy: clinical, radiographic, and endoscopic study. J Oral Maxillofac Surg. 2011;69(2):346–51.
24. Dalston RM, Vig PS. Effects of orthognathic surgery on speech: a prospective study. Am J Orthod. 1984;86(4):291–8.
25. Bowers J, Tobey EA, Shaye R. An acoustic-speech study of patients who received orthognathic surgery. Am J Orthod. 1985;88(5):373–9.
26. Ruscello DM, Tekieli ME, Jakomis T, Cook L, Van Sickels JE. The effects of orthognathic surgery on speech production. Am J Orthod. 1986;89(3):237–41.
27. Kummer AW, Strife JL, Grau WH, Creaghead NA, Lee L. The effects of Le Fort I osteotomy with maxillary movement on articulation, resonance, and velopharyngeal function. Cleft Palate J. 1989;26(3):193–9.
28. Vallino LD. Speech, velopharyngeal function, and hearing before and after orthognathic surgery. J Oral Maxillofac Surg. 1990;48(12):1274–81.
29. Wakumoto M, Isaacson KG, Friel S, et al. Preliminary study of articulatory reorganisation of fricative consonants following osteotomy. Folia Phoniatr Logop. 1996;48(6):275–89.
30. Lee AS, Whitehill TL, Ciocca V, Samman N. Acoustic and perceptual analysis of the sibilant sound/s/before and after orthognathic surgery. J Oral Maxillofac Surg. 2002;60(4):364–72.
31. Ward EC, McAuliffe M, Holmes SK, Lynham A, Monsour F. Impact of malocclusion and orthognathic reconstruction surgery on resonance and articulatory function: an examination of variability in five cases. Br J Oral Maxillofac Surg. 2002;40(5):410–7.
32. Hirano M. Psycho-acoustic evaluation of voice: GRBAS Scale for evaluating the hoarse voice. In: Clinical examination of voice. New York: Springer-Verlag; 1981. p. 81–4.
33. Van Lierde KM, Schepers S, Timmermans LA, Verhoye I, Van Cauwenberge P. The impact of mandibular advancement on articulation, resonance and voice characteristics in Flemish speaking adults: a pilot study. Int J Oral Maxillofac Surg. 2006;35(2):137–44.
34. Chanchareonsook N, Samman N, Whitehill TL. The effect of cranio-maxillofacial osteotomies and distraction osteogenesis on speech and velopharyngeal status: a critical review. Cleft Palate Craniofac J. 2006;43(4):477–87.
35. Niemi M, Laaksonen JP, Peltomäki T, Kurimo J, Aaltonen O, Happonen RP. Acoustic comparison of vowel sounds produced before and after orthognathic surgery for mandibular advancement. J Oral Maxillofac Surg. 2006;64(6):910–6.
36. Chanchareonsook N, Whitehill TL, Samman N. Speech outcome and velopharyngeal function in cleft palate: comparison of Le Fort I maxillary osteotomy and distraction osteogenesis—early results. Cleft Palate Craniofac J. 2007;44(1):23–32.
37. Hassan T, Naini FB, Gill DS. The effects of orthognathic surgery on speech: a review. J Oral Maxillofac Surg. 2007;65(12):2536–43.
38. Pereira V, Sell D, Ponniah A, Evans R, Dunaway D. Midface osteotomy versus distraction: the effect on speech, nasality, and velopharyngeal function in craniofacial dysostosis. Cleft Palate Craniofac J. 2008;45(4):353–63.
39. Sari E, KiliÇ MA. The effects of surgical rapid maxillary expansion (SRME) on vowel formants. Clin Linguist Phon. 2009;23(6):393–403.
40. Jorge TM, Brasolotto AG, Gonçales ES, Nary Filho H, Berretin-Felix G. Influence of orthognathic surgery on voice fundamental frequency. J Craniofac Surg. 2009;20(1):161–4.
41. McComb RW, Marrinan EM, Nuss RC, Labrie RA, Mulliken JB, Padwa BL. Predictors of velopharyngeal insufficiency after Le Fort I maxillary advancement in patients with cleft palate. J Oral Maxillofac Surg. 2011;69(8):2226–32.
42. Bordbar P, Blumenow W, Duncan C, Richardson D. Resonance and speech articulation after midface advancement in craniofacial dysostosis. J Craniofac Surg. 2012;23(2):e100–3.
43. Mishima K, Moritani N, Nakano H, Matsushita A, Iida S, Ueyama Y. Voice characteristics before versus after mandibular setback surgery in patients with mandibular prognathism using nonlinear dynamics and conventional acoustic analyses. J Craniomaxillofac Surg. 2013;41(8):706–9.
44. Knez Ambrožič M, Hočevar Boltežar I, Ihan HN. Changes of some functional speech disorders after surgical correction of skeletal anterior open bite. Int J Rehabil Res. 2015;38(3):246–52.
45. Kim MA, Kim BR, Choi JY, Youn JK, Kim YJ, Park YH. Three-dimensional changes of the hyoid bone and airway volumes related to its relationship with horizontal anatomic planes after bimaxillary

surgery in skeletal Class III patients. Angle Orthod. 2013;83(4):623–9.
46. Enacar A, Aksoy AU, Sencift Y, Haydar B, Aras K. Changes in hypopharyngeal airway space and in tongue and hyoid bone positions following the surgical correction of mandibular prognathism. Int J Adult Orthodon Orthognath Surg. 1994;9(4):285–90.
47. Kawakami M, Yamamoto K, Fujimoto M, Ohgi K, Inoue M, Kirita T. Changes in tongue and hyoid positions, and posterior airway space following mandibular setback surgery. J Craniomaxillofac Surg. 2005;33(2):107–10.
48. Hwang S, Chung CJ, Choi YJ, Huh JK, Kim KH. Changes of hyoid, tongue and pharyngeal airway after mandibular setback surgery by intraoral vertical ramus osteotomy. Angle Orthod. 2010;80(2):302–8.
49. Susarla SM, Abramson ZR, Dodson TB, Kaban LB. Upper airway length decreases after maxillomandibular advancement in patients with obstructive sleep apnea. J Oral Maxillofac Surg. 2011;69(11):2872–8.
50. Sahoo NK, Jayan B, Ramakrishna N, Chopra SS, Kochar G. Evaluation of upper airway dimensional changes and hyoid position following mandibular advancement in patients with skeletal class II malocclusion. J Craniofac Surg. 2012;23(6):e623–7.
51. Raffaini M, Pisani C. Clinical and cone-beam computed tomography evaluation of the three-dimensional increase in pharyngeal airway space following maxillo-mandibular rotation-advancement for Class II-correction in patients without sleep apnoea (OSA). J Craniomaxillofac Surg. 2013;41(7):552–7.
52. Hsieh YJ, Liao YF. Effects of maxillomandibular advancement on the upper airway and surrounding structures in patients with obstructive sleep apnoea: a systematic review. Br J Oral Maxillofac Surg. 2013;51(8):834–40.
53. Hsieh YJ, Liao YF, Chen NH, Chen YR. Changes in the calibre of the upper airway and the surrounding structures after maxillomandibular advancement for obstructive sleep apnoea. Br J Oral Maxillofac Surg. 2014;52(5):445–51.
54. de Sousa MW, de Castro Rocha VÁ, dos Santos Marques KL, Neto AIT, do Prado CJ, Zanetta-Barbosa D. Three-dimensional evaluation of superior airway space after orthognathic surgery with counterclockwise rotation and advancement of the maxillomandibular complex in Class II patients. Oral Surg Oral Med Oral Pathol Oral Radiol. 2015;120(4):453–8.
55. Liu P, Jiao D, Wang X, Liu J, Martin D, Guo J. Changes in maxillary width and upper airway spaces in young adults after surgically assisted rapid palatal expansion with surgically facilitated orthodontic therapy. Oral Surg Oral Med Oral Pathol Oral Radiol. 2019;127(5):381–6.
56. Wiedemeyer V, Berger M, Martini M, Kramer FJ, Heim N. Predictability of pharyngeal airway space dimension changes after orthognathic surgery in class II patients: a mathematical approach. J Craniomaxillofac Surg. 2019;47(10):1504–9.
57. de Souza Pinto GN, Iwaki Filho L, dos Santos Previdelli IT, et al. Three-dimensional alterations in pharyngeal airspace, soft palate, and hyoid bone of class II and class III patients submitted to bimaxillary orthognathic surgery: a retrospective study. J Craniomaxillofac Surg. 2019;47(6):883–94.
58. Jakobsone G, Stenvik A, Espeland L. The effect of maxillary advancement and impaction on the upper airway after bimaxillary surgery to correct Class III malocclusion. Am J Orthod Dentofacial Orthop. 2011;139(4):e369–76.
59. Faria AC, Xavier SP, Silva SN Jr, Trawitzki LV, de Mello-Filho FV. Cephalometric analysis of modifications of the pharynx due to maxillo-mandibular advancement surgery in patients with obstructive sleep apnea. Int J Oral Maxillofac Surg. 2013;42(5):579–84.
60. Kochel J, Meyer-Marcotty P, Sickel F, Lindorf H, Stellzig-Eisenhauer A. Short-term pharyngeal airway changes after mandibular advancement surgery in adult Class II-Patients—a three-dimensional retrospective study. J Orofac Orthop. 2013;74(2):137–52.
61. Li YM, Liu JL, Zhao JL, Dai J, Wang L, Chen JW. Morphological changes in the pharyngeal airway of female skeletal class III patients following bimaxillary surgery: a cone beam computed tomography evaluation. Int J Oral Maxillofac Surg. 2014;43(7):862–7.
62. Kochar GD, Chakranarayan A, Kohli S, et al. Effect of surgical mandibular advancement on pharyngeal airway dimensions: a three-dimensional computed tomography study. Int J Oral Maxillofac Surg. 2016;45(5):553–9.
63. Faur CI, Roman RA, Bran S, et al. The changes in upper airway volume after orthognathic surgery evaluated by individual segmentation on CBCT images. Maedica. 2019;14(3):213–9.
64. Moscarino S, Kötter F, Brandt M, et al. Influence of different surgical concepts for moderate skeletal class II and III treatment on the nasopharyngeal airway space. J Craniomaxillofac Surg. 2019;47(10):1489–97.
65. Hwang DM, Lee JY, Choi YJ, Hwang CJ. Evaluations of the tongue and hyoid bone positions and pharyngeal airway dimensions after maxillary protraction treatment. Cranio. 2019;37(4):214–22.
66. Jiang C, Yi Y, Jiang C, Fang S, Wang J. Pharyngeal airway space and hyoid bone positioning after different orthognathic surgeries in skeletal Class II patients. J Oral Maxillofac Surg. 2017;75(7):1482–90.
67. Ristow O, Rückschloß T, Berger M, et al. Short- and long-term changes of the pharyngeal airway after surgical mandibular advancement in class II patients—a three-dimensional retrospective study. J Craniomaxillofac Surg. 2018;46(1):56–62.
68. Kochar GD, Sharma M, Chowdhury SK, et al. Pharyngeal airway evaluation following isolated surgical mandibular advancement: a 1-year follow-up. Am J Orthod Dentofac Orthop. 2019;155(2):207–15.
69. Marşan G, Öztaş E, Cura N, Kuvat SV, Emekli U. Changes in head posture and hyoid bone position in Turkish Class III patients after mandibular setback surgery. J Craniomaxillofac Surg. 2010;38(2):113–21.

70. Kitahara T, Hoshino Y, Maruyama K, In E, Takahashi I. Changes in the pharyngeal airway space and hyoid bone position after mandibular setback surgery for skeletal Class III jaw deformity in Japanese women. Am J Orthod Dentofacial Orthop. 2010;138(6):708. e1–10.
71. Sataloff RT. Clinical anatomy and physiology of the voice. In: Sataloff RT, editor. Professional voice: the science and art of clinical care. 4th ed. San Diego: Plural Publishing; 2017. p. 157–96.
72. Macari AT, Ziade G, Turfe Z, Chidiac A, Alam E, Hamdan AL. Correlation between the position of the hyoid bone on lateral cephalographs and formant frequencies. J Voice. 2016;30(6):757. e21–757.e26.
73. Sell D, Harding A, Grunwell P. GOS.SP.ASS.'98: an assessment for speech disorders associated with cleft palate and/or velopharyngeal dysfunction (revised). Int J Lang Commun Disord. 1999;34:17–33.
74. Karabekmez FE, Kleinheinz J, Jung S. Dimensions of velopharyngeal space following maxillary advancement with Le Fort I osteotomy compared to Zisser segmental osteotomy: a cephalometric study. Biomed Res Int. 2015;2015:389605.
75. Impieri D, Tønseth KA, Hide Ø, Brinck EL, Høgevold HE, Filip C. Impact of orthognathic surgery on velopharyngeal function by evaluating speech and cephalometric radiographs. J Plast Reconstr Aesthet Surg. 2018;71(12):1786–95.
76. Neeley WW 2nd, Edgin WA, Gonzales DA. A review of the effects of expansion of the nasal base on nasal airflow and resistance. J Oral Maxillofac Surg. 2007;65(6):1174–9.
77. Guenthner TA, Sather AH, Kern EB. The effect of Le Fort I maxillary impaction on nasal airway resistance. Am J Orthod. 1984;85(4):308–15.
78. Haarmann S, Budihardja AS, Wolff KD, Wangerin K. Changes in acoustic airway profiles and nasal airway resistance after Le Fort I osteotomy and functional rhinosurgery: a prospective study. Int J Oral Maxillofac Surg. 2009;38(4):321–5.
79. Seeberger R, Kater W, Davids R, Thiele OC. Long term effects of surgically assisted rapid maxillary expansion without performing osteotomy of the pterygoid plates. J Craniomaxillofac Surg. 2010;38(3):175–8.
80. Magnusson A, Bjerklin K, Nilsson P, Jönsson F, Marcusson A. Nasal cavity size, airway resistance, and subjective sensation after surgically assisted rapid maxillary expansion: a prospective longitudinal study. Am J Orthod Dentofac Orthop. 2011;140(5):641–51.
81. Pourdanesh F, Sharifi R, Mohebbi A, Jamilian A. Effects of maxillary advancement and impaction on nasal airway function. Int J Oral Maxillofac Surg. 2012;41(11):1350–2.
82. Gokce SM, Gorgulu S, Karacayli U, Gokce HS, Battal B. Three-dimensional evaluation of nasal and pharyngeal airway after Le Fort I maxillary distraction osteogenesis. Int J Oral Maxillofac Surg. 2015;44(4):455–61.
83. Marşan G, Hocaoğlu E, Cura N, Emekli U. Nasal profile changes with Le Fort I maxillary advancement surgery. Cleft Palate Craniofac J. 2015;52(2):152–6.
84. Kita S, Oshima M, Shimazaki K, Iwai T, Omura S, Ono T. Computational fluid dynamic study of nasal respiratory function before and after bimaxillary orthognathic surgery with bone trimming at the inferior edge of the pyriform aperture. J Oral Maxillofac Surg. 2016;74(11):2241–51.
85. Ha YC, Han SJ. A 3-dimensional analysis of nasal cavity volume after maxillary Le Fort I osteotomy. J Oral Maxillofac Surg. 2018;76(6):1344.e1–e7.
86. Zaoui K, Kuehle R, Baumann I, et al. Impact of Le-Fort I osteotomy on anatomical and functional aspects of the nasal airway and on quality of life. Eur Arch Otorhinolaryngol. 2019;276(4):1065–73.
87. Baeg SW, Hong YP, Cho DH, Lee JK, Song SI. Evaluation of sinonasal change after Lefort I osteotomy using cone beam computed tomography images. J Craniofac Surg. 2018;29(1):e34–41.
88. Atakan A, Ozcirpici AA, Pamukcu H, Bayram B. Does Le Fort I osteotomy have an influence on nasal cavity and septum deviation? Niger J Clin Pract. 2020;23(2):240–5.
89. Moroi A, Yoshizawa K, Tsutsui T, et al. Assessment of nasal septum after Le Fort I osteotomy with computer tomography. J Craniomaxillofac Surg. 2016;44(9):1187–93.
90. Sivasankar M, Fisher KV. Oral breathing challenge in participants with vocal attrition. J Speech Lang Hear Res. 2003;46(6):1416–27.
91. Sivasankar M, Fisher KV. Oral breathing increases Pth and vocal effort by superficial drying of vocal fold mucosa. J Voice. 2002;16(2):172–81.
92. Marunick MT, Menaldi CJ. Maxillary dental arch form related to voice classification: a pilot study. J Voice. 2000;14(1):82–91.
93. Lammert A, Proctor M, Narayanan S. Interspeaker variability in hard palate morphology and vowel production. J Speech Lang Hear Res. 2013;56(6):S1924–33.
94. Kula K, Cilingir HZ, Eckert G, Dagg J, Ghoneima A. The association of malocclusion and trumpet performance. Angle Orthod. 2016;86(1):108–14.
95. van der Weijden FN, Kuitert RB, Berkhout FRU, van der Weijden GA. Influence of tooth position on wind instrumentalists' performance and embouchure comfort: a systematic review. J Orofac Orthop. 2018;79(3):205–18.
96. Weikert M, Schlömicher-Thier J. Laryngeal movements in saxophone playing: video-endoscopic investigations with saxophone players: a pilot study. J Voice. 1999;13(2):265–73.
97. Macari AT, Abou Chebel N. Upper lip shortening combined with Lefort 1 maxillary intrusion: a novel approach to correct the long face syndrome. Eur J Plastic Surg. 2014;37(4):245–50.

Index

A.-L. Hamdan et al., *Dentofacial Anomalies*, https://doi.org/10.1007/978-3-030-69109-7

MIX
Papier aus verantwortungsvollen Quellen
Paper from responsible sources
FSC® C105338

If you have any concerns about our products,
you can contact us on
ProductSafety@springernature.com

In case Publisher is established outside the EU,
the EU authorized representative is:
Springer Nature Customer Service Center GmbH
Europaplatz 3, 69115 Heidelberg, Germany

Printed by Libri Plureos GmbH
in Hamburg, Germany